Research Techniques for the Health Sciences

Third Edition

Research Techniques for the Health Sciences

James J. Neutens
The University of Tennessee Graduate School of Medicine/Knoxville

Laurna Rubinson
The University of Illinois/Urbana-Champaign

San Francisco   Boston   New York
Capetown   Hong Kong   London   Madrid   Mexico City
Montreal   Munich   Paris   Singapore   Sydney   Tokyo   Toronto

Editor-in-Chief: Paul A. Smith
Editorial Assistant: Annemarie Kennedy
Editorial-Production Administrator: Deborah Brown
Editorial-Production Service: P. M. Gordon Associates
Composition Buyer: Linda Cox
Manufacturing Buyer: Suzanne Lareau
Cover Administrator: Kristina Mose-Libon
Electronic Composition: Galley Graphics, Ltd.

Library of Congress Cataloging-in-Publication Data

Neutens, James J.
    Research techniques for the health sciences / James J. Neutens, Laurna Rubinson. — 3rd ed.
        p. cm.
    Includes bibliographical references and index.
    ISBN 0–205–34096–2
    1. Public health—Research—Methodology. 2. Health education—Research—Methodology.
3. Health promotion—Research—Methodology. 4. Medicine—Research—Methodology.
I. Rubinson, Laurna. II. Title.

RA440.85.R83 2001
610'.7'2—dc21

2001041230

78910   0605
www.aw.com/bc

This book is dedicated to:

*Emily, Elizabeth, and Mary, for their patience,
and to Lori and Mike for showing us what really counts*
J.J.N.

My mother and Susan
L.R.

Contents

Preface

The principal reason for writing the first edition of this volume was to fill the void in our profession for a textbook on how to conduct research in the health sciences. The second edition continued to fill this void while reflecting changes in health science research. This third edition continues to meet that mission and, in addition, it has been tailored to provide greater information in selected areas while reducing the amount of less needed information. For example, evidenced-based health care is introduced as part of the critical review of literature while the discussion of historical research has been reduced, since very little effort has been expended in this research area of health science.

The target audiences for this edition remain the same. The book is intended to assist (1) upper-level undergraduates and graduate students in the health sciences; (2) practitioners in the fields of health education, public health, nursing, medicine, and allied health; and (3) related professionals. As in previous editions, this book focuses on the pragmatic aspects of health science research with a basis in theory. The underlying theory and the research concepts are explained in a commonsense approach, using case studies as examples. The information can be readily adapted to any research course in the health sciences. Most importantly, the content is presented in a "classroom" fashion so that it is understandable and usable to the student.

New to the Third Edition

The chapters in this edition have been rearranged based on comments by those who have been using the text. Those reviewers believed chapter order should be such that the student moves quickly into the research process prior to discussing ethical dilemmas. Consequently, three chapters precede the discussion of ethics in research.

However, each chapter still has case studies throughout the body, with a full discussion at the end.

A second change is that each chapter discusses the use of the Internet or World Wide Web, in either the actual text itself or in the *Suggested Activities*. This combines with a third change, which is the replacement of the previous Appendix B with one entitled *World Wide Web Research*. This appendix provides Web addresses and a brief description of sites applicable to health science research.

A fourth change is the introduction of the use of evidence-based health care to evaluate the existing literature. This stems from medical research efforts and provides the health researcher with a means to rate the level of evidence provided by an article. Extending well beyond a literature review, this new element includes several worksheets to help the student easily determine the level of evidence offered by the research. A fifth change is the reduction of information on attitude-scale construction and the placement of the remaining information on this subject in Chapter 6, *Data Collection Through Surveys and Self-Reports*. In addition, the chapter on historical research in the first two editions was eliminated, whereas an examination of another way to determine sample size was added to Chapter 7, *Sampling Designs and Techniques*. Of course, all chapters have updated references and resources used to illustrate health science research.

Chapter Organization and Descriptions

Chapter 1, *What Is Research?*, provides the basics of research with emphasis on a theoretical foundation so students can understand and appreciate the entire process.

Chapter 2, *Developing the Research Proposal*, offers an overview of the research project, in particular a thesis or dissertation. Discussion of hypothesis development is explained in greater detail than in prior editions.

Chapter 3, *Critical Review of the Literature and Information Sources*, presents information well beyond the usual literature review. Worksheets offer a means to evaluate an article based on the degree of research evidence it provides rather than just on the information it reports. Evidence-based online sources are described to help students find information quickly.

Chapter 4, *Considering Ethics in Research*, discusses several scenarios in which health science researchers can find themselves face-to-face with ethical decisions. The role of IRBs is presented in this chapter.

Chapter 5, *Conducting Experimental and Quasi-Experimental Research*, contrasts experimental designs with quasi-experimental ones. The section on validity was expanded to include diffusion and sequence effects.

Chapter 6, *Data Collection Through Surveys and Self-Reports*, lets the student progress in an orderly fashion to conduct this type of research. Attitude-scale construction is presented as a way to gain information via a survey or self-report.

A new section discusses the use of the World Wide Web as a survey technique. This includes e-mail surveys and related approaches.

Chapter 7, *Sampling Designs and Techniques,* addresses the purposes and uses of probability and nonprobability sampling techniques. Detailed information is presented on how to arrive at a sample size for differing types of research. Power analysis is discussed in some detail, as are formulas to ascertain sample size. Special considerations for survey research sample size are presented in a step-by-step fashion using the case study as an example. Websites that can assist in determining sample size are discussed.

Chapter 8, *Qualitative Research,* deals with a subject that has become increasingly important in health science efforts and appears to be of great interest to the medical field, given changing health care delivery systems and questionable outcomes. Qualitative research is contrasted with quantitative research. Methodologies, including ethnomethodology, are pragmatically discussed. Techniques of collecting qualitative data are detailed, and methods of analyzing and coding such data are presented.

Chapter 9, *Evaluation Research,* outlines the steps in this process and provides several models to the student. Cost analysis is discussed too.

Chapter 10, *Analytical Epidemiologic Studies,* presents the student with cohort investigations followed by case-control studies. Proportional hazards regression has been added as an analysis possibility.

Chapter 11, *Analyzing and Interpreting Data: Descriptive Analysis,* introduces statistics in a nonthreatening manner. It shows students how to calculate central tendencies, measures of spread, and correlations. Use of website power calculators is part of the *Suggested Activities.*

Chapter 12, *Analyzing and Interpreting Data: Inferential Analysis,* carries the discussion beyond descriptive techniques to include detailed inferential data analysis techniques. Both parametric and nonparametric tests are presented, as are advanced data analysis techniques. Meta-analysis is presented in some detail.

Chapter 13, *Techniques for Data Presentation,* suggests the best ways for students to present their data and findings. Table and figure presentations are discussed, as is the use of graphs, charts, and photographs.

Chapter 14, *Writing a Research Report,* is instrumental for students who are defending a thesis or dissertation. The underlying emphasis is that their document is a communication piece. The reader is given a step-by-step approach for developing a sound report for acceptance by other health care professionals as well as the public.

Appendix A, *Common Statistical Procedures,* lists 27 procedures, with a brief explanation of their common usage.

Appendix B, *World Wide Web Research,* is subdivided into three areas. First are statistical sites useful to all health science researchers, including power calculators, sample test calculators, and electronic texts on statistics. The second section provides sites and descriptions for evidence-based health care. These sites offer tremendous amounts of information to health science researchers, regardless of their degree of sophistication in evidence-based approaches. The final section details several government sites relevant to health science research.

Acknowledgments

This third edition, like the first, depended upon feedback from many people. We appreciate the contributions made by professors and students who used the second edition and were kind enough to suggest changes for this one. Special thanks to all the graduate students who have showed us the error of our ways, thereby helping us understand the needs of students and allowing us to address them in the reorganization of this edition.

We are indebted to the editorial staff at Allyn and Bacon, particularly Annemarie Kennedy and Paul Smith. Special thanks to Joseph Burns for his continued encouragement. Finally, we thank our friends and family for their ongoing support and patience.

J.J.N. and L.R.

Chapter 1

What Is Research?

Human beings possess the ability to think rationally and logically, which in turn leads to curiosity. You may have heard of the Philosophy 101 final examination that contained just one question: *"Why?"* Students wrote up to 20 pages, quoting philosophers ranging from Aristotle and Buber, but the correct answer was *"Because."* Research, or the process thereof, answers the question *Why?* There are multiple reasons for a myriad of questions, but how can we know what the best answer is? *Research* and the application of the scientific method will enable us to answer such questions.

Health Science Research

The health science profession had its beginnings at the start of the nineteenth century, when improvement of the health of school-age children provided impetus for the new discipline. In addition, we health science professionals have strived to provide information to those populations of high risk. These have been our primary goals, and we have attempted to use research and evaluation to improve our ability to meet these objectives. However, criticism about the research conducted can be found in the health science literature. With these criticisms in mind, you might be asking: Why study health science research? What can it do? What can we expect? All professionals, including community and school health educators, nurses, physicians, and other health care providers, are involved in the research process.

These questions will be answered as you progress through the text and get better acquainted with the process and product of research in the health sciences. Even though the discipline has been criticized, research in the health sciences has proved to be valuable. In the school setting alone, research has shown that children have increased their knowledge and altered their attitudes in such areas as smoking, human sexuality, dental health, cardiovascular diseases, drug and alcohol abuse, and driver education.

Research endeavors in the schools can inculcate good and acceptable health behaviors in youths if the programs being tried allow for decision-making and problem-solving skills, improve self-concept and self-esteem, and provide additional social interactions. Such programs, under the auspices of rigorous research, can lead to a reduction of risk factors associated with well-being.

Research in the community, conducted by nurses and physicians, can lead to baseline information regarding needs assessments in relationship to health status studies. In addition, public health policies are developed through research in the community. The determination of effective policy strategies can best be accomplished through rigorous and thorough research studies.

Patient education has been the setting for many research projects, including studies on diabetes, hypertension, postsurgical procedures, nutrition, and weight reduction. Many studies, for example, have led to major advances in diabetes control, in which patients are able to self-medicate and be relatively free of hospital regimens. Determination of how overweight patients react to specific weight control programs has had an influence on proper nutrition and exercise for both youths and adults.

For students to gain a thorough understanding of research and its place in the health sciences, they must have a working knowledge of science, scientific inquiry, and the importance of theory in research.

Using Science in the Quest for Knowledge

Knowledge may be gained or accumulated in many ways. Cohen and Manion (2000) classified ways of knowing into three broad categories: experience, reasoning, and research. We are concerned with the scientific method, or science, and how this science helps us know.

> To satisfy our doubts, . . . it is necessary that a method should be found by which our beliefs may be determined by nothing human, by some external permanency, by something upon which our thinking has no effect. . . . The method must be such that the ultimate conclusion of every man will be the same. Such is the method of science. Its fundamental hypothesis . . . is this: There are real things, whose characters are entirely independent of our opinions about them. (Buchler, 1995, p. 42)

Scientists, in their quest for knowledge and truth, use self-correcting devices that serve as built-in checking methods to assure that the conclusions they may reach are factual. Hypotheses are formulated but so too are alternate hypotheses to test the objectivity of the experiment and experimenter. In addition, by publishing the experiment and its results scientists allow for others to replicate and inspect their work.

Each scientific field (physics, engineering, psychology, health, etc.) has a method of arriving at knowledge, which will be discussed later as the scientific approach. Science can be considered a method to solve problems or answer questions that investigators find to be of interest. Scientists acquire specific attitudes that enable them to think and act in a scientific manner. These attitudes are best described by Ary, Jacobs, and Razevieh (1996, p. 14):

1. Scientists are essentially doubters, who maintain a highly skeptical attitude toward the data of science. Findings are regarded as tentative and are not accepted by the scientists unless they can be verified. Verification requires that others must be able to repeat the observation and obtain the same results. Scientists want to test opinions and questions concerning the relationships among natural phenomena. Furthermore, they make their testing procedures known to others in order that they may verify, or fail to verify, their findings.

2. Scientists are objective and impartial. In conducting observations and interpreting data, scientists are not trying to prove a point. They take particular care to collect data in such a way that any personal biases they may have will not influence their observations. They seek truth and accept the facts even when they are contrary to their own opinions. If the accumulated evidence upsets a favorite theory, then they either discard that theory or modify it to agree with the factual data.

3. Scientists deal with facts, not values. They do not indicate any potential moral implications of their findings; they do not make decisions for us about what is good or what is bad. Scientists provide data concerning the relationship that exists between events, but we must go beyond these scientific data if we want a decision about whether or not a certain consequence is desirable. Thus, while the findings of science may be of key importance in the solution of a problem involving a value decision, the data themselves do not furnish that value judgment.

4. Scientists are not satisfied with isolated facts but seek to integrate and systemize their findings. They want to put the things known into an orderly system. Thus scientists aim for theories that attempt to bring together empirical findings into a meaningful pattern. However, they regard these theories as tentative or provisional, subject to revision as new evidence is found.

Science as Static and Dynamic

Conant (1951) describes science in two ways: the static and the dynamic. The emphasis in the *static view* is on the present state of knowledge and of scientists contributing to that state. In addition, the extent of knowledge and the present theories, hypotheses, and principles are considered. In this view science may be used to explain observations and to discover new facts that contribute systematized information to the existing body of knowledge.

The actions of scientists are considered to be the *dynamic view* of science. In this view, the present state of knowledge serves as a base for further inquiry. The *heuristic view* of science (a subset of the dynamic view) means science that discovers or reveals, including the idea of self-discovery. The emphasis here is on discovery of something new that can add to the present base or body of knowledge. In the heuristic method of scientific inquiry, the actual emphasis is on the investigator being imaginative in his or her approach for answering a question or solving a problem.

Science and Theory

The ultimate goal of scientific inquiry is to formulate theories. Theories provide a way to conceptualize, organize, integrate, and classify the facts that scientists accumulate. A theory can describe a tentative explanation of some phenomenon. As scientists, when we ask the question *Why?* and attempt to answer it, we are formulating a theory. It is then verified through evidence obtained by either observation or experimentation.

Several characteristics of a sound theory serve to illustrate the constraints that scientists must work within when formulating a theory:

1. A theory should be able to explain the observed facts relating to a particular problem; it should be able to propose the "why" concerning the phenomena under consideration. This explanation of events should be in the simplest form possible. A theory that has fewer complexities and assumptions is favored over a more complicated one. This statement is known as the principle of parsimony.
2. A theory should be consistent with the observed facts and with the already established body of knowledge. We look for the theory that provides the most probable or the most efficient way of accounting for the accumulated facts.
3. A theory should provide means for its verification. This is achieved for most theories by making deductions in the form of hypotheses stating consequences that one can expect to observe if the theory is true. The scientist can then investigate or test these hypotheses empirically in order to determine whether the data support the theory. It must be emphasized that it is inappropriate to speak of truth or falsity of a theory. The acceptance or rejection of a theory depends primarily on *utility*. A theory is useful or it is not useful, depending on how efficiently it leads to predictions concerning observable consequences, which are then confirmed when the empirical data are collected. Even then, any theory is considered tentative and subject to revision as new evidence accumulates.
4. A theory should stimulate new discoveries and indicate further areas in need of investigation. (Ary et al., 1996, p. 18)

The health sciences have been very slow in achieving theoretical bases, probably because health, along with many other social sciences, is a young science. For the past 40 years, health professionals have been collecting data to gather empirical evidence and build toward theoretical constructs. While several models (such as the Health Belief Model and the Precede Model) have been developed for and by health

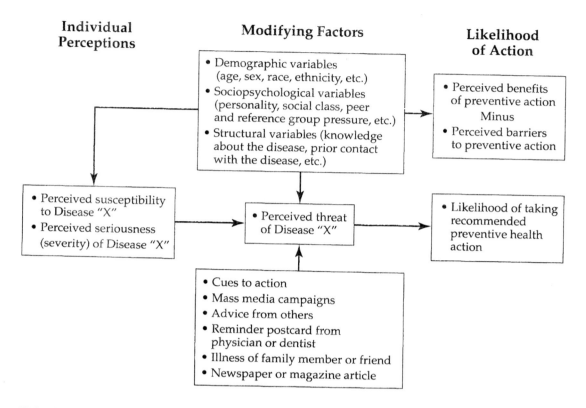

FIGURE 1.1 The Health Belief Model

Source. From Becker, M. (1974). *H. Ed. Monographs, 2*, 409–419. Copyright © 1974. Reprinted by permission of John Wiley & Sons, Inc.

educators, theories that could be directly attributed to the health sciences have been nonexistent.

It must be understood that there is a difference between a model and a theory. Theories provide an understanding of a phenomenon and offer prediction and control. Theories also can provide a way for conceptualizing the world. However, *models* provide perhaps a better way of conceptualizing. Some models are replicas, such as miniature toys; others are symbolic, such as the diagram of the Health Belief Model (see Figure 1.1). Models also can be used in computers, as scientists have been able to program computers to behave in a human-like manner when solving problems. Models provide us with a simplistic way of looking at complex problems or phenomena.

Basic and Applied Research

When we think about research, our initial image is of a laboratory with animals and scientists in white coats. This image is generally true when basic researchers are at work. *Basic research* aims to expand the knowledge base by formulating, evaluating, or expanding a theory. Research in the medical sciences is usually of this type, because biochemistry, biology, and microbiology fall into this pattern. Hence, the primary purpose of basic research is discovering knowledge for the sake of knowledge alone; the practical side of the issue is considered at a later time.

Applied research aims to solve practical problems, although it uses the same characteristics as basic research. Here, theoretical concepts are tested in real situations. Because laboratories cannot be the scene for investigations, the real world (e.g., classrooms, hospitals, clinics) becomes the laboratory for applied health researchers. Most research in the health sciences is applied because it is concerned with testing the processes of health behavior in real-life situations.

Several major health science projects have used the applied research approach. These include the CATCH program, the Healthy Cities program, and the University of Minnesota smoking prevention program. These projects use similar conceptual and theoretical approaches in schools—that is, in the real world. However, whether basic or applied research is being conducted by health scientists, one type of research must depend on the other for the proper research process to take place. Applications of theories help solve some practical problems, such as when social learning theory is used to attempt to explain why children adopt healthful behaviors. This can work the other way as well, as when theoretical concepts are advanced by the practical use of theory. As in the example just mentioned, new light could be shed on social learning theory if it were found to be useful in classroom situations.

The Scientific Approach

To become familiar with the method of scientific inquiry, future researchers should be attuned to several characteristics of the scientific approach (or research process). Rather that reiterate the major traits associated with research, we will use the excellent list provided by Best and Kahn in *Research in Education* (1998, pp. 18–20):

1. Research is directed toward the solution of a problem. The ultimate goal is to discover cause-and-effect relationships between variables, though researchers often have to settle for the useful discovery of a systematic relationship, for lack of enough evidence to establish one of cause-and-effect.
2. Research emphasizes the development of generalizations, principles, or theories that will be helpful in predicting future occurrences. Research usually goes beyond the specific objects, groups, or situations investigated and infers characteristics of a target population from the observed. Research is more than information retrieval, the simple gathering of information. Although many school research departments gather and tabulate statistical information that may be useful in decision making, these activities are not properly termed research.
3. Research is based upon observable experience or empirical evidence. Certain interesting questions do not lend themselves to research procedures because they cannot be observed. Research rejects revelation and dogma as meth-

ods of establishing knowledge and accepts only what can be verified by observation.

4. Research demands accurate observation and description. Researchers use quantitative measuring devices, the most precise form of description. When this is not possible or appropriate, they use qualitative or nonqualitative descriptions of their data-gathering procedures and, when feasible, employ mechanical, electronic or psychometric devices to refine observation, description, and analysis of data.

5. Research involves gathering new data from primary or first-hand sources or using existing data for a new purpose. Teachers frequently assign a so-called research project that involves writing a paper dealing with the life of a prominent person. The students are expected to read a number of encyclopedias, books, or periodical references, and synthesize the information in a written report. This is not research, for the data is not new. Merely reorganizing or restating what is already known and has already been written, valuable as it may be as a learning experience, is not research. It adds nothing to what is known.

6. Although research activity may at times be somewhat random and unsystematic, it is more often characterized by carefully designed procedures, always applying rigorous analysis. Although trial and error are often involved, research is rarely blind, shotgun investigation—trying something to see what happens.

7. Research requires expertise. The researcher knows what is already known about the problem and how others have investigated it. He or she has searched the related literature carefully, and is also thoroughly grounded in the terminology, the concepts, and the technical skills necessary to understand and analyze the data gathered.

8. Research strives to be objective and logical, applying every possible test to validate the procedures employed, the data collected, and the conclusions reached. The researcher attempts to eliminate personal bias. There is no attempt to persuade or to prove an emotionally held conviction. The emphasis is on testing rather than on proving the hypothesis. Although absolute objectivity is as elusive as pure righteousness, the researcher tries to suppress bias and emotion in his or her analysis.

9. Research involves the quest for answers to unsolved problems. Pushing back the frontiers of ignorance is its goal and originality is frequently the quality of a good research project. However, previous important studies are deliberately repeated, using identical or similar procedures, with different subjects, different settings, and at a different time. This process is replication, a fusion of the words repetition and duplication. Replication is always desirable to confirm or to raise questions about the conclusions of a previous study. Rarely is an important finding made public unless the original study has been replicated.

10. Research is characterized by patient and unhurried activity. It is rarely spectacular and researchers must expect disappointment and discouragement as they pursue the answers to difficult questions.

11. Research is carefully recorded and reported. Each important term is defined, limiting factors are recognized, procedures are described in detail, references are carefully documented, results are objectively recorded, and conclusions are presented with scholarly caution and restraint. The written report and accompanying data are made available to the scrutiny of associates or other scholars. Any competent scholar will have the information necessary to analyze, evaluate, and even replicate a study.
12. Research sometimes requires courage. The history of science reveals that many important discoveries were made in spite of the opposition of political and religious authorities. The Polish scientist Copernicus (1473–1543) was condemned by church authorities when he announced his conclusion concerning the nature of the solar system. His theory that the sun, not the earth, was the center of the solar system, in direct conflict with the older Ptolemaic theory, angered supporters of prevailing religious dogma, who viewed his theory as a denial of the story of creation as described in the book of Genesis. Modern researchers in such fields as genetics, sexual behavior, and even business practices had personal convictions, experiences, or observations that were in direct conflict with some of the research conclusions.

Upon reading the above list, you may get a view of researchers that is not realistic but ideal; imaginative, honest, hard-working, very rigid, and probably boring—because all they know is the subject they are so relentlessly pursuing. We can argue that this description is not accurate, especially for the health science researcher. The health professional is usually people-oriented and thus conducts research in real-world settings: hospitals, schools, places of worship, community centers, and so on. However, the good health researcher seeks to be rigorous and to adhere to scientific standards at all times.

Because we have set as one of the goals of this text to provide a basis from which students could conduct research, we will list and briefly explain the stages of the research process. Consideration here should be given to the nature of the research process (i.e., that one component is integral to all others, and that good research becomes almost cyclical). Figure 1.2 points out the various stages of the research process and attempts to show its cyclical nature.

Selecting a Problem.   The health science student will probably decide on a subarea of interest to focus his or her research upon. Selecting a problem involves asking good questions and communicating with others who might be familiar with your research topic. Colleagues, other students, supervisors, and faculty are some people you might ask for assistance in formulating your problem. Below are some examples of research problems that are usually stated in the form of a question:

1. What was the extent of the impact of the reduction of federal aid to dependent children and their families?
2. What factors influence eating disorders among various ethnic/racial groups?
3. What are the effects of a cardiac rehabilitation program?

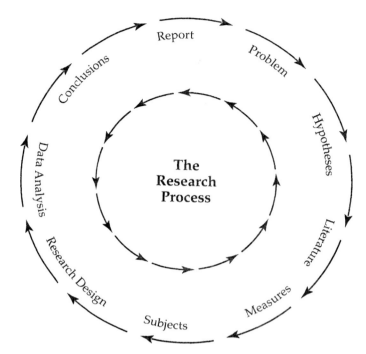

FIGURE 1.2 The Cyclical Stages of the Research Project

Formulating Hypotheses. The hypothesis is the researcher's tentative explanation that will predict the significant results of the research study or process. However, the hypotheses are always supported by theory and/or previous research. Examples of hypotheses that relate to the problems in the previous section are:

1. Dependent children and their families who receive less federal aid will have lowered health status than those dependent children and their families who have not been affected by the reduction program.
2. Disordered eating is more prevalent among Blacks, Asians, and Latinos as compared to Whites.
3. Those patients who complete all phases of a cardiac rehabilitation program will have a better quality of life than those who do not complete the program.

Reviewing the Literature. Relevant literature provides the hypotheses and initial problem selection. In addition, a thorough review of material may lead to suggested investigative methods.

Listing the Measures. Identifying all the possible measures enables the researcher to tighten the hypotheses by eliminating and rethinking those that have no available measure or none that can be developed for use in the study.

Describing the Subjects. The researcher carefully describes and considers the types of subjects necessary for the project. Particular care should be given to the number and availability of the subjects.

Constructing a Research Design. The research design should be fully explained so that the researcher is sure that the design will allow the student to test the stated hypothesis. Chapter 5 discusses the various types of experimental designs.

Constructing and Identifying Measurement Devices. The adoption and/or construction of appropriate instruments is used to measure the selected variables. There are some standardized instruments in the health sciences; however, modification of these instruments, the construction and pilot testing of new ones, or the construction of questionnaires and interview schedules may be necessary.

Analysis of the Data. A plane to analyze the data should be carefully considered, so that the number of subjects, the instruments, and the method of recording the data all coincide to fit the analysis procedure. This is an extremely important part of the stages of the research process, because all too often the instrumentation is not geared for appropriate data analysis, therefore rendering results improper or inadequate.

Generating Conclusions. The data should reveal several conclusions that are directly related to the hypotheses.

Writing the Report of Research. Chapter 14 details report writing, and instruction is offered for each section of the report.

Research Methodologies in the Health Sciences. There are several methodologies that are utilized by the health science investigators, each of which will be described in detail in the subsequent chapters. These methods, in brief, are:

1. **Experimental research** is a study in which the investigator controls and manipulates one or more of the variables. The focus of experimental research is on the relationships between the variables. The major purpose of this type of research is to determine what will happen.
2. **Survey, interview, and observational research** are considered descriptive *methodologies* in which the results reveal what is happening in a particular occurrence. This research involves recording, describing, analyzing, and interpreting conditions that presently exist. Comparisons and contrasts are attempted to reveal relationships between the nonmanipulated variables.
3. **Evaluation research** is a method of assessing a process or program in a specific situation (Wiersma, 1995). Evaluation may establish clear and specific criteria for success. Evidence is collected from a sample of the population, translated into quantitative terms, and compared with the previously set criteria. Conclu-

sions are then drawn about the effectiveness, merit, and success of the program that was studied.

4. **Historical research** describes what has occurred in the past. "The process involves investigating, recording, analyzing, and interpreting the events of the past for the purpose of discovering generalizations that are helpful in understanding the past, understanding the present, and to a limited extent, in anticipating the future" (Best & Kahn, 1998, p. 21).

The type of methodology used is most often determined by the questions asked and the kinds of data that will be collected. Too often, inexperienced investigators will attempt an inappropriate methodology for their convenience. A thorough discussion of these methodologies can be found in the remaining chapters of the text.

The health sciences have grown at a very fast pace since the early 1950s, when they became a separate and valued part of the educational process. During this time, the health field has become increasingly sophisticated in its approach to research. From the early days of one-group, no-control studies, to today's Solomon Four-Group designs, which include correlation of biomedical data, we have seen health science researchers publish and present their work in prestigious journals and meetings.

Summary

Human beings possess the ability to think rationally and logically that, in turn, leads to curiosity. *Why?*, the most asked question, leads researchers to conduct studies to find answers to questions, sometimes simplistic and other times complex.

Research in the health sciences is still in its early years, because the profession is relatively young. Even though they have their critics, and most of them are on target, health scientists have dramatically advanced in the field's research and evaluation efforts in the 1970s and 1980s. Using science in the quest for knowledge, health scientists have become imaginative, rigorous, and conscientious in their approach to research.

The method of science has enabled us to accumulate knowledge in many ways. Scientists assure themselves and the public that their conclusions are based on fact by having built-in checking mechanisms to ensure the accuracy, replication, and inspection of their work. Scientists have very specific attitudes about their work that set them apart from the layperson attempting research. Science has two broad views: static and dynamic, in which the latter describes the actions of scientists—how they think and behave to solve intricate problems.

The ultimate goal of scientific inquiry is to formulate theories. Theories enable us to conceptualize the facts that investigators accumulate. Several characteristics are inherent in a sound theory, each depicting the constraints under which the scientists work. The health sciences have been slow in developing theories, but rely on those of other social sciences such as psychology, anthropology, and education. Researchers in the health field have developed several models (e.g., the Health Belief Model and the Precede Model), which are different from theories. Models provide a simplistic way of looking at complex problems.

There are distinct differences between basic and applied research. However, each may complement the other. Professionals in the health sciences have concentrated upon applying principles and theories for real-world situations. It is difficult to conduct basic research in the settings that are available to health educators: schools, nursing homes, clinics, hospitals, and so on.

The scientific approach is the process investigators use in the quest for knowledge. Several important characteristics of the process enable standards to be scientific and rigorous. Stages of the scientific process begin with the selection of a problem and proceed through the writing of a research report.

Four general methodologies are used in health science research: experimental, survey (interview and observational), evaluation, and historical. The type of methodology required is dictated by the questions that need to be asked and the data that are collected.

Suggested Activities

1. Revise each of the following research topics so that it would be feasible for a research project. Indicate whether the statement is in the form of a hypothesis or a statement of a problem.
   a. Smoking among adolescents
   b. Diabetes control at home
   c. Hypertension in the elderly
   d. Fitness among stroke victims
   e. Cardiovascular rehabilitation for angina patients
   f. Dental health for pregnant teenagers
   g. Alcohol abuse among homemakers

2. Describe in one sentence each of the following characteristics of the research process:
   a. Research is directed toward the solution of a problem.
   b. Research emphasizes the development of generalizations, principles, or theories that will be helpful in predicting future occurrences.
   c. Research is based on observable experience or empirical evidence.
   d. Research demands accurate observation and description.
   e. Research involves gathering new data from primary or first-hand sources or using existing data for a new purpose.
   f. Although research activity may be at times somewhat random and unsystematic, it is more often characterized by carefully designed procedures.
   g. Research requires expertise.
   h. Research strives to be objective and logical.

    i. Research involves the quest for answers to unsolved problems.
    j. Research is characterized by patient and unhurried activity.
    k. Research is carefully recorded and reported.
    l. Research requires courage.

3. Devise your own definition of research and defend it.

4. Discuss how the health sciences have contributed to the body of knowledge concerning one aspect of health behavior.

5. Using the Web, determine five health topics that would be interesting to you in order to complete a research report.

References

Ary, D., Jacobs, L., & Razevieh, A. (1996). *Introduction to research in education.* Fort Worth: Harcourt Brace.

Becker, M. (1974). The health belief model and personal health behavior. *H. Ed. Monographs, 2,* 409–419.

Best, J., & Kahn, J. V. (1998). *Research in education* (8th ed.). Boston: Allyn & Bacon.

Buchler, J. (Ed.). (1995). *Philosophical writings of Pierce.* New York: Dover.

Cohen, L., & Manion, L. (2000). *Research methods in education* (2d ed.). New York: Routledge.

Conant, J. (1951). *Science and common sense.* New Haven: Yale University Press.

Wiersma, W. (1995). *Research methods in education.* Boston: Allyn & Bacon.

Chapter 2

Developing the Research Proposal

Much research ends in futility because the neophyte rushes into research activity—choosing a sample, collecting data, deriving conclusions—with only a meager plan at best. To be successful, the researcher must have a detailed plan as well as an overall conceptualization. The research proposal allows the investigator to specify the problem and related components; elaborate on the significance of the research to the health profession; review related literature; and outline the appropriate methodology within an equitable time frame. The sequence employed throughout this chapter is the format used in most theses and dissertations, although each university, not unlike most requests for proposals in funded research, will have modifications that must be followed by the researcher.

Selection of the Problem

One of the most difficult tasks confronting the beginner is to select a researchable problem. More often than not, the newcomer has a proclivity to tackle an exotic issue, thus making the problem either too broad or too narrow in scope. Some factors that should be involved in the ultimate selection are listed here (Bailey, 1994):

1. **Interest:** The researcher should be interested in pursuing the problem area. It should relate to the background and career interests of the student and help develop useful skills for the future.
2. **Operability:** The nature of the problem should be such that the researcher has both the resources and the time available to complete the subject.
3. **Scope:** While the research problem should not attempt to solve all the health dilemmas of the world, neither should it be so small as to negate the variables necessary for adequate results.

4. **Theoretical and practical values:** The research should contribute to the health field, perhaps through publication, and be of benefit to health practitioners.

5. **Health paradigm:** This is the school of thought or model employed by the researcher. For example, the Health Belief Model (Strecher & Rosenstock, 1997) or the PRECEDE paradigm (Green & Kreuter, 1999) could serve as a source to a problem or as a methodological direction.

6. **Values of the researcher:** The myth of value-free research is just that, a myth. The student of research should be aware that in addition to being unstable, values may prejudice the research effort to the degree that all objectivity is lost. Note that even the selection of a problem is value-laden.

7. **Research methodology:** Every researcher has a philosophy of research that affects procedure. Thus the student must be certain that hypotheses are well written and that appropriate criteria are used to interpret the data to reach conclusions.

8. **Reactivity:** The method of data collection should be scrutinized for reactivity. That is, a reactive technique brings about a reaction on the part of those being studied in a way that affects that data. The reactive effect is commonly labeled the "Hawthorne effect" from the study of the Hawthorne Plant of the Western Electric Company in Chicago, where it was found that worker productivity increased simply because the personnel were being observed.

9. **Unit of analysis:** In health research the unit of analysis may be an individual (such as the health habits of a single anorexic patient) or an entire population (patterns among the hospital anorexic population). The researcher must ascertain which is most appropriate and whether resources are available to collect data.

10. **Time frame:** This is particularly important to the student because only a limited amount of time is usually available. In a cross-sectional study a particular population is involved at a single point in time, whereas in a longitudinal time frame data are gathered over an extended period of time, such as months or years.

11. **Budget:** To ensure that your proposal is feasible, write up a budget for expensive items. These items may include duplicating costs, travel, and postage. Some universities provide modest financial support for research projects, and you should inquire about these sources.

The student should apply all of these criteria to the potential problem to determine the feasibility of the research effort.

Sources of Problems

Now that we have developed some criteria for selecting a problem, the next step is to commence the hunt. It should be kept in mind that the problem must be researchable (i.e., it must meet the requirements of the research process characteristics outlined in Chapter 1).

At the outset, the beginner should look around at the immediate environment; it teems with researchable problems. Many problems in the clinic, the hospital, or the community lend themselves to investigation. Which technique is most likely to bring about a change in smoking behavior? How does the community feel about the establishment of a wellness clinic at the hospital? Does presurgical education reduce the use of analgesics and the number of days of hospitalization?

Technological advances in medicine require continual revision in patient education, as do studies to measure their effectiveness. Similarly, in school health education, the advent of specialized curricula demands research into presentation format, teacher usage, cost benefits, and evaluation. The community health educator can turn in almost any direction to find new drugs, industrial hazards, environmental pollutants, and health fads that need investigation.

The academic experience of college juniors and seniors and of graduate students should serve as a catalyst for a research project. Textbooks, periodicals, seminar reports, and conference proceedings can inaugurate the mind into the research world. Indexes and abstracts such as the *Cumulative Index to Nursing and Allied Health Literature, Social Sciences Index, Hospital Literature Index,* and *Dissertation Abstracts* provide valuable sources for research ideas. Chapter 3 discusses review of literature and offers suggestions for additional library sources.

If possible, the student should attend workshops, national and state conventions, and government-sponsored programs to gather ideas, and more importantly, to meet current researchers in the field. Closer to home, university faculty can be the impetus for health research. Although topics themselves may be provided, consultation with experienced faculty is desirable to check operability, significance, and value.

To stimulate your thinking in the direction of health research, consult the following list from which problems may be defined. It is important to realize that this is simply a list of ideas, not of properly expressed research problems.

1. AIDS education for schoolchildren
2. Patient education and reduction of health care costs
3. Competency-based education
4. Marketing of health education
5. Patient adherence to drug regimens
6. Media effectiveness in community health education
7. Evaluation of health care programs
8. Autonomy of health educators
9. Health policy and health organizations (e.g., ASHA, APHA, SOPHE, AHA, ANA)
10. Patient education and ethics (e.g., informed consent, confidentiality)
11. Health career objectives of students
12. Internship experiences of community health education students
13. Health promotion

14. Content areas (e.g., sex, drugs, nutrition, AIDS)
15. Health locus of control
16. Behavioral change techniques
17. Safe transportation of toxic wastes
18. Health advocacy
19. Employee assistance programs
20. Health education concerns for rural populations
21. Motivation in health-conscious individuals
22. Mental health education in a clinical setting
23. Computer-assisted instruction in health care
24. Diabetes control

Statement of the Problem and Research Questions

The statement of the problem offers focus and direction in the research proposal. The problem statement can be written either as a question or as a declarative statement. In either case, it must be written clearly and concisely. Each word of the statement should be definitive, indispensable, and expressive. On completion, the statement of the problem should be such that it can be read and understood by anyone without the researcher's presence.

Listed here are some examples of poorly written statements that only imply the actual problem:

- Drugs and schoolchildren
- Hypertensive drugs and patients
- The fear of toxic wastes

This indicates to the student that the researcher does not have the problem clearly in mind or at least has not expressed it completely. Needless to say, this would be an inappropriate way to commence a research report.

These three meaningless statements could be refined to show a complete statement of the problem.

- What drug is most frequently abused by those students enrolled in junior high schools in Chatham?
- What factors play a role in the low compliance rate among males and females at an East Tennessee hypertension clinic?
- What are the health fears of residents living near a proposed New Jersey toxic waste dump site?

Research questions are generally used in lieu of hypotheses (discussed below). Sometimes the use of research questions indicates that the research project is not experimental and does not lend itself to the formulation of hypotheses. Some examples of research questions are:

- If African American and Mexican American women have greater body satisfaction and less concerns about diet than their White counterparts, what type of body presentation or image is culturally valued by each group?
- Is an individual's level of self-efficacy predictive of exercise compliance following completion of a Phase II program? (Vidmar & Rubinson, 1994)
- Will self-efficacy scores allow prediction of the likelihood of attrition for subjects of low socioeconomic status who enter an intensive program for poly–drug abuse treatment? (Steinhoff-Thornton, 1994)

It should be realized that these statements are specific as to topic and population. In other words, the parameters have been established within the statement of the problem. The ideas of the researcher must be clearly stated. Clichés, colloquialisms, slang, and professional jargon obscure thought and should be avoided when research is edited.

Subproblems

Frequently, the main problem has inherent components that, if extracted, would serve as minor, related research projects. These are called *subproblems* and as such could be investigated separately; however, the subproblems must add up to the totality of the principal problem. Further, each subproblem must be written in such a manner as to show how the data will be interpreted. Employing these two characteristics—totality and interpretation of data—the researcher may distinguish between subproblems and apparent subproblems.

To identify subproblems, first examine the problem statement itself for the components it contains. For example, inspect the following problem statement:

The purpose of this study is to analyze the wellness practices of Kent County Hospital nurses in contrast to the wellness practice they teach to their patients.

The next step is to demarcate the subproblem areas within the problem statement. This can be accomplished by underlining or bracketing the appropriate sections of the statement. Keep in mind that each subproblem must contain a word or words that imply data interpretation by the researcher:

The purpose of this study is [to analyze the wellness practices of Kent County Hospital nurses] [in contrast] to the [wellness practice they teach to their patients].

Now the subproblems may be written out thus:

1. What are the personal wellness practices of Kent County Hospital nurses?
2. What wellness practices are taught by Kent County Hospital nurses?

3. What will analysis of the wellness practices of these nurses indicate when contrasted with the wellness practices taught in the hospital?

It should be noted that each subproblem implies interpretation of the data, and that the subproblems add up to the totality of the principal problem.

Components Comprising the Setting of the Problem

Though the problem statement offers focus and direction and the subproblems provide a means to stay on course, further delineation is necessary. It is important to indicate what limitations, delimitations, and assumptions surround the problem as well as to define terms that may be new to the reader. Also, if the researcher is making any assumptions, they must be pointed out.

Limitations

Limitations are the boundaries of the problem established by factors or people other than the researcher. For example, in the preceding problem statement the researcher may have wished to investigate five separate counties. However, permission may have been granted by only three of the five counties and subsequently the data limited to those participating counties. Other limitations could be available resources, time, number of survey forms completed, and honesty of the respondents.

Delimitations

Delimitations deal with the boundaries also, but they are set by the researcher. Though the problem statement indicates what the researcher will investigate, it is important to know what will *not* be included. In other words, the delimitations are an answer to the inquiry, *What are the precise limits of the problems?* This is particularly salient to the novice researcher, who is most likely to attempt to solve every problem imaginable. Delimitations rule out the peripheral considerations, allowing the researcher to concentrate on the central effort. The study mentioned may require the researcher to delimit the population to nurses who have a bachelor's degree, not just R.N.s. The researcher may delimit the study by geographical location, the size of the population, a central issue, or similar considerations.

Assumptions

An assumption is a condition that is taken for granted and without which the research effort would be impossible. An assumption is believed to be a fact, but cannot be verified as one. In the Kent County Hospital study on wellness, the researcher may make the assumption that the teachers will answer the questionnaire honestly and thereby submit appropriate data.

Definition of Terms

Many research studies employ terms that may have special meaning to the study itself. To understand the usage of these terms, the researcher must define each term as it relates to the project at hand. Dictionary definitions are usually not adequate or helpful, because they fail to provide the true meaning intended by the researcher. The meaning of "wellness practices" would have to be defined from the Kent County Hospital problem statement. It is recommended that the reader review theses and dissertations to observe the role of the section on definition of terms.

Formulation of Hypotheses

While hypotheses may be included in components that comprise the setting of the problem, they are considered separately because of their significance to the research problem. Simply put, a hypothesis is a logical supposition, a reasonable guess, or a suggested answer to a problem or subproblem. A hypothesis provides further direction for the research effort by setting forth a possible explanation for an occurrence. For example, when the monitor of a personal computer fails to work, the following tentative reasons may be posited:

1. The monitor is not plugged in.
2. The interface cable is not connected.
3. The monitor is not turned on.
4. The picture tube is malfunctioning.

Each of these "guesses" can be tested by checking the plug, the interface cable, the on-off switch, and the picture tube.

Students may have a difficult time deciding how to go about formulating hypothesis statements. The easiest way to think about this problem is to know about two types of approaches that are appropriate for developing hypothesis statements: inductive or deductive reasoning. When using *inductive reasoning,* a generalization is made based on relationships that have been observed. You will discern trends and patterns, and then use these as a basis for your explanation and/or the predictive nature of your hypothesis. An example of an observation in a community setting might be that those who want to stop smoking rarely attend the required number of clinic sessions necessary to complete the smoking-cessation program. Can you now formulate a hypothesis based on this observation?

With the other type of approach used for stating hypotheses, called *deductive reasoning,* the researcher begins with a theoretical tenet and then makes a prediction as to how it can be applied to a specific situation. For example, you might begin by considering what you know about a theory, such as self-efficacy theory, and then make a prediction about how it will effect the behavior or the participants in a study.

Research Hypotheses

Hypotheses are derived from subproblems, and often a one-to-one correspondence is found. However, on other occasions, just one hypothesis may be developed from the problem statement itself or from a single subproblem. Generally, a hypothesis should: (1) be stated clearly and concisely; (2) express the relationship between two or more variables; and (3) be testable. Hypotheses are neither proved nor disproved. The purpose of testing a hypothesis is to ascertain the probability that it is suggested by fact. In other words, the acceptance or rejection of a hypothesis is based on fact rather than a preconceived bias.

In early stages of a study, researchers state a scientific or research hypothesis as a prediction of the outcome of the test. For example, in the medical community it was predicted that as the number of cigarettes smoked increased, so would the incidence of lung cancer. This concise statement expresses the relationship between smoking and lung cancer. Of course, a linear relationship could also be expressed to state that as one variable increases, the other will decrease. The public health educator would predict that as the usage of contraceptives increases among teenagers, the incidence of teen pregnancy would decrease. In some studies there may be a nonlinear relationship between the variables (e.g., as one variable increases, the other increases and then levels off). It might be predicted that as anxiety increases, the ability to perform increases and then plateaus. Hypothesis statements from the above discussions would be written as follows:

1. As the number of cigarettes smoked increases, so will the incidence of lung cancer.
2. Teenagers who utilize contraceptives are less likely to become pregnant.
3. As anxiety increases, the ability to perform on an examination increases and then plateaus.

Null Hypotheses

While research hypotheses demarcate the observations to be made, it is difficult to obtain unequivocal support for them. Subsequently, they are usually rephrased into a negative or null form. This negative or no-difference format is called a *null hypothesis*, symbolized as H_0. The null hypothesis asserts that minor differences between the variables can occur because of chance errors, and thus are not significant differences. In other words, the testing of a null hypothesis reveals either that some force or factor has resulted in a statistical difference, or that it has not resulted in such a difference. When the null hypothesis is rejected, indicating that a statistical difference does in fact exist between the variables, the competent researcher sees this as a red flag and will probe deeper into the problem to discover what has caused the difference and how. For example, a health scientist may find that a particular program alters the attitudes of those exposed to it, thereby rejecting the null hypothesis that the effect of the program would make no difference. This finding leads to another research question: What caused the program to bring about the change, and could this factor or factors be employed in other programs? Note that if the researcher rejects a null hypothesis, then the research hypothesis is accepted.

Returning to the problem of wellness practices of Kent County Hospital nurses at both a personal and teaching level, the null hypothesis may be written as:

> There are no differences in those wellness practices personally employed or taught in the hospital.

Examination of this null hypothesis shows that it is derived from the third sub-problem, and that it expresses the relationship between two variables—practices personally employed and practices taught in the hospital. It is stated concisely and is testable. If the research hypothesis—that there are differences between personal practices and what is being taught—is accepted, then the next step is to explore the dynamics underlying the differences. The research effort should not stop with rejection of the null hypothesis.

Significance and Justification of the Problem

In this section of a research proposal, the researcher has an opportunity to explain why the research effort is so important. The fledgling researcher frequently believes that the significance of the study is self-explanatory, or that, because it is of personal interest, it must be of interest to everyone. Needless to say, that is not usually the case. The relevance of the undertaking to one's peers or community, or to the patients, needs to be stated in a way that the average citizen will comprehend. Although some health researchers may be concerned solely with theory, most health scientists will demand pragmatic value from the research endeavor. Further, with so many areas of health care requiring research, there is no justification for the expenditure of efforts that fail to contribute to the profession.

The researcher must also be able to justify the study by explaining how the project will further knowledge and extend theory. In order to accomplish this, the researcher should be very familiar with and able to articulate any opposing view-points through a thorough review and critical analysis of the literature.

Résumé of Related Literature

Those who conduct an initial research project frequently regard the review of literature as wasted time, because they believe they could be collecting data more appropriately. Skilled researchers, however, realize that the more one knows about similar research, the more likely the study can be conducted in an intelligent, comprehensible fashion.

As a general guide, keep in mind that the problem statement is central, and that everything to be reviewed should serve as an aid in confronting the problem. Similar

TABLE 2.1   Time Schedule: Wellness Research Project

Dec. 1	Dec. 10	Feb. 5
1. Study go-ahead	1. Obtain permission and develop working procedures with Kent County nurses	1. Develop instrument 2. Select pilot sample 3. Select study sample 4. Mail introductory letters to all participants
March 20	**April 15**	**April 30**
1. Mail instrument to nurses in study 2. Revise/complete Chapters I, II, and III	1. Questionnaires returned 2. Data keypunched	1. Fund program 2. Begin data analysis 3. Telephone contact with random sample of participants failing to return questionnaire

studies should be checked for population and sampling techniques; study design, including data-gathering instruments; variables measured; extraneous variables that influenced findings; recommendations for future research; and of course, the findings and conclusions. Though the related literature section of the report follows several other sections, it is important to commence a literature review early so that it can help to define the problem statement, develop components that comprise the setting of the problem, justify the study, and plan the design. Research should be conducted with deliberate speed; otherwise, the only thing accomplished is proof of the adage, "Haste makes waste."

Proposed Research Procedures

Up to the point at which the research procedures are discussed, the report has dealt with the nature of the problem, the significance of the problem, and an explanation of what related studies have found. Now a detailed research plan must be outlined to include sampling techniques, methodological steps, instruments employed, administration of instruments, data required, and method of analyzing data.

Budget Considerations

As mentioned in this chapter, the researcher must carefully consider any financial expenditures that might occur as a result of the proposal. You should review, with an experienced researcher, such expenditures as subject payments, duplication of materials, postage, travel, and software. If these expenditures are not able to be met

Feb. 15	March 10
1. Committee review instrument 2. Mail to nurses in pilot study	1. Revise instrument from pilot study

May 15	June 15
1. Write section on presentation and analysis of data 2. Write summary, conclusions, recommendations	1. Write, edit final report

by you, or with the help from university funds, you should abandon the project and discuss, with your advisor, a more financially viable study.

Time Schedule

Although a time schedule may not be a requirement of an advisor or funding agency, it is an invaluable device to assist in the budgeting of time and energy. Students are advised to develop a time schedule because their time is limited and academic deadlines are rarely negotiable. Moreover, dividing the research effort into operable portions with realistic dates also helps organization and reduces procrastination. Table 2.1 demonstrates how a student may develop a time schedule for the Kent County problem statement:

> The purpose of this study is to analyze the wellness practices of Kent County Hospital nurses in contrast to the wellness practices they teach to their patients.

Research Proposal Checklist

The research proposal is the initial step in developing the research project, and as such the investigator should check each area. The checklist in Table 2.2 offers a series of questions and statements that may be employed for this purpose. It is to serve only as a guide and not as an absolute formula for every research proposal.

TABLE 2.2 Research Proposal Checklist

A. The Problem
  1. The research problem should be able to meet the following criteria: ___ Yes ___ No
     University   ___ Yes ___ No
     Replication   ___ Yes ___ No
     Control   ___ Yes ___ No
     Measurement
  2. In addition, the following factors affecting problem selection must be
     considered and should be checked off once contemplated: ___ Yes ___ No
     Interest   ___ Yes ___ No
     Operability   ___ Yes ___ No
     Scope   ___ Yes ___ No
     Values   ___ Yes ___ No
     Paradigm   ___ Yes ___ No
     Methodology   ___ Yes ___ No
     Reactivity   ___ Yes ___ No
     Unit of Analysis   ___ Yes ___ No
     Time frame

B. Statement of the Problem
  Write out the problem statement.
  1. Is the problem statement clear and concise?   ___ Yes ___ No
  2. Does it focus on one research goal?   ___ Yes ___ No
  3. Does the problem statement set parameters?   ___ Yes ___ No
  4. Is the interpretation of the data implied in the problem statement?   ___ Yes ___ No

C. Subproblems
  Underline or box off the problem statement and then construct and write
  out the subproblem(s).
  1. Is each subproblem written in question form?   ___ Yes ___ No
  2. Is the writing clear and concise?   ___ Yes ___ No
  3. Can each subproblem be investigated separately?   ___ Yes ___ No
  4. Does each subproblem show that interpretation of the data will take place? ___ Yes ___ No
  5. Do the subproblems add up to the totality of the principal problem?   ___ Yes ___ No

D. Delimitations
  Determine the precise boundaries of the problem and write out each.
  1. Are the peripheral considerations ruled out?   ___ Yes ___ No
  2. Is each delimitation established by the researcher?   ___ Yes ___ No
  3. Is the delimitation written clearly and concisely?   ___ Yes ___ No

E. Assumptions
  Consider all the assumptions necessary to conduct the study:
  1. Is each assumption appropriate to the project?   ___ Yes ___ No
  2. Are you assuming too much for the study to be done?   ___ Yes ___ No
  3. Is each assumption really necessary to the study?   ___ Yes ___ No

F. Definition of Terms
  Ascertain which terms require special interpretation:
  1. Is each term defined as it relates to the research project?   ___ Yes ___ No
  2. Are the definitions clear and concise, and do they avoid an abundance   ___ Yes ___ No
     of professional jargon?

TABLE 2.2 *Continued*

G. Hypotheses

Apply the following questions to each hypothesis:

1. Are the hypotheses written in an understandable fashion?	___ Yes	___ No
2. Are they derived from the problem or subproblem(s)?	___ Yes	___ No
3. Are they written in null form?	___ Yes	___ No
4. Does each hypothesis express a relationship between two or more variables?	___ Yes	___ No
5. Is the hypothesis testable? How?	___ Yes	___ No

H. Significance of the Problem

This section is very important to justify a go-ahead for collecting data or to obtain research funding.

1. List the ways in which the research project will contribute to health science.

_____

_____

2. Do others concur that this would be a worthwhile project? Colleagues		
Faculty	___ Yes	___ No
Major advisor	___ Yes	___ No
Related personnel in the field	___ Yes	___ No
Related literature	___ Yes	___ No
	___ Yes	___ No
3. Is this section written in a manner that shows why the study should be conducted without having to make the reader search for an answer?	___ Yes	___ No

I. Related Literature

Whether this segment be brief or lengthy, it should meet the demands listed below.

1. Have all the resources been reviewed?	___ Yes	___ No
2. Does each section relate to the problem statement?	___ Yes	___ No
3. Is this segment well organized?	___ Yes	___ No
4. Is the related literature current?	___ Yes	___ No

J. Research Procedures

All the steps of the research plan should be included in this segment.

1. Where applicable, are the following included?

Sample technique	___ Yes	___ No
Methodological steps	___ Yes	___ No
Instruments employed	___ Yes	___ No
Administration	___ Yes	___ No
Analysis techniques	___ Yes	___ No

K. Time Schedule

This section is suggested for better organization.

1. Is time available to complete the project?	___ Yes	___ No
2. Do all segments or sections surround the problem?	___ Yes	___ No
3. Is the proposal readable, concise, and cohesive?	___ Yes	___ No
4. Does the proposal represent a best effort?	___ Yes	___ No

Summary

An organized and concise research proposal shows that the researcher has a well-developed plan and that the project is likely to be worked through to completion. This chapter explains the factors that affect problem selection and suggests sources of problems suitable to research. Each section of the proposal is overviewed to include the statement of the problem, subproblems, components comprising the setting of the problem, hypotheses, significance of the problem, résumé of related literature, research procedures, and time schedule. Review of the literature and information sources is a step in the process that assists all aspects of the research proposal.

Suggested Activities

1. Explain the errors in each of the following problem statements, and rewrite each to meet the demands of a good problem statement:
   a. The purpose of this study was to examine the relationship between sexual experience and sexual and contraceptive attitudinal responses to a birth control film.
   b. The purpose of this study was to examine which of three different approaches aimed at helping to curb smoking among teenagers enrolled in public schools was most effective: the scare approach, the fact approach, or the attitude approach.
   c. The purpose of this study was to investigate the relationship between emotional maturity and accident involvement of male motorcycle operators in Michigan.
   d. What health education techniques could be used to reduce anxiety in pregnant women who face a cesarean section?

2. Once you have rewritten the problem statements from the first activity, demarcate and write out the subproblems of each.

3. Rewrite each of the following research hypotheses in the form of a null hypothesis:
   a. As patients' involvement in their education increases, so will their knowledge of their health maintenance.
   b. As nutrition knowledge among fifth-graders increases, their selection of junk food will decrease.
   c. As more research information about AIDS is imparted to the community, there will be less anxiety within the community.

4. Read the following problem statement and then develop appropriate definitions, limitations, delimitations, and assumptions for such a study:

What are the preabortion and postabortion attitudes of women experiencing problem pregnancies toward self, contraception, intercourse, and abortion?

References

Bailey, K. D. (1994). *Methods of social research.* New York: Free Press.

Green, L., & Kreuter, M. (1999). *Health promotion planning: An educational and ecological approach.* Palo Alto, CA: Mayfield.

Steinhoff-Thornton L. (1994). *Self-efficacy as a predictor of attrition for African-American and White client populations in treatment for poly–drug abuse.* Unpublished doctoral dissertation, University of Illinois.

Strecher, V., & Rosenstock, I. (1997). The health belief model. In K. Glanz, F. Lewis, & B. Rimer (Eds.), *Health behavior and health education* (pp. 41–59). San Francisco: Jossey-Bass.

Vidmar, P., & Rubinson, L. (1994). The relationship between self-efficacy and exercise compliance in a cardiac population. *Journal of Cardiopulmonary Rehabilitation, 19*(4), 272–284.

Chapter 3

Critical Review of the Literature and Information Sources

A review of relevant literature provides a framework for the hypothesis and statement of the problem. It is usually required in the beginning chapters of a thesis or dissertation. This exercise in reviewing the literature will enable the researcher to formulate ideas and concepts from previous work. We can learn what other investigators have accomplished and have failed to do so that we can make a contribution to the knowledge of health sciences. Many first-time investigators find reviewing the literature a two-sided experience. On one hand it can be a challenging, interesting, motivating exercise. On the other, it can be tedious and painstakingly slow, especially if one allows curiosity to take over: It is easy to get sidetracked into interesting areas that are peripheral to the project at hand.

Purposes of the Review

While the general purpose of reviewing the relevant literature is to gain an understanding of previous work and to generate new ideas and concepts, the process can additionally help the investigator to:

1. Develop an understanding and grounding in theory.
2. Define the problem.
3. Review the procedures and instruments used.
4. Originate new ideas rather than repeat work already accomplished.
5. Use the recommendations for further research.
6. Critique relevant studies.

Understanding Relevant Theory

Too often investigators in the health sciences approach problems from an atheoretical perspective, and, therefore, do not develop a well-defined set of hypotheses. By using the review of literature to search for relevant theoretical perspectives, investigators will gain additional knowledge and confirm hypotheses. This leads to an enrichment of the field in general and builds toward well-founded studies for the future.

Defining the Problem

While reviewing the health science literature, the investigator will be able to develop a concise plan for the study. Often we begin with lofty ideas that are sometimes not workable in the real world of research. The review will enable the investigator to state quite narrowly the relevant hypotheses and research problem.

Reviewing Procedures and Instruments

The review of the literature provides information on, and insight into, proven and unproven methodologies and procedures previously used. Knowing that some research designs are inappropriate, that some sampling frames are inadequate, and that some approaches are unreasonable enables the investigator to improve on his or her research design. In the behavioral sciences, it is especially important to have reliable and valid instruments. The review provides insight into which measures are available and which of those will be useful in the present research study.

Originating New Ideas

Many experimenters have begun the literature search and deduced that their idea would not add any new knowledge or insight to their field of interest. A review of existing research can illuminate interest areas that need subsequent study and indicate useful applications, without reinventing the wheel. While some of us can formulate original ideas and concepts, they also can be manifested by a thorough review of the literature.

Using Recommendations for Further Research

Authors of research studies usually include very specific recommendations for additional research. This is quite helpful to the investigator, because the suggestions provide the valuable insights of an experienced investigator in the same, or similar, areas of research. The list that follows might provide impetus for you to formulate your own specific area of study:

Sample Research Ideas

1. Effects of the menstrual cycle on abstinence in a quit-smoking program
2. The outcome and cost of alcohol and drug treatment in an HMO

3. The intervention trial of a substance abuse program for women of childbearing age
4. The relationship of developmental theories to health education curricula in grades K–8
5. The effect of pregnancy on chronic hepatitis C
6. The role of states in ensuring appropriate public health practices
7. The use of telemedicine as a health education tool
8. Means of altering the attitudes of preschoolers toward family life education
9. Parental knowledge and behaviors regarding immunization of children
10. The use of self-efficacy in behavior change

Criticizing Relevant Studies

In order to adequately understand why there are contradictory results in your specific area of study, you must critically review and analyze other areas of study. Usually, contradictory results among studies arise from differing definitions of important terms, varying instruments and methodologies of science, and utilizing different data analyses. As you review and write the literature section of your proposal with a critical eye, you will certainly be challenged but will also make a very important contribution to your field of study.

Steps in the Review Process

You have decided to embark on a research study, and now the time has arrived to begin searching the literature. A tentative problem statement, centered around a theory, has been determined. Now to the library, the Internet, and beyond!

The following is an outline of the steps to consider when beginning a review of the literature:

1. Reading background information
2. Gathering the necessary tools
3. Listing key words
4. Checking preliminary sources, including databases
5. Conducting a computer search
6. Determining what to read
7. Determining the level of evidence
8. Finding short-cuts to determining the level of evidence

Reading Background Information

At this stage of your search, *secondary sources* are generally used. These are usually textbooks or encyclopedias written by someone who has not directly observed the described event. A good textbook is written by an author who has searched the literature exhaustively and compiled a text based on her or his interpretation of other experiments or events. Of course, the same author may also report on experiments he or she has participated in or witnessed. This would be considered a *primary source* because it was written by someone who has observed or participated in an event. The importance of secondary sources is that they usually have a bibliography, which provides the reader with the primary sources.

After reviewing the few textbooks devoted to your research problem, you realize that primary sources must be read. These include journals, final reports, or books that contain original research. In addition, government publications are good primary sources.

Gathering the Necessary Tools

Systematically gathering data will keep you organized and will prevent you from having to redo what you have already done. Depending upon your computer access and skills, recordkeeping methods can range from notes written on index cards to a computer database. At a minimum, both approaches should contain the name of the author, the title of the reference, and a complete source listing. You should check the format (e.g., American Psychological Association) required for theses and dissertations at your institution to avoid having to recopy bibliographic entries. Additional information, if your approach allows, could be the principal findings and the level of evidence. As discussed below, determining the level of evidence requires critically appraising a source and then categorizing it by the degree to which it supports (i.e., provides evidence for) the topic at hand.

Another necessary tool is a filing system for arranging your bibliography index. Filing systems may be arranged by (1) the authors' names, in alphabetical order; (2) date, with the most recent work first; (3) subheading; or (4) level of evidence. Of course a combination of these techniques could also be used. For example, you may organize by level of evidence and, within each level, by author or topic. Using level of evidence allows you to discern the usefulness of the reference.

Listing Key Words

After you have the background information, which is generally gathered from secondary source materials, you will have an idea of the topic area and be able to generate key words or phrases. Use of a thesaurus has proved valuable in this process. Consult the key word listings in each computer database and contact colleagues and professors who might have related interests.

Key words and phrases are necessary because almost all health science sources are organized by subject, and you should have a list of key words to begin looking in the computer databases. As an example, your topic area may be patient education involving diabetes in outpatient settings. When you complete the general review, your first key word list might include patient education programs, outpatients, hospitals, diabetes, and nursing education. Such a list, although quite incomplete at this stage, will provide a starting point when you begin the actual search through the various computer databases.

Checking Preliminary Sources

The next step in the search process is to check the *preliminary sources*. These include reference books, indexes, abstracts, guidebooks, and periodicals that help the investigator locate primary sources. Most of the sources in the health sciences are available by computer search.

General Indexing and Abstracting Services

Listed below are several databases available through online computer services at most libraries. A growing number of these databases contain full text or direct you to Websites with full text of the document.

- **BIOETHICSLINE** provides bibliographic citations to the literature covering the ethical, legal, and public policy issues of health care and biomedical research. Included are citations to journal articles, monographs, chapters in monographs, newspaper articles, court decisions, bills, laws, audiovisual materials, and unpublished documents derived from the literature of many fields, including the health sciences, law, religion, and philosophy.
- **Biological Abstracts** provides indexing for over 9,000 journals in all areas of life science. Subject areas represented include biology, botany, zoology, microbiology, clinical and experimental medicine, biochemistry, biophysics, instrumentation, and methods.
- **CINAHL** (Cumulative Index to Nursing and Allied Health Literature) provides comprehensive coverage of English-language nursing journals as well as journal titles from 17 allied health disciplines, books, book chapters, nursing dissertations, patient education documents, audiovisual materials, and software. OVID has evidence-based filters that can be used with this database.
- **ERIC** consists of two files: the Resources in Education (RIE) file of document citations and the Current Index to Journals in Education (CIJE) file of journal article citations from over 750 professional journals.
- **HAPI** (Health and Psychosocial Instruments) assists in the identification of measurement and evaluation instruments (e.g., questionnaires, checklists, tests) found in the health and psychosocial literature. The database does not include copies of the instruments.
- **HealthSTAR** (Health Services, Technology, Administration, and Research) focuses on the evaluation/efficacy portion of the medical literature and covers more of the administration and delivery aspects of health care, including the evaluation of patient outcomes; the effectiveness of a procedure, service or program; health care policy and economics; Medicare; and Medicaid.
- **MEDLINE** is the National Library of Medicine's (NLM) premier bibliographic database covering the fields of medicine, nursing, dentistry, veterinary medi-

cine, the health care system, and the preclinical sciences. OVID has evidence-based filters for MEDLINE.

- **MEDLINEplus** is the NLM's Website for up-to-date, private consumer health information.
- **PsycINFO** contains summaries of the world's serial literature in psychology and related disciplines.
- **Social Work Abstracts** contains more than 35,000 records from social work and other related journals, spanning 1977 to the present, on topics such as homelessness, AIDS, child and family welfare, aging, substance abuse, legislation, and community organization. Abstracts of dissertations since 1996 are included.
- **TOXNET** is a collection of both bibliographic and factual databases focused on toxicology and the health risks posed by hazardous chemicals. Included are data related to chemical carcinogenesis, genetic toxicology, and the release of toxic chemicals in the environment (Toxic Chemical Release Inventory).

Evidence-Based Full-Text and Abstracting Services

These database services can save the health researcher an immense amount of time when seeking high-quality evidence-based information. (A full discussion of evidence-based data is provided below in the section entitled *Determining the Level of Evidence*.) Appendix B contains the website addresses of these databases.

- **Bandolier** is a print and Internet health care journal that uses evidence-based medicine techniques. The content is "tertiary," which means that it distills the information from (secondary) reviews of (primary) trials and makes it comprehensible.
- **Cochrane Library** is an electronic publication available on CD-ROM and the Internet. Published by the National Health Service Centre, it is considered the premier site for evidence-based searches.
- **Database of Abstracts of Reviews of Effectiveness (DARE)** is part of the National Health Service Centre's Cochrane Library, and might be searched before MEDLINE for high-quality reviews.
- **National Guideline Clearinghouse (NGC)** is a public resource for evidence-based clinical practice guidelines. NGC is sponsored by the Agency for Healthcare Research and Quality (AHRQ) (formerly the Agency for Health Care Policy and Research [AHCPR]) in partnership with the American Medical Association and the American Association of Health Plans.
- **PedsCCM Evidence-Based Journal Club** is a regular publication of critical reviews of clinical trials pertinent to the practice of pediatric critical care.
- **PERRY** is sponsored by the Centers for Disease Control through the Division of Adolescent and School Health. It is a comprehensive database of abstracts and citations covering all six risk behaviors among adolescents.
- **PubMed,** developed by the National Center for Biotechnology Information (NCBI) at the National Library of Medicine, is based at the National Institutes

of Health (NIH). It provides access to bibliographic information drawn primarily from MEDLINE, PreMEDLINE, HealthSTAR, and publisher-supplied citations. It can be searched by level of evidence
- **TRIP,** a database from the Centre for Research Support, is a meta-search engine that searches across 61 sites of high-quality medical information. It is evidence-based.

Government Documents

The listings below can be accessed as government documents using the website of the Centers for Disease Control for the National Center for Health Statistics (www.cdc.gov/nchs):

- **National Center for Health Statistics (NCHS)** data systems include data on vital events as well as information on health status, lifestyle, exposure to unhealthy influences, the onset and diagnosis of illness and disability, and the use of health care.
- **National Health and Nutrition Examination Survey (NHANES)** has been designed to collect information about the health and diet of people in the United States. It is unique in that it combines home interviews with health tests.
- **National Health Care Survey (NHCS)** provides data on alternative health care settings, such as ambulatory surgical centers, hospital outpatient departments, emergency rooms, hospices, and home health agencies.
- **National Health Interview Survey (NHIS)** provides information on health limitations, behaviors, insurance, health care access, and injuries. In addition, instrumentation that could be very important to survey researchers is available for review.
- **National Immunization Survey (NIS)** is combined with the Survey of Families with Young Children (SFYC) and the Survey of Children with Special Health Care Needs (CSHCN), which collect information on the immunization coverage and health care of children across the United States.
- **National Survey of Family Growth (NSFG)** is based on personal interviews of a national sample of women aged 15–44 in the noninstitutionalized civilian population. The last complete survey was conducted in 1995.
- **National Vital Statistics System (NVSS)** is responsible for the official vital statistics of the United States. Included: state-collected information about such vital events as births, deaths, marriages, divorces, and fetal deaths.

Conducting a Computer Search: Finding the Evidence

After you realize just how many sources are available to you when conducting a literature search, you will want to conduct a computerized literature search. Most major university and college libraries are equipped with the hardware and software that will enable you to conduct that search. Using the computer search will enhance your ability to check the preliminary sources.

Why Conduct a Computer Search?

A computer search enables you to search the literature by using a computer terminal. This terminal will have access to several databases (stored files) of references to literature. These databases are usually broader and more frequently updated than books or periodicals. A computer search is certainly faster and more flexible than a manual one. The computer can scan millions of records in seconds and can combine subject terms in a way that is impossible in a manual search. Searches also can be run on phrases or words that appear in the titles of written materials, which enables you to use the most up-to-date, pertinent terminology.

Full-text electronic journals and abstracts are also available via a computer search. This gives the student a more thorough description of the material and can save time in locating unnecessary or unwanted publications. The printouts of the list of citations will devote a full bibliographic entry, and this can save you time in writing the reference on a note card—just paste or tape it on, or place it in a bibliographic database of your own. (End Notes and Bookends are examples of commercially available databases.)

How to Conduct a Computer Search

In most colleges and/or universities, you will be able to conduct the search yourself. The following hints may aid you in conducting your search:

1. **Specify the research problem:** The more precisely your problem statement is written, the more beneficial your computer search will be. A generalized statement will garner far too many descriptors that will lead to too many citations. A statement such as "self-efficacy in predicting smoking behavior of junior high school students" will provide a focus for the search because the interest is in *self-efficacy, prediction, smoking behavior,* and *junior high school.* These descriptors will limit the number of citations and be precise enough to hone in on the necessary information.

2. **Select the databases:** As we discussed previously, each university or college will have the software it believes necessary to help its users. With the librarian's help, you can decide which database or combinations of databases would be beneficial for your literature search. In the example used above, PSYCINFO and SSCI would be appropriate databases.

3. **Select the descriptors:** With the advice and consultation of the librarian and the procedure provided by the database, you should select the descriptors that best describe your research problem. Return to the example used in Number 1, the descriptors might be *self-efficacy, smoking, junior high school students,* and *prediction.* Dependent on how the particular database is set up, you would combine these

descriptors with *or* or *and* to limit the number of citations. You will also be asked to set the language limits ("English only" is most often requested), and you may also be asked to state a year from which to begin the search.

Many journals now have an electronic format so that the entire article can be retrieved online. While this is convenient, it will save you time only if you know what you should be reading. This is discussed in the next part of this section.

4. Conduct the search: You will be asked to enter the descriptors that coincide with those in the databases and determine how many citations are available in each descriptor. At this time, you will probably want to have a printout of approximately 10 references to see if you have used appropriate descriptors or their combinations. Once you have decided that you are on the right track, then you can tell the computer to print anywhere from 20 to thousands (if available). Some databases also provide abstracts or full text, and you can tell the computer which abstracts you wish to have printed.

5. Increase sensitivity and specificity: If the search renders too many or too few references, it is important to review your descriptors and redo the search. Two terms used in trying to get the right sources and avoid getting the wrong ones are sensitivity and specificity. *Sensitivity* is the likelihood of retrieving relevant items, whereas *specificity* is the likelihood of excluding irrelevant items (Center for Evidence Based Medicine, 1997).

If you get an unmanageably large number of references, you need to increase the specificity of your search. This can be accomplished by:

- Narrowing your question.
- If it is a free-text search, using more specific terms.
- Using a thesaurus/subject search.
- Selecting specific subheadings with thesaurus/subject MeSH (medical subject) headings.
- Using *and* to represent other aspects of the question.
- Limiting by publication type, year, or some other delimiter.

On the other hand, if you retrieve too few references, you need to increase sensitivity by:

- Broadening your question.
- Getting more search terms from relevant records.
- Trying different combinations of terms.
- Using wildcard (?) or truncation (*) features in either free text/text word or thesaurus/subject searches.
- Using *or* to add words of importance.
- Using the explosion feature of thesaurus searches.
- Selecting all subheadings with thesaurus/subject headings.
- Expanding the time frame or publication type.

6. Review the citation list. After you have received the printout, carefully review it and select those published works that you wish to read. You will probably find additional references in the bibliographies of these citations, which may lead to a another computer search.

Determining What to Read: The Information Jungle

The amount of information available today is astonishing, and it is continually growing. The National Library of Medicine database, MEDLINE, contains about 11 million references and abstracts from 4,300 journals. PubMed's retrieval engine links over 700 journals for full text of articles. Needless to say, your goal, like that of other investigators, is to spend the least amount of time finding the best information. As a general rule, useful information must have three attributes: (1) it must be relevant to the research effort; (2) it must be correct; and (3) it must require little effort to procure (Slawson, Shaughnessy, & Bennett, 1994). The formula is:

$$\text{level of evidence} = \frac{(\text{relevance} \times \text{validity})}{\text{work}}$$

Determining the Level of Evidence

Relevance

The relevance component begins with the applicability of the evidence to your problem but goes much further. The information must be critically appraised or evaluated for its validity and research usefulness. This is a crucial step if you are relying on the information to give useful guidance (Rosenberg & Donald, 1995).

Validity

Unfortunately, a large proportion of published health research lacks sufficient methodological rigor or relevance to answer research questions. To overcome this problem in medical research and practice, several investigators at McMaster University in Hamilton, Ontario, Canada developed the concept of *evidence-based medicine* (EBM), a process to systematically find, appraise, and apply research findings to clinical decisions (Oxman, Sackett, & Guyatt, 1993; Rosenberg & Donald, 1995). Specifically, it was designed to provide the best available evidence for patient care involving therapy, diagnosis, harm, and prognosis. Since its origin, it has expanded to include *evidence-based health care* (EBHC), addressing prevention/ therapy, health care recommendations, outcomes in health services, decision analysis, economic analysis, and overview studies such as meta-analysis (Lohr, Eleazer, & Mauskopf, 1998). Much has been written about EBHC, and a multitude of Websites exist to assist health professionals (see Appendix B).

For our purposes, it is important to understand that the health literature can be grouped into a *pyramid of evidence*. The pyramid categories range from expert opinion to double-blind, randomized, controlled studies. Like clinicians, health educators, researchers, and policy-makers want to base their decisions on the best evidence available. For example, if you were considering a communitywide program on smoking prevention for young people, what is the best evidence available to demonstrate effectiveness? EBHC has established categories of evidence as well as approaches to the literature to determine the level of evidence for an article under review. The levels of evidence, beginning with the highest, are:

I	Controlled and randomized
II-1	Controlled but not randomized
II-2	Cohort or case control
II-3	Multiple time series
III	Expert opinion or case study

High levels of evidence will not exist for all research or clinical questions because of the nature of the problems and research and ethical limitations.

To achieve evidence-informed decisions, the health educator or researcher should:

- Develop a focused question concerning the problem(s).
- Search secondary databases and the primary literature for relevant articles.
- Access the validity and usefulness of those articles (determine the level of evidence).
- Judge the relevance of the evidence to the problem.
- Implement the findings in the study or educational program.

The Working Group from McMaster University has published a series of "User's Guides to the Medical Literature" (Oxman et al., 1993). As part of the series, Giacomini and Cook (2000a, b) have applied the questions to qualitative research for interpretation by the clinician. The series offers a step-by-step guide on how to interpret the medical literature in terms of accuracy or validity. The following information is based on this work but has been modified to fit the needs of the health educator and researcher rather than the clinician.

For all articles reviewed, three basic questions must be asked:

1. Are the results of the study valid?
2. What are the results?
3. Will the results help me in conducting my study or educational endeavor?

The first question addresses the accuracy of the results. That is, are the results accurate and correct or incorrect due to bias or chance? As discussed in Chapter 5, on experimental research, study design attempts to decrease bias as much as possible. Dolan (1998) ordered study designs on the basis of increasing susceptibility to bias. From least biased to most, they are: controlled, randomized trials, cohort studies, case control studies, case series, case reports, and expert opinions. Chance, of course, involves the choice of statistical tests.

The second question is addressed only if you have determined that the results are unbiased or not a result of chance. If the results are valid, you should next consider the results themselves. This includes the precision of those results.

The third question considers the relevance of the results to your presenting problem. Using our previous example of a communitywide smoking prevention program, you would want to know if the article under review really answers the question of effectiveness.

These three questions should be expanded or modified when reviewing an article on specific health issues to help you determine its level of evidence or validity. The five principal areas of concern to health educators and researchers are: (1) prevention, education, or therapy; (2) overview studies (such as meta-analysis); (3) health or educational service outcomes; (4) clinical utilization; and (5) health care recommendations. The following worksheets offer questions that can be used to determine the relevance and validity of articles in each of these areas.

Relevance and Validity Worksheet for Articles on Prevention, Education, or Therapy

This worksheet is for articles on controlled studies, cohort and case-control investigations, and related research methodologies (Guyatt, Sackett, & Cook, 1993, 1994; Dolan, 1998).

Relevance (Is it worth taking the time to read this article?)

1. Does this information pertain to your central problem or question of prevention, education, or therapy?
2. If this information is true, will it change your way of approaching prevention, education, or therapy methodology and content?

Validity (Study design, flaws, and accuracy of information)

1. Are the results of the study valid?
    1.1. Was the assignment of subjects randomized?
    1.2. How were the cases and controls chosen in case-control studies?
    1.3. Were all subjects accounted for at the conclusion of the study?
    1.4. Were all subjects analyzed in the groups to which they were assigned?
    1.5. Was the sample size large enough to detect a meaningful difference in outcome?
    1.6. Were the subjects and/or investigators "blind" to the prevention, education, or therapy technique under investigation?
    1.7. Were the groups similar at the beginning of the study?
    1.8. Were the groups treated equally except for the prevention, education, or therapy treatment?
    1.9. In cohort and case-control studies, was exposure status clearly defined?

1.10. Was the follow-up time adequate to assess the outcome of interest?

1.11. What did the investigators do to control for bias?

2. What are the results?

    2.1. How large was the effect from the prevention, education, or therapy treatment?

    2.2. How precise were the authors in estimating the treatment effect?

3. Will the results help you conduct your research or carry out your educational endeavor?

    3.1. Can the results be applied to your research or education question?

    3.2. Were all the important outcomes considered?

    3.3. Are the likely benefits demonstrated in this article worth their potential harm, efforts, and costs?

Relevance and Validity Worksheet for Articles on Overview Studies

This worksheet is for articles that summarize the literature and meta-analysis articles that use quantitative methods to summarize the results (Oxman, Cook, & Guyatt, 1995).

Relevance (Is it worth taking the time to read this article?)

1. Does the article propose to answer a specific question? (The question addressed by the summary must be very focused, or you will be forced to guess at whether it is pertinent to your investigation or endeavor.)

2. Will this information, if true, change your way of doing things (research or educational methodology, community intervention, and the like)?

Validity (Study design, flaws, and accuracy of information)

1. Are the results of the study valid?

    1.1. Were the methods used to locate relevant studies comprehensive and clearly stated?

    1.2. Were the criteria used to select articles for inclusion appropriate?

    1.3. What is the likelihood that important studies were missed?

    1.4. Did the authors appraise the validity of the included studies?

    1.5. Did more than one reviewer decide (a) which studies to include; (b) the validity of each study; and (c) which data to extract from the study? (Each of these is judgment decision, and having two or more reviewers involved in the decision decreases the possibility of bias or random errors. There should be agreement among the reviewers.)

    1.6. Was variation between the results of the relevant studies analyzed? (This is a test of homogeneity.)

2. What are the results?

    2.1. What are the results of the review as they pertain to your question or problem?

    2.2. How precise were the results?

3. Will the results help you conduct your study or educational endeavor?
   3.1. Can the results be generalized to your investigation or population?
   3.2. Were all the research or educationally important outcomes considered?

Relevance and Validity Worksheet for Articles on Health or Educational Service Outcomes

Changes in health care delivery have made outcomes a strong force in redesigning public health policy. This worksheet is for articles on the outcomes of health or educational services, which have become principal "markers" for politicians, administrators, health care professionals, and researchers (Naylor & Guyatt, 1996).

Relevance (Is it worth taking the time to read this article?)
   1. Does this article include or focus on the health or educational service outcomes that you are investigating?
   2. What is the base perspective of the article? In other words, is it from the point of view of an administrator, health care provider, health care deliverer, politician, researcher, or educator?

Validity (Study design, flaws, and accuracy of information)
   1. Are the results of the study valid?
      1.1. Are the outcome measures accurate and comprehensive?
      1.2. Were the comparison groups clearly identified and logically chosen?
      1.3. How similar are the comparison groups in regard to important determinants of outcome other than the one under investigation?
      1.4. How did the authors handle factors that could affect outcomes?
         1.4.1. What was the exact health or educational service provided?
         1.4.2. Who provided the service under question?
         1.4.3. Where was the service provided?
         1.4.4. When was the service provided?
      1.5. Is the difference in outcome attributable to differences in prognosis rather than intervention?
         1.5.1. Were all important prognostic issues measured?
         1.5.2. How accurate or reproducible were measures of patients' or learners' prognostic factors?
         1.5.3. Did the authors employ multivariate analysis to adjust for differences in prognostic factors?

   2. What are the results?
      2.1. Do the results have a logical basis?

   3. Will the results help you conduct your research or carry out your educational endeavor?
      3.1. Can the results be applied to your research or education question?

Relevance and Validity Worksheet for Articles on Clinical Utilization

Health care administrators and providers observe clinical procedures to make sure they are within the usual range of usage. This worksheet is for articles that discuss decisions related to clinical utilization (Naylor & Guyatt, 1996a, b).

Relevance (Is it worth taking the time to read this article?)

1. Is the clinical utilization review directly related to the one you are studying?
2. Will the information provided, if true, support a change in clinical utilization at your institution?

Criteria Validity

1. Are the criteria valid?
   1.1. Did the authors employ a sensible, detailed, and rigorous process to identify, choose, and combine evidence for the criteria?
   1.2. What is the quality of the evidence used in framing the criteria? Are the criteria based on evidence from controlled studies, observations, or expert opinions?
   1.3. If expert opinions were used, did the authors have an explicit, systematic, and reliable process for choosing panelists and collating their opinions?
   1.4. Did the authors address the role of values in influencing the panelists' opinions? (Not all clinicians—for example, generalists versus subspecialists—value the same things.)
   1.5. How well are the criteria correlated with patient outcomes? Expect criteria from controlled studies to be highly correlated. When using weaker evidence, the authors should have checked for this correlation.
2. Were the criteria appropriately applied?
   2.1. Were the criteria applied in a reliable, unbiased fashion? Was inter-rater reliability used?
   2.2. How did the authors handle the uncertainty associated with evidence and values on the criteria-based ratings of process of care? For example, when panelists disagreed, did the authors present alternative results based on harsher or more lenient raters, or did they see uncertainty as either adequate or inadequate care?
3. Can the criteria be used in your own practice or institutional setting?
   3.1. Do the criteria in the review really fit your setting? How do the medical culture, values, and circumstances compare? There is less to worry about if the criteria are based on strong evidence such as controlled studies.
   3.2. Have the criteria been field-tested for diverse settings, including one or more like your own?

Relevance and Validity Worksheet for Articles on Health Care Educational Recommendations

Applied health research has become a major emphasis for governmental and nongovernmental entities. This is particularly true for health care and, in some instances, educational recommendations (Guyatt et al., 1995). This worksheet is for articles on these issues.

Relevance (Is it worth taking the time to read this article?)

1. Do the recommendations directly apply to the health care or educational intervention you are considering?
2. Will implementation of the recommendations improve your health care or educational outcomes?

Validity

1. What is the strength of the evidence? In other words, are the recommendations based on strong evidence such as randomized, controlled trials (RCTs) or more on observational studies?
    1.1.   If there was a systematic review of RCTs, were the results consistent from study to study?
    1.2.   Did the overview of studies reveal a differing treatment effect? If so, is it due to differences in students/patients, administration of the intervention, outcome measurement, study methodology, or chance? Check for homogeneity of the intervention effect.
    1.3.   Is the difference between the confidence interval (CI) boundaries for the two most disparate studies greater than 5%? If so, heterogeneity may exist. However, such heterogeneity should be reviewed for both educational and clinical importance as well as statistical significance before claiming that heterogeneity had a bearing on the recommendations.
    1.4.   Was the evidence based on cohort, case-control, or other observational studies and thus weakened?

2. How large an impact is needed to warrant use of the educational or health care intervention?
    2.1.   Does the educational/clinical intervention have a great enough effect to warrant its financial, administrative, and perhaps student-teacher or patient-provider burdens?
    2.2.   What is the incidence of an unwanted outcome for the group if not treated? If treated?
    2.3.   What is the threshold number of students or patients that needs to be treated (NTT)? (A full explanation of this issue is in Guyatt et al., 1995.)

3. How well does the intervention or treatment work?
    3.1.   If meta-analysis was used, what is the effect from pooling all the results from the various studies? What is the CI around this point estimate? Is the CI range large or small?

4. Where would you grade the recommendations using the evidence scale below?
    A1   RCTs with homogeneity and CIs all on one side of the NTT
    A2   RCTs with homogeneity and CIs overlap the NTT

B1   RCTs with heterogeneity and CIs all on one side of the NTT
B2   RCTs with heterogeneity and CIs overlap the NTT
C1   Observational studies with CIs all on one side of the NTT
C2   Observational studies and CIs overlap the NTT

Finding Short-cuts to Determining the Level of Evidence

The third part of the formula for determining the usefulness of information (presented in the *Determining What to Read* section above) is work. While the worksheets are invaluable tools for assessing the relevance and validity of an article, they do take time to complete. In the field of evidence-based medicine or health care, some databases do allow the researcher to search by level of evidence. Databases that conduct systematic reviews are preferred because they locate, appraise, and synthesize evidence from scientific studies in order to provide informative empirical answers to scientific research questions. Systematic reviews differ from other types of reviews in that they adhere to a strict scientific design in order to be more comprehensive, to minimize the chance of bias, and so to ensure their reliability.

Several evidence-based databases are listed in the *Evidence-Based Full-Text and Abstracting Services* section of this chapter. The Cochrane Library is now the premier resource for information on the effectiveness of health care interventions. It is an electronic publication designed to supply high-quality evidence. It is published quarterly on CD-ROM and the Internet, and is distributed on a subscription basis. Explicit criteria are used to include or exclude articles, and data are often combined statistically, using meta-analysis, to increase the power of numerous studies, each too small to produce reliable results individually. The complete reviews are exceedingly detailed (some as long as 25 pages) and include background material on the subject, criteria used, computer search strategies, methods of review, description of studies, methodological quality, detailed results, outcome measurements, discussion, implications for both clinicians and researchers, and an extensive reference list.

The Internet has several excellent sites that address evidence-based health care in detail. They range from simple descriptions to resources that benefit health science investigators and practitioners. Appendix B contains a section listing these Websites.

Writing the Section on Related Literature

You now have gathered all, or most, of the information necessary to begin writing the review of literature section of your paper, research report, thesis, or dissertation. It is important to note here that at this point you will have already written the introduction (discussed in detail in Chapter 2), which must be related to the review of literature. In addition, you should develop a plan for the review, be sure to have the proper theoretical orientation, and summarize the entire section.

Relating the Review

As we discussed, the purpose of doing the review of literature is to develop an understanding of the background for the study; to delineate very clearly the problem; and to provide an empirical basis for the hypothesis or research questions. To present a clear and concise rationale for attempting the study, the information in the literature review should always relate to the introductory material. This will enable the introduction to flow coherently and present an organized approach to theory and research related to your topic. The literature should be related to the purpose of the study, the generated hypotheses, and the population in question. Recall that the literature search is done with a critical eye toward reviewing previous, similar studies and using that information to distinguish between the various kinds of problems your area of interest might encounter.

Developing a Plan

We have stressed that being organized is of paramount importance in preparing for the review and in gathering the materials. That organization will help you in writing the review, as you have already established subheadings. Subheadings are usually based on the variables and their relationship to the problem of your study. To make it easier for the reader, we suggest that each subtopic begin with an introductory sentence to explain the relevance of the section and end with a summarizing section that depicts the conclusions or insights gleaned from this subsection.

Deriving a Theoretical Orientation

Each literature review in the health sciences must have a theoretical orientation, as discussed in the beginning of this chapter. The theory is usually derived from any of the social sciences, and tends to build on the theoretical perspectives of the health-related literature. The central theme to the review is a theoretical core; from it emanate the subheadings, topics, and even subtheories. During the writing of the review, the theoretical orientation becomes part of the organizing framework, as shown in Figure 3.1.

Summarizing

At the conclusion of the review of literature, a separate subheading entitled *Summary* should be included. This section recaps the relevant information relating to theory, previous research, new insights, and the stated hypotheses. Generally, one or two paragraphs should suffice, if presented cogently.

Summary

This chapter told you about the tools and information necessary for a review of literature for a paper, research report, proposal, thesis, and/or dissertation. The

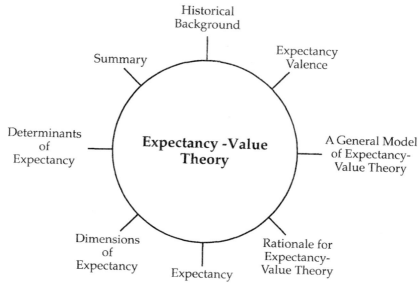

FIGURE 3.1 Theoretical Core and Subheadings

benefits of the review include being able to limit the problem, develop an understanding and grounding in appropriate theory, review previously used procedures and instruments, originate new ideas, use the recommendations for further research, and critically review the material. A discussion of the steps in the research process included: (1) reading the background information; (2) gathering the necessary tools; (3) listing key words; (4) checking preliminary sources; (5) conducting a computer search; (6) determining what to read; (7) determining the level of evidence; and (8) finding short-cuts to determining the level of evidence.

The list of indexing and abstracting sources presented in this chapter included evidence-based sources, which allow you to select related studies that offer varying degrees of support to your research effort. Further, those databases can be searched in an evidence-based manner. Several worksheets were provided so that you can ascertain the level of evidence of an article when such sources are not available. Finally, a strategy for actually writing the review was devised so that you can integrate the literature with the introductory materials described in Chapter 2.

Suggested Activities

1. Go to the website entitled *Explore the Internet: Library of Congress* (http://lcweb. loc.gov/global/explore.html). Under the section *Internet Search Tools*, click on *Read Comparisons and Reviews of Search Tools*. Select at least two links and read their evaluations of various search tools. Do you agree with their evaluations and believe that this site can help researchers?

2. Go to the website of the Centers for Disease Control (http://www.cdc.gov) and check out PERRY. Be thorough in your review. Would you recommend this site to other health researchers? Justify your answer.

3. Develop a problem statement and list the key words you would use in a computer database search. Select at least two databases available at your university and conduct a search. Check your results for specificity and sensitivity. Using the directions in this chapter, increase or decrease your search yield as needed. Compare the results of your second search with those of your first.

4. From the list obtained in Number 3, select two articles that can be reviewed using two of the evidence-based worksheets presented in this chapter. Apply the criteria for relevance and validity. Where would you place the articles on the level of evidence chart?

5. Access the PubMed database at your university. In the search line, enter the key words *interventions* and *cervical cancer* and *sex*. What is the number of items (articles) returned? Next, click on *Limits*, immediately below the search line. In the boxes, limit the publication type to *Randomized Controlled Trials*, the language to *English*, the research to *Human Studies*, and the gender to *Female*. Click on *Search*. What is the number of items returned?

6. Access the Cochrane Library and conduct a search using the following key words: *intervention* and *sexual lifestyle* and *cervical cancer*. Look at the list of complete reviews and select the study by Shepard, Weston, Peersman, and Napuli entitled *Interventions for Encouraging Sexual Lifestyles and Behaviours Intended to Prevent Cervical Cancer*. Review everything provided in this Cochrane review and compare it to what is provided in reviews from other databases. Based on your review, why is the Cochrane Library referred to as the premier database for evidenced-based health care?

References

Center for Evidence Based Medicine. (1997). Searching for the best evidence in clinical journals. Available at: http://cebm.jr2.ox.ac.uk/docs/searching.html.

Dolan, M. S. (1998). Interpretation of the literature. *Clinical Obstetrics and Gynecology, 41*(2), 307–314.

Giacomini M. K., & Cook, D. J. (2000a). Users' guides to the medical literature, XXIII: Qualitative research in health care. A. Are the results of the study valid? *JAMA, 284*(3), 357–362.

Giacomini, M. K., & Cook, D. J. (2000b). Users' guides to the medical literature, XXIII: Quali-

tative research in health care. B. What are the results and how do they help me care for my patients? *JAMA, 284*(4), 478–482.

Guyatt, G. H., Sackett, D. L., & Cook, D. J. (1993). User's guides to the medical literature, II: How to use an article about therapy or prevention. A. Are the results of the study valid? *JAMA, 270*(21), 2598–2601.

Guyatt, G. H., Sackett, D. L., & Cook, D. J. (1994). User's guides to the medical literature, II: How to use an article about therapy or prevention. B. What were the results and will they help me in caring for my patients? *JAMA, 271*(1), 59–63.

Guyatt, G. H., Sackett, D. L., Sinclair, J. C., Hayward, R., Cook, D. J., & Cook, R. J. (1995). User's guides to the medical literature, VIII: How to use clinical practice guidelines. A method for grading health care recommendations. *JAMA*, 274(22), 1800–1804.

Lohr, K., Eleazer, K., & Mauskopf, J. (1998). Health policy issues and applications for evidence-based medicine and clinical practice guidelines. *Health Policy*, 46(1), 1–19.

Naylor, C. D., & Guyatt, G. H. (1996a). User's guides to the medical literature, X: How to use an article reporting variations in the outcomes of health services. *JAMA*, 275(7), 554–558.

Naylor, C. D., & Guyatt, G. H. (1996b). User's guides to the medical literature, XI: How to use an article about a clinical utilization review. *JAMA*, 275(18), 1435–1439.

Oxman, A. D., Cook, D. J., & Guyatt, G. H. (1995). User's guides to the medical literature, VI: How to use an overview. *JAMA*, 272(17), 1367–1371.

Oxman, A. D., Sackett, D. L., & Guyatt, G. H. (1993). User's guides to the medical literature, I: How to get started. *JAMA*, 270(17), 2093–2095.

Rosenberg, W., & Donald, A. (1995). Evidence based medicine: An approach to clinical problem solving. *British Medical Journal, 310,* 1122–1126.

Slawson, D. S., Shaughnessy, A. F., & Bennett, J. H. (1994). Becoming a medical information master: Feeling good about not knowing everything. *Journal of Family Practice*, 38(5), 505–513.

Chapter 4

Considering Ethics in Research

Case Study

Emily, a nurse on Six East, was hoping that she could combine her clinic work with a research project needed for her master's degree. A good part of her job is to take complete medical and sexual histories as well as physical exams on patients referred to the colposcopy clinic. In this clinic a colposcope is used to evaluate patients who have an abnormal Papanincolaou (Pap) smear, and a punch biopsy is taken together with an endocervical curettage. Emily follows up on many patients, explaining the results to them—normal or varying degrees of dysplasia. In cases of severe dysplasia or invasive cervical cancer, she helps the patient schedule surgery.

In collecting her information and following the patients, Emily has observed that several things in their history appear to be related to cervical cancer. Some of the more significant events appeared to be early first intercourse, multiple sexual partners, young at marriage, young or early pregnancy, smoking, and having a partner who has had multiple sexual partners. She wondered if her perceptions were accurate and if there may be other precursors to cervical cancer that she was missing.

As a research project, Emily decided to review patient records for the last six months and to collect data for another six months. At that time, she would look at all of her data and do a multiple regression analysis of those risk factors. Since this was part of her work, Emily knew this project would save herself time and would not require informed consent. The patients would be simply following their usual course of action and no harm could befall them. While this wasn't a perfect project, it came very close.

In speaking with her project advisor, it was pointed out that several breaches of ethics were contained in her proposal. What ethical problems do you see in her proposed research? If you were Emily's advisor, what would you suggest she do to remedy the problems?

General Ethical Dilemmas in Human Research

Research on human subjects has been conducted since the time of the ancient Greeks. However, not until the atrocities of Nazi research became known was an effort made to protect research subjects. The Nuremberg medical trials documented such charges as:

1. From August 1942 to May 1943, some Dachau prisoners were severely chilled or frozen in either a tank of ice water for three hours or forced to stand outside, naked, at below freezing temperatures.
2. From December 1941 to February 1945, prisoners at Buchenwald and Natzweiler were injected with spotted fever virus to keep it alive.
3. From July 1942 to September 1943, prisoners were deliberately given wounds infected with *Streptococcus*, tetanus, and gas gangrene, which were then irritated by forcing wood shavings or ground glass into them. After the blood vessels to the wounds were tied off, the wounds were treated with sulfanilamide to check for its effectiveness.

Yet even as the Nuremberg trials of 23 physicians were being conducted in postwar Germany, the U.S. Public Health Service supported a research project in the rural South with complete disregard for the rights of subjects.

The study, known as the Tuskegee syphilis study (Brandt, 1978), commenced in 1929 in Macon County, Alabama, where Tuskegee is located. This county was found to have the highest syphilis rate in the United States, and it was believed that it merited special attention. The project was regarded as a study in nature rather than an experiment because the purpose was to follow the natural course of the disease. The researchers at the time felt that because so many Blacks had syphilis anyway, it was simply a matter of taking advantage of a natural situation. No formal protocol was written, but letters between Dr. Taliaferro Clark, Chief of the U.S. Public Health Service (U.S. PHS) Venereal Disease Division, and his colleagues revealed that, in addition to observing the natural course of the disease, the researchers desired to show that antisyphilitic treatment was unnecessary. This was speculated because many Blacks experienced a spontaneous cure, and because 70% of the remainder were not inconvenienced by the disease. It was admitted that 30% of the subjects were highly contagious and seriously affected. Nevertheless, the U.S. PHS chose not to treat the disease with arsenic and bismuth, which was recognized as a treatment at the time.

The male subjects, between the ages of 25 and 60, were not told about the nature of the study but believed they were being treated for the disease. The study continued indefinitely so subjects could be watched until they died and an autopsy could be performed. Incentives were used throughout the 40-year period to keep everyone participating. Moreover, the U.S. PHS gave the U.S. Army a list of 256 men who were in the study and subsequently drafted, requesting that they not be treated for syphilis. The Army complied.

Although articles about the Tuskegee syphilis study appeared in the medical press as early as 1936, news about the study did not reach the national public press until 1972—when the study was still ongoing. The U.S. Department of Health, Education, and Welfare (DHEW; now called the Department of Health and Human Services) formed a committee to investigate criticisms. Three basic issues arose: (1) should the study have been conducted and should the men have been informed; (2) should the men have been treated when penicillin became available; and (3) should the study be terminated? Needless to say, many still believe that the incident was handled too casually and that a myriad of ethical issues were not addressed.

More recently, information has come forth about radiation research conducted in the 1940s and 1950s. In one investigation at Fernald State School in Waltham, Massachusetts, from 1946 to 1956, mentally disabled boys were given radioactive milk as part of a research project on the digestive system. The boys believed they were in a science club and were administered low-level radioactive forms of calcium and iron in their breakfast milk. Although consent forms were sent to parents and guardians, they failed to disclose information about the radiation. The former Atomic Energy Commission helped sponsor the research ("Retarded kids fed radiation," 1993). In a related study, women attending a free prenatal clinic at Vanderbilt University in the 1940s were given a mildly radioactive isotope to determine how iron was absorbed. This was done under the guise of a nutritional experiment. The follow-up revealed a small, yet significant, increase in cancer in the children born of these women. No documentation of informed consent has been found (Gribben, Norvell, & Van Vorst, 1994). In other experiments, prisoners in Oregon had their testicles irradiated without their consent. In September 1995, President Clinton, reacting to a 925-page government report documenting the extent of experimental radiation treatments since WWII commented, "The United States of America offers a sincere apology to those of our citizens who were subjected to these experiments" (Powelson, 1995). He believed that many persons were due compensation from the government.

The beginning researcher should realize that the Tuskegee study and many of the radiation studies were carried out by supposedly forthright Americans through branches of the federal or state governments. Oftentimes, they were supported through tax dollars and generally accepted by portions of the medical community. In the case of the Tuskegee study, only with the hue and cry from the public did it stop. As a health scientist, like Emily, you should scrutinize the objectives, justification, and methodology of your study with ethical eyes. Any researcher may mean well, but failure to consider ethical dilemmas is inexcusable.

Some of the major issues are (1) justification to experiment on humans, especially children, the handicapped, the elderly, and prisoners; (2) informed consent of the subject; (3) confidentiality through the right to privacy; (4) truthtelling and deception; (5) the degree of organization that qualifies a procedure as experimental;

(6) the researcher's responsibility for harmful consequences; (7) the duty to continue a successful experiment or research effort; (8) the relationship of therapeutic to nontherapeutic research; (9) sponsored research; and (10) the publication of unethical research. As to be expected, these ten issues hold inherent ethical problems that tend to compound the research endeavor. This chapter addresses these major issues as well as the institutional review process.

Justification to Experiment on Humans

In any research effort, there must be substantial justification for the need to experiment with humans, including the implications for usage of results. The *Nuremberg Code* was devised as a result of the trials at Nuremberg to prevent future atrocities in human research (Fromer, 1981). It suggests ten principles to be addressed in justification and methodology. Simply, they are:

1. Voluntary consent of the participant is absolutely essential. The subject must be capable of giving consent without coercion, and full responsibility for obtaining consent rests with the principal investigator.
2. The experiment must be designed to bring forth results that will benefit society and that cannot be obtained in any other manner.
3. Human experimentation should be based on animal research results as well as knowledge of the natural course of events, disease, or problems.
4. All unnecessary mental or physical harm should be avoided.
5. When there is reason to believe that death or disabling injury may occur, no experiment should be conducted except, perhaps, when the experimenting physicians also serve as subjects.
6. The degree of risk should never exceed the humanitarian importance of the problem to be solved.
7. All precaution should be taken to protect subjects from even remote possibilities of injury or death.
8. Only qualified personnel should be allowed to conduct experiments.
9. The subject must be able to withdraw from the experiment at any time if a point is reached that may bring about physical or mental harm.
10. The principal investigator must be ready to terminate the experiment at any stage if it appears that injury or death will result.

On the surface the Nuremberg Code appears to embrace all the necessary components. However, at least three flaws are evident. First, too much onus is given to the principal investigator, especially in regard to informed consent. Concomitantly, the overall tone is that as long as the investigator possesses positive intentions, no harm will come to the subject. It may be asked, who knows what is good for society, and who knows how much risk is worth that good? Finally, no one monitors the principal investigator to determine whether his or her actions and decisions are in fact ethical ones. Nevertheless, the Nuremberg Code provided a start in protecting the rights of the human subjects.

Frequently, argument about justification revolves around the interests of (1) the health sciences; (2) the subjects or patients; and (3) the community (Beecher, 1970). While it may be noted in the first issue that acquisition of knowledge and full understanding of any truths are not morally objectionable, it must be realized that not every method is allowable simply because it potentially increases knowledge and understanding. Health sciences, like other sciences, must be placed in line with other life values. When this is done, it can be readily witnessed that the interests of the health sciences are not the highest values to which all others must be subordinated.

Regarding the interests of the subject or patient as justification, the health science researcher must be cognizant of the myriad of questions raised through consent. For example, what limits should a competent adult be allowed to take? Should the subject or the researcher set the limits? These inquiries become more complex when a researcher deals with special target groups such as children, the ill, the elderly, or prisoners.

The third issue, the interests of the community (i.e., human society, the common good) as justification, introduces more questions. Can public authority endow the researcher with the power to experiment on the individual in the interests of the community when such experimentation may transgress individual rights? Does the person exist for the community, or does community exist for the person? Keep in mind the experiments in Germany in World War II as well as those conducted in Tuskegee. Was there a well-meaning community in both instances?

In Emily's study on risk factors for cervical cancer, what would be an acceptable justification? Is the acquisition of knowledge about such risk factors adequate? Is there benefit for the patients? Is potential benefit for others appropriate justification?

Vulnerable Target Groups: Children

Justification of research on human beings is always demanding, but particularly so for those target groups who are especially vulnerable. Children are often selected for studies in the health science field because they are a captive audience in the school system as well as in pediatric wards across the country. Neither the 1947 Nuremberg Code nor the 1949 International Code of Medical Ethics mentions the use of children or other "incompetents" in nontherapeutic research. The 1964 Helsinki Declaration requires parental or guardian consent for nontherapeutic research on children. This was endorsed by the American Medical Association in 1966. Although it appears plausible on the surface, giving parents or guardians total freedom to submit children to experiments is somewhat frightening. Further, there may be direct or indirect coercion on the parents to "volunteer" their children.

The most famous example of experimentation on children is the Willowbrook experiment (Veatch, 1977). Willowbrook State Hospital in Staten Island, New York, is an institution for the care of people with mental retardation (i.e., having an IQ of less than 20). Dr. Saul Krugman was appointed as consultant in pediatrics and in infectious diseases in 1954. He noted that several infectious diseases, especially hepatitis and measles, were prevalent within the institution. In 1956, Dr. Krugman and his associates commenced research on hepatitis and did not stop their research effort until 1970. During that period, four times each year approximately 12 to 15 children were admitted into the research unit, for a total of 700 to 800 children out of the 10,000 admissions to Willowbrook.

In order to gain a better understanding of the disease and hopefully to develop a method of immunization against hepatitis, the researchers injected live hepatitis serum into the subjects to produce the disease. This research effort was approved by the Armed Forces Epidemiological Board, the Committee on Human Experimentation of New York University, and the New York State Department of Mental Hygiene. Justification was based on the grounds that (1) the children were bound to be exposed to the same strains under the natural conditions existing in the institution; (2) they would be admitted to a special, well-equipped and well-staffed unit where they would be isolated from exposure to other infectious diseases that were prevalent in the institution—namely, shigellosis, parasitic infections, and respiratory infections—and thus their exposure in the hepatitis unit would be associated with less risk than in the institutional setting where multiple infections could occur; (3) they were likely to have a subclinical infection followed by immunity to the particular hepatitis virus; and (4) only children with parents who gave their informed consent would be included (Krugman, 1967).

The ethical issues in this "experiment" are numerous. Parents were put in the difficult position of having their children placed either in unsanitary and poor social conditions or in the research unit, where high-quality health care and better social conditions existed. There was at least indirect if not direct coercion by Krugman and his associates. Should parental consent have been enough in this case? The fact that these subjects were children, mentally disabled and institutionalized, made them particularly vulnerable. Why did these agencies fund such a project? Why was the money not diverted to improve conditions at Willowbrook so that disease would be less rampant for all children? If better conditions had existed within the institution, the justification offered by the researchers would collapse.

Veatch (1977) presents both extremes of ethical alternatives by stating:

> At one extreme one could argue that the moral duty of any researcher encountering a group of subjects who will volunteer only because of their social condition is to improve that condition rather than take advantage of it. . . . One might argue from a morally rigorous position that there is always a duty to alleviate social conditions producing suffering when one has the skill and is directly involved with those suffering.
>
> At the other extreme is the argument that one can trade off a medical service to the general group in need of medical help for the privilege of experimenting. . . . This proposal has crassness, however, suggesting that the individual may be sacrificed for the good of the group. The end results might benefit the whole

group, but the benefit to the subject certainly cannot justify the experimental risk. (p. 277)

Even when considering the moral trade-off, which occurs in some prisons and with individuals such as the mentally disabled who are incapable of giving consent, such a trade-off is difficult to support. Dr. Krugman and others at Willowbrook were dealing with two evils—poor social conditions within the institution and an intentional personal risk of harm.

Partially as the result of the Willowbrook incident, in 1974 Congress mandated that the National Commission for the Protection of Human Subjects and Behavioral Research (hereinafter the Commission) establish guidelines to protect vulnerable populations, including children, from exploitation as research subjects (McCartney, 1978). In brief, the Commission's recommendations to the Secretary of the DHEW in 1977 were as follows:

1. Research involving children is important and should be conducted according to these recommendations.
2. Research may be conducted providing that the Institutional Review Board (IRB) determines that the research is scientifically sound, has been conducted on animals or adult humans first (where appropriate), has minimal risks in design and procedure, provides for privacy of children and parents, and makes selection in an equitable manner.
3. Research that does not involve greater than minimal risk to children may be conducted if the risk is justified by the anticipated benefit for the subjects; if the risk is no greater than alternative approaches; and if consent is given by parents and, when possible, by the children themselves.
4. Research that involves more than minimal risk and holds a prospect of direct subject benefit may be conducted only if such risk is justified by the anticipated results; the risk is at least as favorable to the subjects as that presented by alternative approaches; and consent is given.
5. Research that involves more than minimal risk and fails to hold out the prospect for direct benefit for individual subjects may be supported if the IRB determines that such a risk is only a minor increase over minimal risk; that generalizable knowledge about the condition will be obtained; that the anticipated knowledge is of vital importance for understanding or ameliorating the condition; and of course, that consent is given.
6. When research cannot be approved under the preceding conditions, it can only be conducted provided that it presents an opportunity to understand, prevent, or alleviate a serious problem affecting children; that a national ethical advisory board has reviewed the proposal and determined that it would not violate respect for persons or the principles of beneficence and justice; and that consent is given.
7. In addition to these recommendations, the IRB should solicit the assent of both children and parents or guardians when appropriate; involve at least one parent or guardian in the conduct of the research; and accept a child's objection as

binding unless the intervention via research provides direct benefit to the health or well-being of the subject.

8. Parental consent may be waived if it is not reasonably required to protect the subjects. However, there must be an adequate alternative mechanism for protecting the children, depending upon the nature of the research protocol.

9. Children who are wards of the state should be included in research only if it is related to their status as orphans, abandoned children, and the like, or conducted in a setting wherein the majority of the children are not wards of the state. An advocate for each child must be appointed and given the same opportunity to intervene as would a parent.

10. Children who reside in institutions for the mentally disabled or correctional facilities should participate in research only if the conditions regarding research are fulfilled in addition to the aforementioned conditions.

In 1978, the DHEW adopted all the Commission's recommendations but also declared that: (1) a child's objection to participation is binding; (2) no specific age should be set for a child's consent to be mandatory; and (3) the Secretary may appoint an ad hoc panel rather than a national commission to review difficult proposals. The Department of Health and Human Services (DHHS) continues to operate with these guidelines.

The general rule of thumb set by the DHHS is that anyone below the age of 18 is considered a child. If a researcher wishes to treat subjects under 18 years of age as adults in a research project, complete rationale has to be provided, including any laws, legal precedents, agency rules and regulations, and the like. If the children are wards of the state, an advocate with appropriate background should be appointed for each child. The section in this chapter entitled *Exempt and Nonexempt Review Status* provides further information about research with children.

In regard to Emily's investigation of cervical cancer, if the patient were 16 years old, is informed consent required for either the medical procedure or the research effort? Does the age of the patient make any difference in collecting this type of data?

Informed Consent: Truthtelling and Deception

Informed consent essentially entails making the subject fully aware of the research project (a detailed explanation is presented later in this section) and obtaining permission from the subject to go ahead with the project. Over time, informed consent has also come to mean the written document signed by the potential research subject, although oral permission is granted in some cases. The requirement of informed consent is designed to protect the inviolability of the subject. Specifically, Capron (1974) views the functions of informed consent as (1) to promote individual autonomy; (2) to protect the patient-subject's status as a human being; (3) to avoid fraud and duress; (4) to encourage self-scrutiny by the researcher; and (5) to foster rational decision-making.

A classic case of research in which there was great disregard for informed consent is a doctoral dissertation by Laud Humphreys (Beauchamp & Childress, 1994). He believed that the general public and law enforcement officials held several myths and misconceptions about homosexual males and their behavior in public places, especially bathrooms—known as "tearooms." To research behavior, he placed himself in various bathrooms and offered his services as "watchqueen," the person who watches out for police. Through this method of research he was able to observe hundreds of acts of fellatio, eventually gaining the confidence of some of the regulars. To many of them, he explained his role as a researcher and persuaded them to disclose their motivations for tearoom sex and to talk about their lives in general.

In other instances, however, Humphreys was not so open, secretly following the men outside, where he copied their license plate numbers and thereby learned names and addresses. A year later he showed up on their doorsteps, posing as a health services interviewer, and questioned them about their lives, jobs, marriages, and so on. Overall, it was found that over one-half of the subjects were married, living with their wives, and leading good lives. About 38% of the men were neither bisexual nor homosexual, but had poor marriages and subsequently sought sex without emotional entanglements and without jeopardizing their current community positions. These men felt masturbation was too lonely. Another group, comprising 24%, were bisexual, happily married, and economically successful; still another 24% were single and covertly homosexual; and only 14% were openly homosexual. In conclusion, he showed that not just gay men were involved but he did so with unethical research.

The research effort managed to eliminate many myths and did alleviate harassment of homosexual men by police authorities. Nonetheless, informed consent was not obtained, and the men did not know they were part of a study. The research proposal had been reviewed by dissertation committee members only, and when the issue came to light, the entire sociology department at Washington University was in a furor. After publication (*The Tearoom Trade: Impersonal Sex in Public Places* [Chicago: Aldine] in 1970, there was considerable outrage about research methodology, informed consent, and privacy. While the topic of Emily's research in the case study may not be this explosive, her thesis committee will have to review the proposal thoroughly.

As a result of a Canadian study (Pappworth, 1969) in which a University of Saskatchewan student suffered cardiac arrest and subsequent decrease in memory and concentration during an experiment to test a new anesthetic, the DHEW formulated the guidelines for informed consent. According to the DHHS, the basic requirements of a written informed consent for adults should include:

1. Fair explanation of the research effort—its purpose, expected duration of participation by the subject, and experimental procedures, including exactly what the participant will do
2. Description of any attendant discomforts and risks reasonably to be expected
3. Description of any benefits reasonably to be expected

4. Research projects involving treatment, therapy, or a service must disclose alternative procedures or courses of treatment that might be advantageous to the subject
5. Explanation of how confidentiality will be maintained
6. When more than minimal risk is anticipated, informed consent must include an explanation of compensation (if any) and a statement about whether medical treatments are available in case of injury. (Note that "minimal risk" means a risk that is not greater than the risk encountered in daily life or during the performance of routine physical or psychological examinations.)
7. An offer to answer any inquiries concerning the procedures or whom to contact if problems should arise
8. Instruction that the person is free to withdraw consent and to discontinue participation in the project or activity at any time without prejudice to the subject

Some types of research in the health sciences require additional elements of consent. These elements are:

1. **Unforeseeable risks:** If any exist, these need to be pointed out to the potential research subject. For example, pharmaceutical experiments may have unforeseeable risks to a fetus that must be explained to a subject who is, or is likely to become, pregnant.
2. **Additional costs:** If the subject should require medical assistance, therapy, or some other service, who will pay for it and exactly how much it will cost must be stated.
3. **Investigator termination:** The circumstances under which the investigator would terminate the subject's participation without the subject's consent must be explained.
4. **Termination procedures:** The subject must be told how to withdraw from the research project and what consequences, if any, may result.
5. **New findings:** If new findings are likely during the course of the research project, subjects should be informed of those findings that relate to their willingness to continue participation.
6. **Number of subjects:** When appropriate, subjects should know the number of participants involved in the whole study.

When research involves children (under 18 years of age), written parental permission should be obtained, unless exemption is given by the IRB. Beginning in about junior high or middle school, the child's written consent is needed in addition to parental consent. Children in lower grades should provide oral consent—a positive statement of willingness to participate—in addition to parental consent. Age-appropriate explanation should be given to preschool children in addition to obtaining parental consent. In all cases, but especially for preschoolers, if children experience undue stress, their participation should be discontinued.

While the guidelines provide a basis for informed consent, the researcher still faces several research and ethical dilemmas. For example, how much does the subject need to know before consent can be given? If too much detail is given, the subject may not understand or perhaps may skew the data by acting the way the researcher hopes. In some instances the researcher may not be aware of the potential discomforts that could occur even a year after the research (e.g., guilt from participating in sexual research that then affects a marital relationship). How would you have altered Humphrey's study of homosexual males to incorporate informed consent?

Should Emily have informed consent in her study? What are the pros and cons of informed consent in her research effort? If informed consent is to be present in her study, how should she go about it? Would informed consent be different if her patient were 15 years old? 18 years old? What forms and procedures are required by your university or IRB to determine that informed consent has been fairly applied in studies dealing with human subjects?

Informed Consent and Double-Blind Studies

The design of double-blind studies is simple and logical. One-half of the subjects are randomly selected to receive the experimental product, and the other half is given a placebo, and the results are compared. Neither the researcher nor the subjects know who obtains the active substance or the placebo; hence the term *double-blind*.

Although the researcher values this methodology to earn accurate results, it possesses many ethical dilemmas. A study conducted by Goldzieher of the Southwest Foundation for Research and Education displays many of the ethical problems encompassed in double-blind research (Veatch, 1971). The purpose of the experiment was to discover whether some of the reported side effects of the contraceptive pill were physiological or psychological. The subjects were primarily poor, multiparous, Mexican American women who had come to a San Antonio clinic for contraception to prevent further pregnancies. Seventy-six of the women were given placebos, and another group got various hormone contraceptives. None were told that they were involved in a research project or that they were receiving placebos. All were instructed to employ vaginal cream because the contraceptive pill might not be "completely effective."

The results of the experiment showed that the women taking placebos had many of the same side effects—depression, breast tenderness, and headaches—as those on the contraceptive pill. However, 13% (10) of the 76 women taking placebos became pregnant. Needless to say, these women were deceived; yet, a request for full informed consent would have made the study impossible, because the women came to the clinic for pregnancy prevention. Could some information have been given without ruining the research? If deception is part of the research process, should the experiment be cancelled? In other words, what justification is required to approve deception? Were the results of the Goldzieher study worth 10 women getting pregnant? Who is to decide whether the results of an experimental procedure are potentially worthwhile? Moreover, if such studies are even contemplated, how should the population for the study be chosen? In this case, why were poor, Mexican American women selected, particularly individuals who could not afford medical care as clinic patients?

In short, the double-blind methodology is excellent for some research objectives, particularly if a placebo is employed; however, it is fraught with ethical dilemmas that should be addressed by the principal investigator.

Overall, recent trends indicate that the requirements for informed consent are becoming more and more rigorous. There are many special circumstances regarding persons who speak foreign languages and other minority groups. It is believed that a long consent form attached to a mail survey will reduce the number of returns. Just reading the form will take more time and thereby reduce returns, and the usual ominous tone is likely to decrease responses even further. Singer (1978) has shown that informed consent procedures lower response rates for interviews. Thorne (1980), in speaking about sociological research, has complained that federal regulations are based on the biomedical model of research and as such are not workable in research that is observational field research. He states that

> the requirement that one obtain signed consent forms from everyone one studies may violate anonymity and actually increase risks for some groups of subjects. In the end the procedures may result in meaningless ritual rather than improving the ethics of field research. (p. 285)

The problem of informed consent for the researcher is difficult, with the major problem being that of application—how much information, how much consent.

Right to Privacy and Confidentiality

All participants in human research have the right to privacy in that they have the right to request that their individual identities remain concealed. While the charge of invasion of privacy can be made in all methodologies, it is most likely to occur with survey research, audiotaping, and videotaping. The question of what constitutes invasion of privacy is quite subjective and may imply something different to the subject than the intent of the researcher. For example, in a drug survey the participant may have used cocaine but felt very guilty about it and may have not admitted it to anyone. Such a person may understandably feel that his or her privacy is being invaded when asked if cocaine had been taken at any time. This feeling of "invasion" may be underscored if the interview was either audiotaped or videotaped.

To ensure anonymity it is important to explain to the subject that most researchers are interested in group data and that individual scores are compiled with others. Further, individuals are identified by number rather than by name. Perhaps most importantly, the subject needs to understand the importance of the data being gathered; if the project is deemed important enough, the subject may be willing to sacrifice some privacy.

The principle of confidentiality is related to the right to privacy. Who will be able to see the data? In school systems, both teachers and students are concerned that research data may be used to evaluate performance. The health science researcher should treat all data confidentially and ensure that (1) all data is returned anonymously and directly to the research office; (2) all data is rostered by number; and (3) unneeded material is destroyed upon completion of the project.

Of course, there are several other ways in which confidentiality could be broken. It may occur if a subject is a relative or friend of a member of the research team who has even limited access to the data. Research records can be stolen. A questionnaire may be found by a spouse, friend, parent, or colleague, or a telephone message could be taken that identifies the participant. Even the participant may break confidentiality by writing a name on the questionnaire that reveals the illicit use of drugs. These breaks may occur no matter how careful the investigator.

Review the case study at the beginning of the chapter. What has Emily done to ensure the right to privacy and to maintain confidentiality? If her study were conducted as presented, might she violate the right to privacy? What suggestions could be given to Emily?

Audiotapes and Videotapes

Audiotaping and videotaping subjects preclude anonymity. This does not mean that they should not be employed in research; however, it does mean that:

1. Complete justification of use must be given by the researcher to the IRB.
2. If confidentiality is threatened more by use of tapes than nonuse, the researcher must have more reason than simple convenience.
3. The researcher must be very specific about how the tapes will be used and information analyzed; who will have access to them; where and for how long they will be stored; and the method of disposal.
4. If the tapes are to be used for purposes other than the research (e.g., an oral history interview used for teaching), complete explanation must be given, and the informed consent must reflect this additional use, including the length of time (e.g., two years) that it will be used. Note that a separate release form should be given to subjects regarding the use of the tapes outside of the research project. This separate form gives the rights of ownership to another individual, group, or institution.
5. If a panel of judges or the like are to review the tapes, the IRB should be informed as to their names (if available), credentials, and functions in regard to the research and tapes. The subjects need to receive this same information.
6. Subjects should be permitted to listen or view their tape upon completion to affirm their permission for use of the material. In the case of children (or other vulnerable groups), parents should be permitted to review the tape. They may

not want a video of their child's antisocial behavior or an audiotape of family "secrets."

7. In some instances consent to participate may be given on the tape. This is especially true when the investigator uses the subject's voice without name or identification. Generally, this approach requires approval from the IRB because it is a departure from the written form.

Responsibility for Harmful Consequences

Subjects have a right to expect the health science researcher to prevent harm from befalling them and to be sensitive to their need for human dignity. Further, as discussed under the *Informed Consent* section, DHHS guidelines require that each subject be told of any "attendant discomforts and risks reasonably to be expected." Once again, however, how much need be explained so as not to frighten the subject? What one subject finds disquieting, another might not. The researcher must find a common ground for explanation and answer all inquires honestly.

Dava Sobel (1981), a science reporter for the *New York Times*, described her experience as a subject in an experiment at Montefiore Hospital in the Bronx. The purpose of the study was to observe how certain bodily functions change in the absence of timing devices—clocks, calendars, natural light cues, and social regimentation. As the seventeenth volunteer and the first female, she was placed in a special environment (room) and allowed to set her own schedule according to the dictates of her body for 25 days. Her account of informed consent from the subject's viewpoint is quite noteworthy but perhaps more so is her view of harm to the subject:

Within hours, I realized that I had not quite understood what subjecthood entailed. First came the insertion of the catheter which was extremely painful. The procedure had to be done in both arms, since the doctor mistook the lack of blood flow from the right side for a defective or improperly inserted needle. [Blood samples were part of the experiment.]

. . . The frequency of those samples was my second shock. . . . I feel I should have been warned that the samples would be taken "very" frequently [every 20 minutes], interfering constantly with my work, my meals, and the time I expected to be alone in the bathroom. . . .

Feeling tense, I wrote a letter to my husband date "Day 1," stamped it, and gave it to the white-coated technician who came in for a blood sample. He waved it almost tauntingly and said, "This will go out, but I won't say *when* it will go out. Maybe in a few days." I panicked. (Sobel, 1981, pp. 5–6)

There is no doubt that research of this nature will cause some discomfort, but how much? From Sobel's vantage point, there was too much.

To complicate matters further, she was given very little help in reorienting herself to the "real" world. After 25 days in which she would sleep and eat at any desired interval, Sobel found her normal patterns so disrupted that she "might as well have been living inside a stranger" (p. 7). It took her approximately two weeks to readjust to her former schedule, and she missed work most of that time. Should it be the responsibility of the researcher to reimburse a subject who misses that much work? Overall, her account offers the researcher insight into harms, or at least risks, that the subject should be told of. As a point of note, these researchers did change their protocol somewhat.

Kolodny (1977) cautions of potential long-term consequences of study participation. In sexual research, a subject who is observed in some type of sexual activity may experience no problems while the study is underway, but may discover feelings of guilt years later. Perhaps, a potential spouse may refuse marriage when he or she learns of the participation.

In the case of Emily, could harmful consequences occur to any of her subjects? What would be the reaction of the patients if they discovered their medical and sexual histories were being used as part of a research project? What would happen to the trust level among the patients going to the colposcopy clinic? Would future research efforts be placed in jeopardy? Could Emily's proposed research have negative connotations for nursing?

Though the health science researcher cannot hope to predict all risks and consequences, he or she should make an effort to communicate all known ones.

The Duty to Continue a Successful Research Effort

Researchers in the health science discipline frequently embark upon research efforts to improve the health of people suffering chronic conditions such as obesity, smoking, hypertension, and others. The underlying question is whether contemporary health scientists have an obligation to continue successful programs.

For example, if Emily successfully demonstrates that five variables serve as risk factors for cervical cancer, is she obligated to plan, implement, and evaluate clinic educational programs warning women of the dangers? What if she found that only two variables contributed? Who would be responsible for the costs of the program?

In another example, if a health scientist finds that a stress reduction program does in fact lower physiological tension, improves work satisfaction, and augments productivity when compared to a control group, should the program be offered to all workers? What if only two of the three variables are positive? Who would be responsible for continuing costs? The obligation of the researcher to the subjects subsequent to the research effort are debatable but should be addressed before the project commences.

Therapeutic and Nontherapeutic Research

If the research objective is to acquire information, should the justification be different than if the objective were to develop a cure or behavior pattern to improve health? In other words, is a different justification required for nontherapeutic research than for therapeutic research? In nontherapeutic research there may be no apparent benefit for the human subjects, while in therapeutic research at least the experimental group may benefit. Of course, in therapeutic research the question arises as to the right of the participant to request placement in the experimental group so that potential benefits may be obtained.

Is the nature of Emily's proposed study more nontherapeutic or therapeutic? If she is only attempting to gain knowledge about risk factors for cervical cancer, should her justification be different than if she were in fact planning a therapeutic study? Should health scientists who research in the behavioral field be held accountable for subjects' health behavior? All in all, therapeutic and nontherapeutic research efforts differ in objectives, but differences in justification are a moot point.

Sponsored Research

More often than not health science researchers cannot afford to pay for a project out-of-pocket. The myriad of expenses—drawing a large sample; training interviewers; paying for postage, offices and overhead, and computer time—must be met by a sponsor. Usually a government agency such as the U.S. Department of Public Health or a charitable foundation may provide funds and allow the researcher to conduct the project with no strings attached. However, previous examples throughout this chapter have illustrated how some agencies attempt to inflict their views on the project.

Bailey (1994) presents three major areas in which ethical conflict arises between the sponsor and the researcher. First, the sponsor may tell the researcher how to conduct the study or what findings are to be expected. Second, the sponsor may request suppression of findings, which could range from total falsification to manipulation of statistics. Third, the actual sponsor may be concealed or the true purpose of the study hidden. The latter has occurred in several research efforts for which the Central Intelligence Agency served as sponsor (Sjoberg, 1959).

The source of sponsorship in Emily's study is very subtle in that it is her employer. Would it make any difference if a pharmaceutical company supported her efforts by paying for such things as data analysis, computer time, and the like? How much support is too much?

In writing grants or procuring funding from outside sources, the health science researcher must be cognizant of these potential ethical breaks. The researcher must be prepared for compromise in some instances, but in such cases should examine all ethical questions so as not to end the project with results that have been questionably attained.

Publication of Unethical Research

A research project does not become ethical because it produces valuable data; it is ethical or unethical from its inception. Subsequently, researchers, editors, and editorial boards must look beyond the results of an investigation into all the ethical aspects involved in research. Only then can a fair and just decision be made about possible publication.

One option that may be chosen is the decision not to publish. Ingelfinger (1978), former editor of the *New England Journal of Medicine*, stated that "reports of investigations performed unethically are not accepted for publication" (p. 791). His belief is that researchers should not be involved in unethical acts, directly or indirectly. Subjects are not to be used as a means to an end. Moreover, failure to publish such research should serve as a caveat to other researchers. While some very worthwhile information will be lost to the profession, proponents of this position feel that more good consequences than bad will occur in the long run.

Beecher (1970) suggested a modification of this view by stating that "such material *ordinarily* should not be published" (p. 31). If unethical circumstances exist, Beecher believes that the researcher should report, in the text, where the dilemmas existed. In a parallel position, Levine (1973), former editor of *Clinical Research* and professor of medicine at Yale University, advocates that "manuscripts describing research conducted unethically but which satisfy the usual scientific criteria for acceptability should be published along with editorials on which the ethical deficiencies are exposed and criticized" (p. 763). This plan raises the ethical issues to a level of debate and still allows the results to be received by other professionals. Nevertheless it raises questions, too. Does such publication indicate that the editor or journal approves of such actions or at best frowns upon them? Will it function as a deterrent to unethical research?

In essence, no matter what position is taken, the majority of the responsibility rests with the researcher. As a professional, the health scientist must act in a fashion that is conducive to subject protection and growth of the professional. Publication is both a responsibility and a privilege.

Research or Just a Look-See?

A major question is, when does research become research or an experiment an experiment? Most researchers have "pet" ideas or theories they would like to test a "little bit" before taking on a full-blown study. However, when human subjects are involved, is it fair to include them in such tryouts without informed consent? What if data are collected when the health scientist is functioning as a clinical person and the data are later incorporated into research? For example, if a master's candidate serves as a counselor in local clinic for patients seeking an abortion and then records the anxiety and psychological trauma experienced by each patient for his or her own growth as a counselor, is that ethical? If at a later date the same candidate wishes to incorporate the patients' reactions into a master's thesis, is that ethical? The patients were not informed about the use of the data, because at the time a research project was not planned. Should consent be obtained even at this late date?

"The borderline between being a human being with whom we work, play, and exchange information and being a human subject of research is not a line at all. It is a misty frontier" (Committee on Research Participation, 1995). These statements reflect the difficulty in identifying boundaries on some occasions. If you were Emily's research advisor, would you consider her proposed effort as research or a "look-see"? What criteria did you use to arrive at your answer?

From a broad perspective, whenever a person plans a systematic inquiry to gain generalizable knowledge, the effort must be considered research. To clarify this statement, if you can answer "yes" to any of the following questions, you are doing research.

1. Are you planning to procure subjects? (This would be in contrast to people seeking you out for normal, professional services.)
2. Will the data collected be analyzed, interpreted, and disseminated?
3. Do you think the knowledge you will gain can be generalized to similar situations or perhaps lead to new processes or procedures?

In contrast, if the data gathered are to be used in the classroom only, for administrative purposes alone, or for a contractor's project in which there is no dissemination of data, then the effort might be considered nonresearch. Once you determine that your project is indeed research involving human subjects, the next step is to decide whether your project is exempt from review by the full IRB.

Role of the Institutional Review Board

Two federal agencies, the DHHS and the Food and Drug Administration (FDA), have complete sets of regulations about the review of research involving human subjects. To ensure compliance with the regulations, the government requires each institution conducting research to establish an IRB. In addition, investigators using disease registries usually have to obtain permission from private physicians before contacting patients at home. Researchers using deceased cases generally have to get approval from the state health department and the vital statistics bureau to procure death certificates. As a side note, regulations exist for animal research and research with recombinant DNA, too.

Although IRBs may vary slightly from institution to institution, some functions common to all are:

- To review all research efforts involving human subjects except those projects exempted from review according to regulations
- To develop policies for research with human subjects

- To provide education to investigators and departments regarding policies, procedures, and related issues
- To maintain records in accordance with federal regulations. These are usually kept for a minimum of three years after the termination of a project.

The review process may vary slightly from institution to institution. Box 4.1 highlights the general review process for graduate work. In reviewing the submission, the IRB employs the following criteria:

1. *Risks:* These must be kept minimal by design.
2. *Risks versus benefits:* Any risks must be reasonable in relation to potential benefits received and to the potential knowledge gained via the research. Keep in mind that only those risks and benefits involved in research are evaluated, not those obtained from services or therapies subjects would receive even if they were not in the research.
3. *Subject selection:* Selection methodology must be considered in light of research purposes and settings as well as the nature of the population from which the sample is to be drawn. As to be expected, children, pregnant women, the mentally disabled, prisoners, and other vulnerable groups are given special attention.
4. *Informed consent:* Complete documentation must be given to ensure that each participant (or the legal representative) has been sought out. The IRB has the right to observe (or have observed) the consent process.

BOX 4.1 The Review Process

Be certain to review the guidelines particular to your own institution. Generally the review process includes the following steps:

1. **Research investigator:** Completion of the proposal and forms for IRB review is the responsibility of the investigator. The investigator must monitor the progress of the proposal and forms as they go through each level of review.

2. **Graduate students:** Thesis and doctoral committees usually have to approve the research project before the appropriate forms are forwarded for IRB review at the departmental level.

3. **Departmental review:** Although a department head holds the responsibility for signing-off on IRB forms, an advisory departmental review committee may be in place. Stu-

dents should inquire as to how long this process takes.

4. **University review:** If the research project has been approved at the departmental level, it is then forwarded to the university (or institution) for review. If the project is deemed to be "exempt from full review," then the full committee does not have to review it. This takes much less time than a full review. If a full review is required, the investigator should inquire as to the next meeting date and the date for submission of materials. Depending upon the institution, this could easily be a one-month wait.

5. **Schedule:** It is important to plan time for the review process when designing your study. Upon review, the IRB may approve, disapprove, request minor modifications, or request an external review.

5. *Safety and privacy:* The proposal should show how the data will be monitored during collection to ensure subjects' safety and to maintain both privacy and confidentiality of the data.
6. *Additional considerations:* These are tailored to the specific research project and can include standards of professional conduct, local laws and regulations, the mission of the institution, and so forth.

After its review, the IRB may approve, disapprove, request minor modifications, or request an external review. Accepted submissions require an annual review. The intent of the annual review is to determine whether changes requested in the past review have taken place. The IRB has the right to terminate or suspend the research based upon the annual review.

Exempt and Nonexempt Review Status

When preparing a research proposal you should get information from your IRB or committee on research participation (CRP). Following their guidelines will increase your chances for approval. In reading the guidelines, you will find that some studies require review by the entire IRB, while other studies are exempt from full review. "Exempt from review" means that you must notify your IRB and complete forms to exempt your project from a full IRB review. It does not mean you can ignore the IRB and simply do what you want. Five areas of research that are often, but not always, exempt from review are:

1. Research about normal educational practices—instruction strategies, effectiveness, classroom management, curricula
2. Educational tests with information recorded in a way to protect the identity of the children
3. Observation of public behavior as long as subjects cannot be identified and the researcher is not involved in the activities being observed
4. Use of existing data (documents, pathological specimens, diagnostic specimens) if they are publicly available or if the information is used in a way that the subjects cannot be identified
5. Surveys and interviews wherein the data are recorded so that subjects cannot be identified, directly or indirectly. If there is any likelihood that the subject's responses could place him or her at risk of criminal or civil liability or be detrimental to his or her employability or financial standing, a full review is necessary.

Although surveys and interviews are often exempt for adults, they need to be reviewed when used with children.

When a review by the IRB is required, two routes are available. One route is an expedited review, which is only available to projects involving no more than minimal risk to subjects. If it is determined that greater than minimal risk is present, then a full committee review is required. Box 4.2 illustrates an example checklist for completing forms for IRB review.

BOX 4.2 Example Checklist for IRB Review Forms

Project director(s): Full name, mailing address, phone number, department or affiliation

Project: Title, external funding agency and identification number, grant submission deadline, starting date, estimated completion date

Exempt research: Category of exempt research (usually on the form)

Objectives of project: This is as they apply to the exact procedures involving human subjects.

Subjects: Description of subjects, criteria for inclusion and exclusion, population from which sample will be taken, duration of subject participation, special components if vulnerable populations are being used, age range of children (if applicable), source and selection of the control group (if any)

Methods or procedures: Research methods involving human subjects, voluntary participation, explanation of no penalty for refusal or early withdrawal

Specific risks and protective measures: List of potential risks to subjects; list of protective measures; explanation of risks (stresses, drugs, experimental manipulations, photos, recordings, and so on) and, if none, an explanation

of why; full explanation of anonymity of identities and confidentiality of data; location of where materials having subjects' names will be stored and who (by name) will have access to them; how materials will be destroyed at the appropriate time

Risk versus benefits: Reasonableness of risks compared to benefits for current subjects, future populations, and for knowledge gained. If risks are minimal, be certain to indicate.

Informed consent: Detailed explanation of your method to obtain informed consent, written consent form to be signed by subject (when necessary)

Investigator qualifications: Education and special training (if appropriate), past research efforts of a similar nature regarding human subjects, training of personnel

Adequacy of facilities: In some instances, information about the facility which will support the research must be given. This is especially true when children or other vulnerable groups are involved.

Signatures: Principal investigator, co-investigators, advisors (for students), department head and chair of departmental review committee

---

Case Discussion

This section highlights some of the issues raised throughout the chapter regarding Emily's research discussed at the opening of this chapter. The following points apply:

1. Emily's proposed project constitutes "research." She will collect data to gain generalizable knowledge and will be using human subjects.
2. Using her work setting as an opportunity for research is feasible; however, she must be extra careful in her planning, especially with regard to informed consent.
3. A review of literature supports her selection of variables: range of dysplasia, early first intercourse, multiple sexual partners, young age at marriage, young or early pregnancy, smoking, and a partner who has had multiple sexual

partners. These variables can all be continuous in nature, allowing for multiple regression.

4. The results of the study may be of great benefit in reducing severe dysplasia through education.
5. If Emily decides to engage patients 18 years of age or younger, she would need special consent from a parent, guardian, or other person who has the authority to give permission.
6. Informed consent is a must for her research for all the reasons outlined in this chapter.
7. Information gained combines behavioral and medical data. As such, confidentiality is of the utmost importance, and Emily should be able to demonstrate appropriate storage of data as well as destruction of such when her research is completed.
8. Emily may have to go through two IRBs—university and hospital—for her project.

Summary

This chapter offered viewpoints on ethical dilemmas that confront the research effort. It was seen that unethical research has been conducted in the past with and without approval of recognized government bodies. One of the initial issues to be reviewed by any investigator is the justification to experiment on human subjects rather than on animals or by computer simulation. Frequently, justification revolves around (1) the interests of health sciences; (2) the interests of the subjects or patients; and (3) the interests of the community. All can be questioned.

Justification for research on vulnerable target groups, particularly children, was seen to be more complex. DHHS guidelines were reviewed because they are employed by IRBs.

Another major issue was informed consent, involving truthtelling and deception. This area is of particular importance to both the researcher and the subject and is well scrutinized by professionals. Double-blind methodology presents unique problems to the informed consent issue.

Privacy and confidentiality are two issues highly regarded by subjects. Concomitantly, fear of harm, albeit subjective, is a point of concern to subjects and researchers alike.

Another issue was the degree of organization required to designate an experiment as an experiment. When an experiment or research effort, such as the reduction of smoking, has been proven to be successful, the question of whether it should be continued was discussed. This is particularly so if the nature of the study is therapeutic rather than nontherapeutic.

Sponsorship and publication of results were also seen to be fraught with ethical decisions. Overall, the major responsibility rests with the researcher.

Obtaining permission for research with human subjects requires approval from an IRB. While review boards may vary somewhat from institution to institution, general guidelines were presented.

Suggested Activities

1. Paco is planning his informed consent form to use in his study of patients who come to the Family Medicine Clinic in his community. His thesis deals with adults who have diabetes mellitus, and he will be randomly assigning them to either an experimental education group or a control group. His list of points to include in the consent form is below. What, if anything, is he missing from his list?

   a. Fair explanation of the research effort
   b. Description of any discomforts and risks
   c. Explanation of confidentiality of test scores and attitude scales
   d. His name and phone number for subjects to call if questions or concerns arise
   e. Instructions on how to withdraw from the study and a notation that no penalty will be incurred from leaving the study before it is finished

2. Sarah, an instructor at the local community college, teaches three classes in health education. She is very curious as to the knowledge and attitudes of her students regarding HIV/AIDS. The only way to obtain this information, she believes, is by using a questionnaire—one that has both a cognitive test and an attitude scale. She plans to use the information for planning her lessons on the same subject. If you were her department chair, would you classify her plans as research? Justify your answer.

3. Jo, a nurse practitioner in obstetrics, proposes to research the efficacy of fetal monitoring. Her research would require the use of a fetal scalp monitor during delivery. Having done this hundreds of times in the labor and delivery section of the hospital, she knew it was not too intrusive a procedure. Therefore, she requested exempt status from the IRB. If you were a member of the IRB for her institution, would you grant it? Explain your answer.

4. Go to your IRB office and get the forms for both exempt and nonexempt status. Compare the two forms. Also, get information about an expedited review versus a full review. Apply this information to research you are plannning.

5. Search the Internet for five university Websites to ascertain where the IRB office is located in each university. Download a current IRB form and compare it with your university's form.

References

Bailey, K. D. (1994). *Methods of social research* (2d ed.). New York: Free Press.

Beauchamp, T. C., & Childress, J. F. (1994). *Principles of biomedical ethics* (4th ed.). New York: Oxford University Press.

Beecher, H. K. (1970). *Research and the individual: Human studies*. Boston: Little, Brown.

Brandt, A. (1978). Racism and research: The case of the Tuskegee syphilis study. *The Hastings Center Report, 8*(6), 21–29.

Capron, A. (1974). Informed consent in catastrophic disease research and treatment. *University of Pennsylvania Law Review, 123*(20), 364–376.

Committee on Research Participation. (1995). *Working with human subjects: CRP Flyer #2.* Knoxville: Research Administration, The University of Tennessee.

Fromer, M. J. (1981). *Ethical issues in health care.* St. Louis: C. V. Mosby.

Gribben, S., Norvell, S., & Van Vorst, B. (1994, January 17). The widening fallout. *Time.*

Ingelfinger, F. J. (1978). Ethics of experiments on children. *New England Journal of Medicine, 288,* 791.

Kolodny, R. (1977). Ethical requirements: Informed consent. In W. H. Masters, V. E. Johnson, & R. Kolodny (Eds.), *Ethical issues in sex therapy and research.* Boston: Little, Brown.

Krugman, S. (1967, May 8). Experiments at Willowbrook State School. *The Lancet, 1971,* p. 321.

Levine, R. J. (1973). Ethical considerations in the publication of the results of research involving human subjects. *Clinical Research, 21,* 763.

McCartney, J. J. (1978). Research on children: National commission says "yes, if. . . ." *The Hastings Center Report, 8*(5), 26–31.

Pappworth, M. H. (1969). Ethical issues in experimental medicine. In D. R. Culter (Ed.), *Updating life and death.* Boston: Beacon Press.

Powelson, R. (1995, October 4). Radiation victims to be compensated. *Knoxville News-Sentinel,* p. 1.

Retarded kids fed radiation in '50's. (1993, December 27). *Chicago Tribune,* p. 14, Section 1.

Singer, E. (1978). Informed consent: Consequences for response rate and response quality in social surveys. *American Sociological Review, 43,* 144–162.

Sjoberg, G. (1959). Operationalism and social research. In L. Gross (Ed.), *Symposium on sociological theory.* New York: Harper & Row.

Sobel, D. (1981). Time out of joint: 25 days in a sleep lab. *The Hastings Center Report, 11*(1), 5–7.

Thorne, B. (1980). You still takin' notes? Fieldwork and problems of informed consent. *Social Problems, 27,* 284–297.

Veatch, R. M. (1977). Medicine, biology, and ethics. *The Hastings Center Report,* Supplement 2–3.

Chapter 5

Conducting Experimental and Quasi-Experimental Research

Case Study

Carol was given a golden opportunity by her employer, the Kent School District. Her board, which is in full support of Comprehensive School Health Education, directed her to select a K–12 curriculum that would be most effective for the district. Throughout her years as a health education coordinator, she had reviewed many curricula. Like the board, Carol's objective was to find one that was most suitable for the Kent School District. Her superiors gave her one year to choose an effective curriculum and then two years to implement it. Which curriculum would be most effective? That was the principal problem facing her right now.

Characteristics of Experimentation

The experimental method of conducting research is an attempt to account for a factor in a given situation. It is generally considered to be the most highly regarded research method for hypothesis testing. The experiment carried out by the investigator is really a plan to garner evidence concerning the stated hypotheses. The natural environment is controlled and manipulated so that the researcher can observe and measure the results. When a true experimental situation is determined, the investigator is measuring the relationship between two or more variables in an attempt to discover the effect one variable might have on others.

Scientists began experiments with observation of the natural setting but realized that extraneous events were not being controlled. The next step was to perform experiments in the laboratory, where these extraneous factors could be controlled or at least taken into account. Physical and biological scientists used the laboratory method, and when, in the latter part of the 1800s, psychologists began using experiments in the laboratory, experimental psychology was born. However, experiments are not limited to the laboratory; they are achieved in the classroom and elsewhere, but with much caution. It is understandable that children in classrooms cannot be randomly assigned to groups and randomly exposed to different teaching styles, because doing so may lead to nonequivalent groups. Although there are some problems inherent in "real-world" research, our behavior takes place in the real world, and thus experimentation should occur in lifelike situations. Behavioral scientists must exercise extreme caution and regard for variables and controls because of these limitations.

An experiment has three characteristics: (1) a manipulated *independent variable*; (2) control of all other variables (*dependent variables*); and (3) the *observed effect* of the manipulation of the independent variable on the dependent variables. In our case study, if Carol wanted to examine the effects of a health science curriculum on the increase in knowledge of students, she would manipulate the curriculum (the independent variable) to determine the effect on achievement (the dependent variable). As can be deduced from the preceding discussion, the major issue in an experiment is the control of the independent and confounding variables.

Graziano and Raulin (2000) make two distinctions in experimental research designs. First is the difference between independent-group (or between-subjects) designs and correlated-group (or within-subjects or matched-subjects) designs. Independent-group designs have different participants in each group. In correlated-group designs, identical or closely matched subjects are in each group. Their second distinction is between univariate (or single-variable) designs and multivariable (or factorial) designs. The former have a single independent variable, while the latter have two or more independent variables.

Control in Experiments

Without controlling variables, the experimental method cannot exist. Therefore control is of utmost importance in an investigation. Control allows the scientist to arrange the experiment so that the effect of the variables can be studied. Because health scientists deal with humans outside of the laboratory, not *every* variable can be controlled. However, it is acceptable to attempt to control those variables that might have a significant impact on the experiment. For example, if Carol wanted to test the effects of a health science curriculum, she would need to have two groups of children who were exactly alike, except that Group A would be exposed to the new curriculum, and Group B would not. These students should be alike in respects that are likely to have an impact on the health science curriculum: reading ability, morale, and motivation. However, other variables, such as artistic ability, height, and vocal ability, would be variables that could be ignored. Carol would seek to choose two groups of students who would be most similar in the *significant variables*.

In Carol's example, the experimenter is attempting to study the relationship between the independent and dependent variables. To do this, Carol would have to control for *confounding variables*. An extraneous variable is one that may affect the dependent variable and is not related to the major purpose of the experiment. Here Carol would have to control for the extraneous variable of intelligence, because it would have an influence on the dependent variable. If the students in Group A were more intelligent than those in Group B, and Group A performed better on the health science achievement tests, those gains could not be directly attributed to the new health science curriculum but to the higher intelligence level of the students in Group A. In this experiment, we have a *confounding variable*. A confounding variable is one in which independent and extraneous variables may each have an effect on the outcome of the experiment, and these effects cannot be separated.

When an experiment is carried out, the investigators must take precautions to be sure that there is as much equivalence as possible among the groups in the study. Several procedures are used to ensure equal groups: random assignment to group, randomized matching, and analysis of covariance.

Random assignment is the assignment of experimental subjects to groups such that every member of the population has an equal chance of being assigned to any of the groups. The investigator numbers all the subjects in the population, and uses a table of random numbers to draw the necessary number of subjects for each group. These groups are then considered to be *equivalent* in a statistical sense. In other words, the groups are so equal that if there is any difference between the groups, then it must be the result of chance alone and not of bias on the part of the investigator. Can Carol use this method in her study of health science curricula?

Randomized matching occurs when subjects are matched on as many extraneous variables as could possibly affect the dependent variable. Then the matched pairs are assigned to an experimental condition. Variables used for matching usually include sex, age, socioeconomic status, and reading or pretest score. In a school situation where groups preexist (classrooms), investigators match groups on the extraneous variables. The researcher will determine that scores of groups on standardized tests (IQ, reading, pretest scores) are not significantly different in terms of means and standard deviations. Although group matching is not as ideal as individual randomization in certain real-world situations, this is the best method left to the investigator.

Analysis of covariance (ANCOVA) can be used to control for differences among the groups in the experiment. ANCOVA is a statistical method that analyzes differences of the experimental groups on the dependent variable only after initial differences on the pretest measures are taken into account. ANCOVA would probably be used in our case study of Carol, because the method is very useful for intact groups (classrooms). However, ANCOVA only partially controls the extraneous variables that may confound the independent and dependent variables, and attempts at random assignment should be made.

The Hawthorne Effect in Controlling Situations

The experimental situation itself must be controlled to ensure that the differences observed are caused by the dependent variable and not the extraneous situational variables. In the famous Hawthorne experiment, it was determined that any attention paid to subjects in experiments may cause them to behave in a way that they believe is expected of them. At the Hawthorne plant of the Western Electric Company, a group of investigators wanted to determine the effects of the intensity of light and working hours on the productivity of a group of women factory workers. The workers *increased* their productivity no matter what the experimenters attempted. The study team eventually deduced that the increased productivity was caused by the attention the workers received as subjects in a study.

Investigations involving the use of drugs routinely use a placebo (nonchemical look-alike) so that all subjects believe they are taking the drug. Otherwise, subjects might only react to the fact that they are taking a drug and act as might be expected, which would confound the results of the study. Again, control becomes a large part of the experiment. There are several methods to attempt to control situational variables: (1) hold the variables constant; (2) manipulate the variables systematically; and (3) randomize the situations.

Holding the variables constant is achieved by treating all subjects alike, regardless of group assignment, except for their exposure to the treatment. Ideally, the same teacher should teach the experimental health science curriculum in Carol's case study. Additionally, all tests, instructions, and general procedures should be as identical as possible for each group.

Manipulating the variables systematically includes controlling the order in which the experiment is given to the subjects. If the subjects were to take a series of achievement tests in relation to the health curriculum, it might be beneficial to split the group in half. One group would receive the decision-making tests first. This is an attempt to separate the groups from the main independent variable.

Randomizing the situational variables can provide a method to deal with the extraneous condition of having the same teacher for each group. The investigator could randomly assign half the experimental group and half the control group to each teacher. In this manner, extraneous conditions are not able to affect the dependent variable.

Advantages and Disadvantages of the Experimental Method

It is important to recognize the benefits and pitfalls you might encounter when conducting experimental research. In our case study, Carol might discuss these issues with her superiors so that they, as well as she, would be aware of the possible effects an experiment might have on the school system. *Advantages* include: (1) convenience; (2) replication; (3) adjustment of variables; and (4) establishment of cause-and-effect relationships.

1. *Convenience:* The investigator may decide to carry out the experiment whenever or wherever feasible. Of course, real-world research puts some limitations on convenience, but nonetheless, the experimenter may choose the time and location.

2. *Replication:* By repeating the experiment, or parts of it, the validity of the results increases. This is because the results are based on several observations, rather than just one.

3. *Adjustment of variables:* Being able to vary an aspect of the experiment allows the investigator to attempt several steps at a rather rapid pace. For example, in the previously mentioned Hawthorne experiment, the investigators were able to vary the aspects of the workers' environment in succession.

4. *Establishment of cause-and-effect relationships:* This can be accomplished because the experimenter manipulates the independent variables and then observes the effects on the dependent variable. A caution here: Make sure your independent variable is valid, because if it is not the effects may not be attributable to that variable.

Disadvantages of the experimental method include: (1) cost; (2) inability to generalize; and (3) securing the cooperation of those involved in the project.

1. *Cost* can at times be a hindrance to experimental research. Many times, the training of experimenters and obtaining of equipment are expensive. When this happens, investigators must either carry out a bare-bones experiment, or not conduct the study at all.

2. *Inability to generalize* the results of a study usually occurs because the samples used were not representative of the population. In our case study, if Carol used a group of private school students in her experiment, it would be an inappropriate sample, because the results of the experiment could not be generalized to public schools.

3. *Securing cooperation* from those in the experiment and from significant others (parents, administrators, supervisors) can be a major stumbling block for conducting a study.

Internal and External Validity

When designing an experiment the investigator must be certain that the study is technically sound. This is called the *validity*—internal and external—and should be dealt with to prevent problems that may cast doubt on the implications derived from the results of the study. Two other types of validity are statistical and construct (Graziano & Raulin, 2000). *Statistical validity* refers to the accuracy of the conclusion drawn from a statistical test. *Construct validity* addresses the degree to which the underlying theory of the research effort explains the observed results.

G R O U P A	Values Clarification Method
G R O U P B	Didactic Method

FIGURE 5.1 Internal Validity Design

Internal Validity

Internal validity can be defined as control for all influences between the groups being compared in an experiment, except for the experimental group. In our case study, Carol would be comparing two methods of teaching the health science curriculum to two groups. The only differences between these two groups would be the teaching method (values clarification or didactic). Figure 5.1 illustrates this concept.

Internal validity is extremely difficult to achieve outside of the laboratory because there are too many extraneous variables to control. As we attempt to control for internal validity and tighten those controls, external validity (to be discussed later) suffers. As is so often true of the research in the real world, the investigator must compromise. Not all extraneous variables can be eliminated, but the experimenter, in designing a study, should take into consideration the many confounding variables. Confounding occurs when the independent variable varies with at least one other variable. These confounding variables, or threats to the research design, were originally discussed by Campbell and Stanley (1963) and include the following:

Maturation refers to factors that may influence subjects' performance because of the time that has elapsed. The change that has occurred within the participants is the problem, because people normally change over time, regardless of interference (e.g., an experiment). This threat is especially apparent in longitudinal studies of young or adolescent children. Usually this problem can be attenuated by including a control group in the research design. The members of this additional group should be as comparable to the subjects in the experimental group as possible—they should have similar characteristics in their maturational development.

History is defined as those events that occur at the same time as the study. These external events can interfere with the subjects' performance in the experiment. Sometimes these events are unpredictable, such as a catastrophe in the community (e.g., a tornado). Events such as this make history very difficult to control. In our case study, Carol has decided to pretest the students on a day when they are having an examination in mathematics. Undoubtedly, the subjects will be under stress, and this may interfere with their performance on the pretest. One way Carol could attempt to limit the effect on the internal validity of the experiment would be to use a control group, which would be exposed to the same historical experiences during the time of the study. While this may not account for an unexpected event (e.g., a lunchroom fight), it can control for some historical events.

It also should be noted here that the concept of history is within the experiment, including the procedures and materials used to conduct the study. All methods, test instruments, and situations should be the same for every subject in the study, regardless of group assignment.

Testing at the onset of an experiment, or actually before it begins, can have an effect on the subjects' performance at the time of the posttest. What is thought to occur is that the subjects practice taking the test and thus are "test-wise." Pretests may even give the subjects information (e.g., about cardiovascular health knowledge instruments), and thus threaten the internal validity of the experiment. This occurs because the investigator does not know if the results of the posttest resulted from the dependent variable (e.g., health science curriculum), from the practice or knowledge gained from the pretest, or even from a combination of both situations.

To eliminate this test practice threat, two suggestions are offered: (1) use a comparison group that is exposed to the dependent variable but does not receive the pretest; and (2) increase the length of time between the administration of the pretest and posttest. While neither of these plans is absolutely foolproof in reducing the threat to the internal validity of the experiment, they do lessen the chance that the results of the study are suspect to testing practice.

Instrumentation can be a cause for concern in the internal validity of an experiment. The term refers to any changes in the instrument or measuring device used to test the effect of the dependent variable. In addition, changes in those who might be observers or raters in an experiment could unknowingly change their rating system. When considering a written instrument, the posttest should remain the same as the pretest, and procedures for recording the data (e.g., use of scanner sheets) should remain the same each time data are collected.

When observers or interviewers are used to collect data, they must be cognizant that they are fallible to fatigue, boredom, and awareness of the "right" answers. It is advisable that investigators check for intrarater and interrater reliability (Rubinson, Stone, & Mortimer, 1977; Graziano & Raulin, 2000) of these types of data collectors, to alleviate the possible threat to internal validity.

Statistical regression presents a threat to internal validity when subjects are assigned to a group because of their extreme scores on tests. As an example, students who scored in the highest and lowest quartile on a nutrition knowledge test were chosen as subjects for the experimental group, and those in the middle 50% were eliminated from the study. At the time of the posttest, the scores of the highest quartile would decrease toward the mean, while the scores for the students in the lowest quartile would increase toward the mean. This condition would produce differences between the groups on the posttest measures regardless of the intervention. So this will not occur, the investigator should make sure that the groups are composed of subjects whose scores represent the full range of possible scores.

Differential selection is actually a bias in selecting individuals for group selection. This usually occurs when participants volunteer for experimental group membership. In this case they usually are more highly motivated, which may cause them to be a biased group. Selection bias can also occur when intact classroom groups are assigned to either an experimental or control group. For example, the students in the seventh-hour science class also may be in the advanced algebra class, hence introducing a bias to the study. One of the best ways to avoid this particular threat to internal validity is to randomly assign subjects to each group. However, this usually cannot be facilitated in a school, for obvious reasons. Then the investigators must limit their generalization of findings to the particular sample in the study.

Experimental mortality is the loss of subjects in an experiment (also called *attrition*), especially if there is a differential loss between the experimental and control group. Many times subjects involved in studies in schools will be "lost" due to absence on the day of a test, or they will have moved out of the school district. If this happens equally between the groups, experimenters can select replacement subjects. Other methods to ensure against biased samples resulting from attrition are to choose large groups of subjects and make sure they are representative. In addition, it is wise to follow a sample of those who left the study to obtain comparison data.

Selection-maturation interaction occurs when the maturation of subjects becomes the confounding variable. As an example to explain this threat to internal validity, let us use our case study. The seventh-grade students selected for the experimental group to test the health science curriculum were from Carol's school district. The control group of seventh-graders was selected from another school district where, because of the different ages of the beginning students, the seventh graders were nine months younger than those in Carol's school district (the experimental group). If the experiment were to proceed and results indicated that the experimental group's gains in knowledge were not as great as those in the control group, how could we interpret this data? The extraneous variable of maturation has confounded the results of Carol's experiment. To avoid this situation, investigators must be sure to select groups of comparable maturity levels.

Diffusion of treatment takes place when participants in a particular research condition communicate with participants in a different research condition. Those in an experimental group may inadvertently discuss events with participants in the control group, when the latter did not even know they were in such a group. This could affect how they might respond.

Sequence effects can be confounding because participants' performance in later conditions may be the result of their role in a previous condition of the study. Within-subject designs are prone to this confounding. A study in which participants are exposed to three different conditions is conducive to this type of validity problem (Graziano & Raulin, 2000).

Another threat to internal validity, not discussed by Campbell and Stanley (1963), is that of *contamination*. This bias occurs when the researcher has previous knowledge concerning the subjects in the experiment. The investigator may inadvertently treat the groups differently, or even give the subjects hints as to correct responses on surveys. In medical research, the subjects do not know who receives the experimental medication and who receives a placebo; this is known as a blind study. A double-blind experiment is an even better safeguard against contamination. In this case the person who administers the treatments and records which subjects are in either the placebo or experimental group is not the experimenter, but rather an aide in the study. In our study, Carol would have to make sure not to involve herself in the teaching and/or testing of the curriculum.

External Validity

External validity is the researcher's ability to generalize the findings of an experiment. In an attempt to control threats to internal validity in research in the behavioral sciences—real-world research—the investigator runs the risk of creating an unreal situation from which generalization to other settings is impossible. Most researchers outside of the laboratory tend to compromise and set up a rigorous experiment in a realistic situation.

Campbell and Stanley (1963) suggested four threats to external validity: (1) the reactive effect of testing; (2) the interaction effects of selection biases and the experimental variable; (3) the reactive effects of experimental arrangements; and (4) multiple-treatment interference. Bracht and Glass (1968) delineated Campbell and Stanley's four factors into a more specific set of threats to external validity. The following discussion is based on their work.

Population validity refers to the extent to which the results of an experiment can be generalized from the sample used in the study to a larger group of similar people. There are two types of population validity, according to Bracht and Glass. *The extent to which results can be generalized from the experimental sample to a defined population* is the first type. In our case study, if Carol randomly selected a group of seventh-graders to expose to the experimental curriculum and found positive gains in terms of skills in decision-making, she would like to generalize these findings to all seventh-grade students. However, she can only generalize to those students from whom the sample was drawn: seventh-grade students in her school district. This sample is defined as the *experimentally accessible population*. When we read reports of experiments, we sometimes, without thinking, generalize the sample to include all subjects (e.g., seventh-grade students in all junior high schools in New York). The latter group (seventh-grade students in all junior high schools in New York) is called the *target population*. When making these generalizations, the researcher must be sure that the two groups are representative of each other. This can be accomplished, although with intact classrooms in schools it is virtually impossible. However, large-scale studies, such as the one conducted by Ireson, Hallam, Mortimore, Hack, and Clark (1999), can be generalized to the target population. The schools in this experiment were truly representative of a cross-section of the schools in the United States.

Bracht and Glass wrote about a second type of population validity: *the extent to which personological variables interact with treatment effects.* Personological variables such as ability, sex, anxiety level, extroversion-introversion, and independence can have an effect on students' performance. Hence if Carol wanted to generalize the findings to another grade level (e.g., eighth grade), it would be unwarranted. This phenomenon has gained support as its own branch of research called *aptitude-treatment interaction (API) research.*

Ecological validity is the second major type of threat to external validity that Bracht and Glass described. They define ecological validity as the *extent to which the results of an experiment can be generalized from the set of environmental conditions in the experiment to other environmental conditions.* If the results can be obtained only under a very limited set of conditions, those results have low ecological validity. Bracht and Glass described several factors that may contribute to the ecological validity of an experiment:

1. *Explicit description of the experimental treatment:* Researchers must describe the experimental treatment in exact detail, so that it can be replicated by other experimenters.
2. *Multiple-treatment interference:* When it appears that subjects will be exposed to more than one experimental treatment that may affect the generalizability of the findings of the study, the investigator should choose an experimental design in which one treatment is assigned to each subject.
3. *Hawthorne effect:* This phenomenon, which was discussed earlier, can prevent the findings in a study from being generalized because subjects simply reacted to being in a study.
4. *Novelty and disruption effects:* An experimental treatment may be effective just because it is different from what the subjects normally receive. This can cause low generalizability, because as the novelty wears off, so does the effectiveness of the treatment.
5. *Experimenter effect:* This refers to the inability of the person who administers the treatment (physician, teacher, nurse practitioner) to be involved in subsequent investigations. This is also an area of concern for low generalizability.
6. *Pretest sensitization:* Just as the pretest can affect internal validity, so can it act in an adverse way on the posttest performance of subjects. The usual occurrence is that the pretest positively affects the scores on the posttest.
7. *Posttest sensitization:* As in the case with pretest sensitization, at times the posttest can affect the subjects' scores and thus cause concern for generalizability of the experiment.
8. *Measurement of the dependent variable:* When instruments are used to measure the effects of a treatment, they may limit the generalizability of the results to the other tests if they are particularly well adapted to the dependent variable.
9. *Interaction of time of measurement and treatment effects:* Experiments may use two or more posttests to measure the effects of an intervention. Usually, the first posttest is administered immediately after the intervention is concluded, and then again several weeks or months later to measure the subjects' retention.

These second measurements have changed the effects of the intervention and therefore pose a threat to ecological validity.

Investigators must take into account the many threats to internal and external validity when they design an experiment. Because most behavioral scientists work in the real world, some threats must remain, while others can be minimized and even excluded. If investigators find that a discrepancy exists between the experimental condition and real-world setting, then they should note this in the report as a limitation to the generalizability of the study.

Constructing Experimental Designs to Control Variables

The major purpose in constructing an experimental design is to control as many extraneous variables as possible. Because experimental research in the health sciences is usually conducted outside a laboratory, the investigator must take great pains to ensure that the proper controls are employed. However, in attempting to control for so many variables, real-world research can produce artificial results. This occurs because the environment and/or the subjects are sometimes put into unnatural situations. Snow (1974) has developed an alternative called *representative design*, whereby experiments accurately reflect real-life environments and the natural characteristics of the learners. In our case study, Carol would then attempt to conduct her experiment in an environment in which she could easily generalize the findings of the research.

We shall discuss several experimental designs, which can be divided into the following categories: preexperimental, true experimental, factorial, and quasi-experimental designs. To simplify this process, we will include symbols and terms to describe designs. These symbols are widely used in the literature and include:

X: Independent variable that is manipulated
O: Process of observation or test
R: Random selection of subjects to groups
Xs and Os across a given row: Apply to the same people
– –: Dashed lines between groups indicate no random assignment to groups.

The left-to-right dimension indicates the temporal order, and the Xs and Os, when vertical to one another, are given simultaneously.

Preexperimental Designs

The least adequate experimental designs fall into this group; there is no control group, and extraneous variables can cause threats to internal validity. As we progress from these types of experiments to those that do not have such weaknesses, you will be able to build an experiment that will avoid such problems.

The One-Shot Case Study Design

$$X \qquad O$$

In this type of experiment, a treatment is given to one group. Then observations (O) are made on the subjects in that group to detect the effects of the treatment. Those observations are made in the form of a posttest. There is no control group, but rather the investigator makes inferences or comparisons of the results based on what the results would have been had the intervention not been given. In our case study, Carol would introduce a health science lesson to a class of sixth-graders and then give a posttest to determine the treatment effects. What might she deduce from this one-shot case study experiment?

This is the very weakest of experimental designs and should be avoided. As we have discussed, the sources of invalidity in this instance would be history, maturation, selection, and mortality. If Carol has only one group to use, then it is recommended that at least a pretest be given to the subjects to provide a measure of change.

The One-Group Pretest-Posttest Design

$$O_1 \qquad X \qquad O_2$$
$$O_1 = \text{pretest}$$
$$O_2 = \text{posttest}$$

Although this design improves the one-shot case study experiment, it is still considered to be weak. The group is administered a pretest to measure the dependent variable and then the treatment is introduced. The same test is readministered at the conclusion of the intervention (posttest). Carol, in attempting to test the new health science lesson, did give the students a pretest and posttest. She found that the students increased their knowledge significantly after being exposed to the intervention. Is she correct in believing that the gains in scores resulted from the new lesson? Probably not, because this design does not control for student maturation, history, the testing situation, or statistical regression.

The use of the one-group pretest-posttest design is sometimes necessary in school systems that will not allow their students to be treated differently. In other words, some school districts insist that a new or experimental program must be made available to all students. In this case, it is necessary for the investigators to make estimates of the gains the subjects would make and then set their experimental significance levels against that standard. Therefore, this type of design can be safely used because most of the extraneous factors that cause threats to validity have been estimated to reach certain levels by the investigators. To test the differences of scores between the pretest and posttest, the usual method of analysis would be to employ the *t*-test for correlated means, because the same subjects take both tests.

The Static-Group Comparison Design

$$X \qquad O$$
$$\text{-} \text{-} \text{-} \text{-} \text{-} \text{-} \text{-} \text{-} \text{-}$$
$$O$$

The static-group comparison experiment includes two treatment groups (experimental and control) in which each is given a posttest only. However, the subjects are not randomly assigned to the treatment groups, indicated by the – – – lines above. Here, selection and mortality interfere with the internal validity of the experiment because the results of the experiment may not be attributable to the intervention but to the differences in the subjects in each group. It is necessary that the groups be equivalent, and because random assignment was not employed, the investigator cannot ensure that the groups are equal.

In our case study, Carol selected Ms. Evans's class as the control group and Mr. Jackson's class as the experimental group, and each group would be given a posttest after a series of new health science lessons were introduced. She analyzed the data using a *t*-test of the posttest mean scores and found that Mr. Jackson's class did score significantly higher on the achievement tests than Ms. Evans's class. Does this mean that the new health science lessons are better than the usual science series that Ms. Evans used? Not necessarily so, because Mr. Jackson's students may have had more science knowledge than Ms. Evans's students. They may not have been equivalent at the start of the study, a serious limitation of this type of experimental design.

True Experimental Designs

In these types of real experimental designs, control groups and experimental groups are involved in the study, and subjects have been randomly assigned to each group. These are the strongest types of designs, but Carol will have difficulty using them because she is dealing with intact groups (i.e., subjects in classrooms). However, she can assign *classrooms* randomly to groups, and then check students' records for standardized test scores to determine the homogeneity of the classes.

The Posttest-Only Control Group Design

$$R \qquad X \qquad O_1$$
$$R \qquad \qquad O_2$$

In this true experimental design, the experimental group experiences the intervention, but the control group does not. In addition, subjects are randomly assigned to each group, and they both receive the same posttest. This is a very powerful design because it controls for all threats to internal validity with the exception of mortality. This is especially useful when the researcher has a large group of subjects, because random assignment of the subjects allows for equivalence of the groups.

The pretest is not used in this design, which can be useful in several ways. There is no interaction between the pretest and the independent variable, and therefore the design should be used when there is likelihood that pretest reactivity would occur. In addition, there are cases in which pretests are not appropriate (studies of very young children in whom learning has not yet happened) or not available. A disadvantage of this design is that you cannot determine if change has occurred. Carol would have to use a table of random numbers to select subjects to be assigned to experimental and control groups. Sixty students were chosen from an initial pool of 400 seventh-graders. The experimental group would receive the new health science curriculum, while the control group would be taught the regular curriculum. All factors would be equated, and at the end of the intervention both groups would be posttested. The data would be analyzed by using a t-test comparison of the mean posttest scores of the groups. If Carol had used more than two groups, she would use analysis of variance. The results of the statistical scores show that the experimental group's scores were significantly higher than those of the control group. What can she conclude in regard to the new health science curriculum?

The Pretest-Posttest Control Group Design

$$R \quad O_1 \quad X \quad O_2$$
$$R \quad O_3 \quad \quad O_4$$

This design includes a pretest addition to the previously discussed true experimental design: posttest-only control group design. The subjects in the experimental and control groups are randomly assigned, and each group is given both a pretest and posttest. This design eliminates all threats to validity and thus provides an excellent setting for conducting a study. Randomization of the subjects will ensure that there was no systematic bias in the groups, but in some cases, there *may be* initial differences between groups, as shown on pretest scores. Once again, Carol randomly selected her subjects, assigned them to groups, administered the pretests, had the appropriate teacher introduce the new health science curriculum, and posttested each group. She analyzed the data by using analysis of covariance. The posttest mean scores were compared with the pretest scores as a covariate. In this experiment, no significant differences were found on the scores between the groups, but there were some that increased, showing positive changes in the experimental group's scores. See if you can interpret these results.

The Solomon Four-Group Design

$$R \quad O_1 \quad X \quad O_2$$
$$R \quad O_3 \quad \quad O_4$$
$$R \quad \quad X \quad O_5$$
$$R \quad \quad \quad O_6$$

This is a very sophisticated experimental design that takes into account factors associated with external as well as internal validity. The design is set up to determine several factors at once: assess the effect of the treatment in relation to the control group, determine the effect of the pretest, and explain the interaction between the treatment conditions and the pretest. Random assignment of subjects to groups and inclusion of groups that are not pretested add to the significance of the results of the experiment. This results from combination of the previously discussed designs: posttest only and pretest-posttest. The design actually has two experiments going on at once and thus provides replication of the study.

However, there is a major disadvantage to this design: finding enough subjects to complete the four equivalent groups and randomly assigning them into groups. Even if enough subjects can be located, the time to conduct two experiments may not be available to the investigators. Because several school health science studies (Peterson & Rubinson, 1982; Huss & Ritchie, 1999; Haight, Michel, & Hendrix, 1998) have been conducted using the Solomon four-group design, Carol has some frame of reference from which to conduct her investigation.

The analysis for this design is not simple but with today's computers can easily be handled. Campbell and Stanley (1963) suggest disregarding the pretests, except as a treatment, and analyzing the posttest scores with a simple analysis of variance design of 2 (pretest) × 2 (treatment), as shown:

	No X	X
Pretested	O_4	O_2
Unpretested	O_6	O_5

From the mean scores in the columns, one estimates the main effect of X, and from the mean scores in the rows, the main effect of pretesting. The cell means provide an estimate of the interaction of testing with X. If the main and interactive effects of pretesting are negligible, an analysis of covariance of O_4 versus O_2, with the pretest scores as the covariate, should be performed.

Factorial or Multivariable Designs

Factorial designs are more complicated than the previously discussed designs in which there was a single variable and one independent variable that was manipulated to have an effect on the dependent variable. A factorial design is one in which two or more variables are manipulated simultaneously to allow study of the independent effect of each variable on the dependent variable. In addition, the effects caused by the interaction among the several variables are assessed. The effect of each independent variable on the dependent variable is called a *main effect*, while the effect of the interaction of two or more independent variables on the dependent variable is termed an *interaction effect*:

R	O_1	X	Y_1	O_2
R	O_3		Y_1	O_4
R	O_5	X	Y_2	O_6
R	O_7		Y_2	O_8

		Pretest	Curriculum	Posttest
Workshop group	R	O_1	XX	$O_{2,3}$
Orientation group	R	O_4	XX	$O_{5,6}$
	R	O_7		$O_{8,9}$

FIGURE 5.2 Four-Solomon Group Design of the Health Science Curriculum Experiment

The above diagram illustrates a factorial design where *Y* is the second variable to be manipulated. In our case study, suppose Carol were to set up her experiment to determine if a group of randomly assigned sixth-graders learned more after being exposed to a new health science curriculum. Two methods of instruction for teachers were used: a three-day workshop and a two-hour orientation session. She set up a modified four-Solomon group design that looked like Figure 5.2.

The data were analyzed with a two-way analysis of variance using the posttest knowledge scores. The factors considered were training (Treatment I, II, or III) and test sequence (pretest or no pretest). Figure 5.3 illustrates the results of the analysis of the mean knowledge scores showing an *interaction* between the variables. The data revealed that there were significant *main effects* and a significant training X sequence *interaction*.

Quasi-Experimental Designs

There are times when researchers cannot control all sources of internal and/or external validity. These occasions call for the investigator to use a quasi-experimental design, which although not as strong as the true experimental designs, is certainly preferable to the pre-experimental designs. Experiments in this group use designs in which random assignment of subjects to groups has not been accomplished. These experiments are usually carried out where intact groups are available (i.e., schools). In our case study, Carol would have to use a quasi-experimental design, as she had determined that school officials in her district will not allow students to be reassigned from their original classes.

Campbell and Stanley (1963) originally described 13 quasi-experimental designs; however, we have decided to explain only those that would have a direct bearing on the health sciences: time series, equivalent time samples, nonequivalent control groups, and counterbalances. Each design has strengths and weaknesses that enable investigators to choose the design that would be most appropriate for a particular setting.

The Interrupted Time Series Design

$$O_1O_2O_3O_4 \qquad X \qquad O_5O_6O_7O_8$$

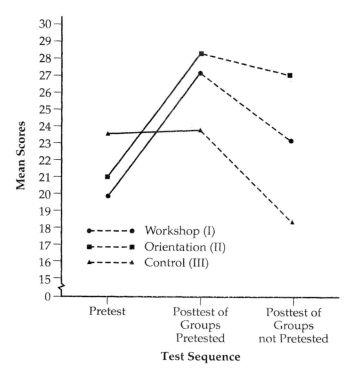

FIGURE 5.3 Interaction Between Variables

If Carol wished to have the entire school system involved in her study, she would want a comparable school district to serve as a control group. Unfortunately, she cannot find one that is both comparable and willing to join in the experiment. Therefore she decides to use the interrupted time series design, as diagrammed above.

As evidenced, there is one experimental group in which observations occur before and after the intervention. Several sources of validity are not threatened when using this design, but the general weakness includes a threat to the effect of history; other influences might have an effect on the dependent variable after it is introduced. This can be controlled by adding a control group, but in our case study this is impossible. Another minor weakness of interrupted time series designs is that of the effect of instrumentation. During this experiment, there are many points at which data are collected, and those who administer the tests may do so differently and even score them improperly. This is especially true of data and recordkeeping in hospitals, where many different personnel may be involved in this activity.

A caution that all researchers should consider when using interrupted time series designs is the cyclical nature of performance and attitudes, which may be attributed to seasonal variations. For example, more hospital admissions occur during the Christmas holidays, and schoolchildren will not respond well to serious interventions the day before a vacation. Several other interrupted time series designs may be used. (For a thorough discussion of these, refer to Cook and Campbell, 1979; and Graziano & Raulin, 2000.)

There are a few limitations associated with interrupted time series designs. They include:

1. Treatments are rapidly implemented, but rather slowly diffused.
2. Effects are not instantaneous.
3. Data observations are too few—50 are recommended.

The statistical analysis for interrupted time series designs depends on the number of observations within the experiment. If 50 to 100 observations are available, it is recommended that the *autoregressive integrated moving average* (ARIMA) models be used. Refer to Box and Jenkins (1976) for a complete description of this technique. However, if fewer than 50 observations occur and the errors are independent, *analysis of variance* (ANOVA), with repeated measures, should be used to analyze the data. If the errors are correlated and the number of observations is small, *multiple analysis of variance* (MANOVA) is a satisfactory statistical technique.

The Equivalent Time Sample Design

$$X_1O \qquad X_0O \qquad X_1O \qquad X_0O$$

The equivalent time sample design is similar to the time series design; however, the treatment is not introduced once but rather introduced and reintroduced to the subjects. In addition, another experience is introduced (X_0), and it too is reintroduced at predetermined intervals. To fully implement this design, the investigator needs large and representative samples and should have a random sample of time periods. In our case study, Carol would introduce a new health science lesson, using a behavioral approach, to 100 sixth-grade students and reintroduce this lesson or an equivalent follow-up. At the same time, another group of 100 sixth-graders would be exposed to a different health science lesson that used a values clarification approach and followed the proper or same intervals.

The equivalent time series design controls for all threats to internal validity, therefore covering the threat of history, which the time series design does not. In other words, extraneous events should not have an effect on the outcome of the experiment.

Two types of generalizations occur in this type of experiment: (1) across occasions; and (2) across subjects. Analysis of the data may be accomplished by comparing the two experiences against a between-occasions-within-experience error term. This provides information about the changes that occur over time.

The Nonequivalent Control Group Design

$$O_1 \quad\quad X \quad\quad O_2$$

$$O_3 \quad\quad\quad\quad O_4$$

In this design, both groups are pretested and posttested, no control group is exposed to the intervention, and none of the subjects have been randomly assigned to groups. This design and its many variations (adding nonpretested experimental and control groups) are frequently used in situations such as our case study. As mentioned previously, classrooms are intact, as are other groups: prisoners, some patients in hospitals (dependent on illness), and so on. However, what does become random is the assignment of the intervention. While this design can appear weak, it does become sound in that subjects are usually chosen from a pool of those with somewhat similar characteristics (e.g., age, experience, grade in school). This homogeneity can be tested by comparing scores of the groups on the pretest. The interaction of selection and maturation can be a threat to the validity of the nonequivalent control group design.

To statistically analyze this design, the investigator should use ANCOVA, which would reduce the effects of initial differences between the groups because it makes adjustments to the posttest scores of each group. If you use ANCOVA, remember that only the *measured* variables are used as covariates. There is the possibility that subjects in the groups may differ on other, nonmeasured variables that have not been used in ANCOVA. The investigator also can use multiple regression to analyze the data from the results of the experiment. This method is advantageous compared to ANCOVA only because it has less stringent assumptions than ANCOVA. In multiple regression, the posttest scores would be the criterion variable, and the investigator could then decide if the treatment was significant to the prediction.

The Counterbalanced Design

	$Time_1$	$Time_2$	$Time_3$	$Time_4$
Group A	X_1O	X_2O	X_3O	X_4O
Group B	X_2O	X_4O	X_1O	X_3O
Group C	X_3O	X_1O	X_4O	X_2O
Group D	X_4O	X_3O	X_2O	X_1O

Counterbalanced designs, also called Latin squares, are usually used when two or more interventions are to be tested. All the subjects will receive all the treatments for a specific time period. The order of administration of treatments is varied between subjects, so that order effects are not confounded with treatment effects.

These have been called *rotation experiments.* In our case study, Carol would use counterbalancing to test the effectiveness of two methods of teaching a health unit to eighth-grade students. The two units, however, must be equal in all aspects—difficulty, age-relatedness, factual information, and the like. After each class completed the unit, a cognitive test would be administered to the subjects. This design is especially useful for intact groups, and actually is slightly better than the nonequivalent control group design in that it might "rotate out" differences that could exist between groups. In addition, students are matched to themselves, making statistical analysis more discriminatory.

There are some weaknesses in carrying out an experiment like the one just described. A carryover effect from one teaching method to another may affect the scores on the tests. In addition, it is sometimes very difficult to determine that units of study are, in effect, equal in all aspects as prescribed. Also, it could be possible that students would tire of taking as many tests as required in the counterbalanced design.

Case Discussion

Carol's objective was to find the best health science curriculum for the Kent School District. We can assume that she wants a curriculum that will increase health knowledge and foster positive health attitudes and behavior. Carol understands the difficulty in measuring the latter, so she decides to measure the curriculum effects on both knowledge and attitude. Knowing that the middle school years are probably the most important regarding students' acquisition of some very unhealthy behaviors, she can focus on a curriculum that is most likely to influence students at these grade levels. This helps narrow her sample.

To select her sample, Carol reviewed her sampling frame of all public middle schools in the Kent district. Note that she has elected not to go outside of her school district in order to have better control. Her design choice was the pretest-posttest control group design. She decided to use randomized matching of schools to control for as many extraneous variables as possible. From the matched pairs, she randomly assigned one (from the pair) of the schools to the experimental group, which would receive the new curriculum. The teachers of the new curriculum will receive an extensive in-service prior to commencement of that program. The in-service is to present information about the curriculum as well as about implementation, fidelity, and the experiment. Another in-service will be held for the teachers in the control school classrooms.

The teachers will administer the knowledge and attitude instruments, which were selected for their reliability and validity for this population and for the content, respectively. The initial testing would be in the first week of the new semester, with the second testing at the conclusion of the semester. In her analysis, Carol will compare the scores obtained from the schools receiving the new curriculum to those from the traditional curriculum.

Summary

This chapter attempted to introduce and explain the very important concept of *control* in conducting experimental research. Good research studies ensure and take into account the advantages and disadvantages of conducting an experiment. While experimentation originally began in the laboratory, it has been successfully conducted in naturalistic settings such as schools, factories, ships, and hospitals. When conducting an experiment, the investigator must be concerned with several threats to internal validity, including variables, history, selection, instrumentation, testing, differential selection, experimental mortality, selection-maturation interaction, and contamination. Another type of validity, external validity, was discussed with specific reference to population validity and ecological validity.

Experimental designs can be classified into four categories: preexperimental, true experimental, factorial or multivariable, and quasi-experimental. Ten designs were discussed with respect to controlling extraneous variables: the one-shot case study, one-group pretest-posttest, static-group comparison, posttest-only control group, pretest-posttest control group, four-Solomon group, interrupted time series, equivalent time samples, nonequivalent control group, and counterbalanced. Investigators may use each of these designs based on need, availability of subjects, proposed hypotheses, and suitable data analysis capabilities.

Suggested Activities

1. Explain the differences and similarities in the following designs:

Design 1					Design 2		
R	O_1	X	O_2		R	X	O_1
R	O_3		O_4				O_2

2. You are conducting a stop-smoking program, which has three groups of smokers. Each meets on a different evening once a week for a total of six weeks. You pretest each of the intact groups prior to implementing the smoking-cessation program. Upon completion of the program, you immediately administer a posttest and then repeat it eight weeks later. The design would look as follows:

Monday group	O_1	X_1	O_2	O_3
Tuesday group	O_4	X_2	O_5	O_6
Thursday group	O_7	X_3	O_8	O_9

What is the meaning of each of the following sets of data?

a. $O_1 = O_4 = O_7 = O_2 = O_3 = O_5 = O_8$, but O_6 is greater than O_5, and O_9 is greater than O_6.

b. O_1, O_4, and O_7 are not equal because O_1 is greater than O_4, which is greater than O_7; and O_2 is greater than O_5, which is greater than O_8. However, O_3, O_6, and O_9 are equal.

c. Are you able to check for the effect of pretesting using this design? Explain your answer.

d. Does the lack of randomization make any difference in your study since you are pretesting the groups?

3. You have developed the following design to compare the effects of two different drugs for hypertension on three groups, all of which are randomized and pretested; all are then given two posttests, three months apart:

Group 1	R	O_1	X_1	O_2	O_3
Group 2	R	O_4	X_2	O_5	O_6
Group 3	R	O_7		O_8	O_9

a. What is the advantage of using randomized subjects versus intact groups?

b. Why did you decide to pretest rather than posttest only?

c. Explain these results: $O_3 = O_6 = O_9$ but $O_2 > O_8$ but $< O_5$.

d. Interpret this: $O_2 = O_5$ but $> O_8$; $O_3 > O_6$ and O_9.

e. How would you explain the results if O_7, O_8, and O_9 were not equal as observations in the control group?

References

Box, G., & Jenkins, G. (1976). *Time-series analysis: Forecasting and control.* San Francisco: Holden-Day.

Bracht, G., & Glass, G. (1968). The external validity of experiments. *American Educational Research Journal, 5,* 437–474.

Campbell, D., & Stanley, J. (1963). *Experimental and quasi-experimental designs for research.* Chicago: Rand McNally.

Cook, T., & Campbell, D. (1979). *Quasi-experimentation.* Boston: Houghton Mifflin.

Graziano, A. M., & Raulin, M. L. (2000). *Research methods: A process of inquiry.* Boston: Allyn & Bacon.

Haight, B. K., Michel, Y., & Hendrix, S. (1998). Life review: Preventing despair in newly relo-

cated nursing home residents. *International Journal of Aging and Human Development, 47*(2), 119–142.

Huss, S. N., & Ritchie, M. (1999). Effectiveness for a group for parentally bereaved children. *Journal for Specialists in Group Work, 24*(2), 186–196.

Ireson, J., Hallam, S., Mortimore, P., Hack, S., & Clark, H. (1999, April 19–23). *Ability grouping in schools: An analysis of effects.* Paper presented at the annual meeting of the American Educational Research Association, Montreal. (ERIC Document Reproduction Service No. ED 430989).

Peterson, F., & Rubinson, L. (1982). An evaluation of the effects of the American Dental Association's dental health education program on the knowledge, attitudes, and health locus of control of high school students. *Journal of School Health, 52*(1), 363–369.

Rubinson, L., & Stone, D. (1975). An evaluation of the positive aspects of the American Dental Association's oral health program, level II. *Proceedings of the National Symposium on Dental Health Education in Schools*, 1–16.

Rubinson, L., Stone, D., & Mortimer, R. (1977). Statistical reliability of NPI administered to a sample of sixth grade children. *Dental Hygiene, 51*(3), 109–113.

Snow, R. (1974). Representative and quasi-representative design for research on teaching. *Review of Educational Research, 44*, 265–291.

Data Collection Through Surveys and Self-Reports

Case Study

Elizabeth was recently hired by the community hospital as the Director for Outreach Education to plan, implement, and evaluate hospital-sponsored health education programs in rural Tennessee. Her immediate administrator explained that resources would be available to her for one year and that after that her outreach programs would have to stand alone—at least economically. In other words, Elizabeth had one year in which to make her programs self-sufficient. Although some programs had been conducted in the past for the two-county catchment area, no one knew if they were successful or if they were what the people really wanted or needed. Elizabeth knew that she had to find out a lot about (1) her catchment area including the nature of residents—demographics and health needs, (2) the resources available to her in terms of both personnel and money, and (3) the best way to deliver her programs so that she could reach the greatest number of people and remain within her budgetary constraints. She realized that research was necessary if she was to be successful.

Characteristics of Survey Research

One kind of research that often appears in the health science literature is survey research. For many, this type of descriptive investigation is viewed as being unworthy and misusing funds. Not unlike other research methods, this perception is correct if the survey is conducted in poor fashion. Trow (1967) observed the following about this form of research:

The errors and inadequacies of survey research in education appear at many points from the way problems are initially chosen and defined to the choice of the subject population, the selection of the sample, the design of the individual questions and the questionnaire as a whole, and the analysis of the resulting body of data. (p. 89)

Johanson, Green, and Williams (1998) have found similar blunders in survey research. They point out errors and offer correction for many of them, including nonresponse and interpretation.

To prevent such problems, the survey approach should include (1) a clearly delineated research problem; (2) appropriate questions to respondents to gain information; (3) a well-systematized data collection technique; (4) a generation of group-level statistics; and (5) results that are generalizable to the larger population (Aday, 1989). These characteristics are very similar to those of other types of research. The major differences are in type of data collection—existing data, participant or nonparticipant observation, and case studies.

Researchers who plan to use survey methodology should review existing health surveys to learn about good designs for small and large budgets and to become familiar with secondary analysis of health survey data sets. At the national level, the National Center for Health Statistics–National Health Interview Survey (NCHS-NHIS) or the Youth Risk Behavioral Survey conducted by the Centers for Disease Control (CDC) could be reviewed. The School Health Policies and Programs Study (SHPPS) carried out by the Division of Adolescent and School Health at CDC illustrates questionnaires for the following components of comprehensive school health: health education, physical education, school food service, school health services, and school health policies (CDC, 2000). Elizabeth, from our case illustration, may want to review data from any Health Hazard Appraisal (HHA) or Health Risk Appraisal (HRA) that has been conducted in her community. These two survey instruments have been used at state and local levels in the United States as indicators of people's health. In summary, the survey approach to research is widely used and oftentimes serves as the basis for program planning, just as Elizabeth wishes to do.

Survey Flow Plan

A flow plan is used to outline the design and subsequent implementation of a survey. It begins with the objectives of the survey, lists each step to be taken, and concludes with the final report. In short, the flow plan is an organizational device. Keep in mind that several decisions may have to be made at the same time. The major components of this process are:

1. *Planning the survey:* This section includes (a) survey objectives, (b) monetary resources, (c) time resources, and (d) personnel resources. This section should be completed in detail.

2. *Overall design:* A survey should be designed to match the objectives and be in concert with data needs, sample size requirements, data collection, resources, interviewer selection, data analysis, budget, and method of reporting the results.

3. *Method of data collection:* The method chosen should match the survey objectives and fit within resource constraints.

4. *Planning data analysis:* This step describes how the data are to be analyzed.

5. *Drawing the sample:* From the survey objectives and design come (a) the questionnaire population, (b) the sample size and selection, and (c) interviewers, when appropriate.

6. *Questionnaire construction:* The questions formulated for a survey are of the utmost importance and require detailed attention. All questions should match the objectives.

7. *Pretest questionnaire:* The survey should be pretested with a sample comparable to the intended population to be surveyed.

8. *Questionnaire revision:* Revisions should be based upon the findings from the pretest. If they are extensive, a second pretest should be conducted.

9. *Administering the survey:* The method chosen (e.g., regular mail, e-mail, telephone, personal interview, or even the Internet) should fit the nature of the data to be gathered and, of course, the objectives.

10. *Code preparation:* This is the initial step in data reduction. It is the translation of question responses and respondent information to specific categories for analysis. The coding should be consistent and conventional. A precoded questionnaire should be used if at all possible.

11. *Verification:* This is an important step to check for bias, particularly when interviewers are employed. According to Aday (1989), the two principal means of cleaning the data are range-checking and contingency-checking. As the name implies, range-checking looks for the valid range of numbers/codes used for a particular answer. For example, if the codes are to be "1" or "2" and a "3" shows up, then a mistake has been made. Contingency-checking cleans data for related questions. For example, if a question were to be skipped by certain respondents, this approach would check to be sure they were omitted from the survey. For example, the respondent's age may be recorded as 12 years old but the educational level may be recorded as college graduate. For interviewers, the answers collected by one interviewer can be compared with those of others to see if bias is present. Some respondents could be reinterviewed. Also, the researcher could check with some outside criterion, such as whether the respondents really did what they said they would do (e.g., get an annual Pap exam). The errors should be located, and when appropriate, the responses should be sent back to field operations for corrections.

12. *Data entry:* This will vary according to resources, but in most instances data will be entered into a software database program on a PC, laptop, or mainframe. The key here is to use a program that is user-friendly, advantageous for analysis, and can be "watched" for errors.

13. *Tabulation:* Initially, a frequency count should be conducted to ascertain how many answers are in each of the categories for every question.

Planning the Survey
Objectives and Resources

↕

Overall Design
Descriptive, Analytical, Experimental

↕

Method of Data Collection
Self-Administered Questionnaire, Telephone or Personal Interview,
Computer-Assisted Telephone Interview (CATI) or Personal Interview (CAPI)

↕

Planning Data Analysis
Determined by Research Questions and Survey Design

↕

Drawing the Sample
Population, Sample Size, Sample Selection, Interviewers

↕

Questionnaire Construction
Prequestionnaire Planning, Researcher-Respondent Considerations,
Type of Questionnaire, Nature of Questions

↕

Pretest Questionnaire
Pretest with a Group Similar to Intended Target Audience

↕

Questionnaire Revision
Base upon Evaluation from the Pretest and Retest if Necessary

↕

Administering the Survey
Implementation at Target Level

↕

Code Preparation
Established at Outset and Carried Out Now for Data Reduction

↕

Verification
Range-Checking and Contingency-Checking

↕

Data Entry
Resource Driven–PC, Laptop, or Mainframe

↕

Tabulation
Initial Frequency Count for Categories

↕

Analysis
Percentages, Means, Relational Indices, Tests of Significance

↕

Recording and Reporting
Emphasis on Hypotheses, Testing, Reliability of Results, Implications

FIGURE 6.1 Survey Flow Plan

14. *Analysis:* This varies according to the purpose of the study, but it generally includes percentages, averages, relational indices, and tests of significance.
15. *Recording and reporting:* All the prior steps should be outlined in the report, with special emphasis on hypotheses, hypothesis testing, reliability of results, and implications of results for the subjects and further research.

Figure 6.1 summarizes the flow plan steps.

Survey Design

The nature of the research questions should determine the research design. The research questions should address the what, who, where, and when of the survey. On occasion, the researcher may wish to incorporate what findings are to be expected. Research design falls into two broad categories: descriptive and analytical.

In Elizabeth's case, one of her objectives is to determine the health needs of the bicounty residents. Let's suppose that an overview of hospital data shows that a high accident rate is one of the major reasons for emergency room visits and hospital admissions for children. However, she would like, as part of her survey, to find out more about injury and injury prevention. Table 6.1 illustrates the relationship between her research questions and descriptive designs. As shown in Table 6.1, she may use any of three types of descriptive designs: cross-sectional, longitudinal, or group comparison. The primary difference among the three choices are time dimension and group focus. Cross-sectional occurs at one point in time, whereas longitudinal takes place over a period of time. Group comparison simply compares groups on the issue, in this case childhood injuries. Descriptive designs emphasize what characteristics the group or groups possess.

TABLE 6.1 Research Questions for Descriptive Survey Designs

Elements of the Research Question	Descriptive Designs		
	Cross-Sectional	Longitudinal	Group Comparison
What	What is the prevalence of injuries	What is the incidence of injuries	Is there a difference in characteristics between those who suffer injuries and those who do not
Who	among children	among children	among children
Where	in the bicounty area	in the bicounty area	in the bicounty area
When	in the last month of summer (no school)?	during June, July, and August?	in the last month of summer (no school)?

TABLE 6.2   Research Questions for Analytical Survey Designs

Elements of the Research Question	Analytical Designs		
	Cross-Sectional	Case Control	Prospective
What	Are injured children more likely than non-injured children	Are injured children more likely than non-injured children	Is the incidence of injury greater
Who	among children	among children	among children
Where	in the bicounty area	in the bicounty area	in the bicounty area
When	in the last month of summer	in the last month of summer	during June, July, and August
Why	to be at home?	to have a history of injuries?	for those who attend summer camps?

On the other hand, Elizabeth may want to make her design analytical rather than descriptive. Table 6.2 shows how three analytical designs relate to research questions. The nature of the design—cross-sectional, case control, or prospective—must fit the research question asked. Analytical designs go beyond description to address the relationship of the variable in question (here injuries) to other factors or variables. Analytical designs, like experimental ones, explore why certain groups have particular characteristics.

In addition to these designs, there is the experimental study design. If using this design, Elizabeth would want to find out the impact her program has on injury reduction. Her research question might read as follows: "Is the incidence of injury less among children in the bicounty area during the summer break for those children who attended the injury control program?" This implies pre- and postmeasurement or data collection. Obviously several variables would have to be controlled.

Data Collection Methods

The method of data collection should be linked with the objectives and research questions (including sample coverage). In addition, the availability of the method and the budget for the study impact methodology selection. If Elizabeth finds that migrant workers who speak little English come into the counties during the summer months to help on the farms, neither mail questionnaires nor telephone interviews would be good methods. Instead, personal interviews would be necessary. In contrast, in seeking very sensitive data about health issues, it would be best for her to use a mail questionnaire to ensure anonymity. Telephone interviewing is to her advantage if the questions are not too sensitive and her target audience is readily accessible. Of course personal and telephone interviews require a large number of well-trained personnel, which can be prohibitive to many programs. The price tag is of concern to most graduate students, also.

Issues to Consider in Mail Surveys

Whether to use a mail survey or an interview technique should be determined before sample selection and questionnaire design and construction are done. Subsequently, Elizabeth should have made this decision some time ago in her survey of the two counties. This section will deal with some of the advantages, disadvantages, and factors involved with mail surveys.

Advantages of Mail Surveys

Briefly, some of the advantages of a mailed questionnaire are (1) a savings of money and time, especially as compared with the interview technique, (2) no interviewer bias, (3) greater assurance of anonymity, (4) completion by the respondent at his or her convenience, (5) accessibility to a wide geographic region, (6) accurate information because respondents can consult records before answering, and (7) identical wording for all respondents. In short, there are some definite pluses for using the mail survey technique. On the other hand, drawbacks do exist.

Disadvantages of Mail Surveys

While a mailed questionnaire may appeal to Elizabeth, she should consider its disadvantages: (1) lack of flexibility, (2) likelihood of unanswered questions, (3) low response rate as compared to interviewing, (4) inability to record spontaneous reactions and/or nonverbal responses, (5) lack of control over the order in which questions are answered and over the immediate environment, (6) no guarantee of return by the deadline date, and (7) inability to use a complex questionnaire format.

Factors Influencing Mail Surveys

Further consideration of whether or not to do a mail survey should include the seven variables enumerated by Sellitz, Jahoda, Deutsch, and Cook (1959), which affect the adequacy of data and the number of questionnaires returned.

One factor is sponsorship of the questionnaire. The organization or individuals involved may enhance or detract from the legitimacy of the study, thereby influencing questionnaire completion. A second variable is questionnaire color. It appears that color makes little or no difference in the rate of return. A third factor is questionnaire length; it seems that a less cluttered questionnaire, although longer, will bring a higher return rate than a shorter version. Ease of completion and return serves as a fourth factor. It is suggested that directions be explicit and that a stamped, self-addressed envelope be supplied. Incentives, which can range from money to a copy of the survey results, usually increase the response rate. However, monetary incentives should be seen as a goodwill gesture and not payment for time (O'Connor, Sharp, & Olson, 1999)! Moreover, incentives should be sent on the first mailing. The nature of the respondents also affects the number of questionnaires returned and the adequacy of data collected. If a highly select group is used, such as directors of mental health centers, responses tend to be more favorable than if the general public is used. Sellitz et al. (1959) also noted that the cover letter (discussed later) is of great importance.

The time and type of mailing as well as the nature of the follow-up also play a role in the success of mail surveys. As may be expected, first-class mail provides a greater return than any other class of mail. Concomitantly, using a hand-stamped envelope rather than a business-reply envelope may increase the return slightly. This difference seems to be shrinking, however, and with rising postal rates, the researcher should seriously consider the use of business-reply envelopes to save money.

Mailings must be well timed. Obviously major holidays should be avoided. Surveys received during the latter part of the week are more likely to receive quick response than those received early in the week. The months of February and April offer the lowest rate of return and March the highest, although for school surveys September may be the best month.

As a final note on factors influencing mailed questionnaires, follow-up letters or telephone calls should be employed. This should be standard procedure. The literature reveals that an increase of 20% can be expected with one follow-up or more. Frequently the researcher may send out a reminder letter, followed by an additional questionnaire and letter, and then either another letter or a phone call.

A reasonable rate of return is a highly questionable topic because so many factors affect it. Some researchers hold that a 90% return rate is needed, others claim that 50 to 60% is permissible, and still others believe that a lower rate is acceptable depending on the target population. Whatever the response rate, it is important that there be a demonstrated lack of response bias. Of course, the greater the return, the less opportunity for response bias. The amount of time and money available to the researcher will dictate response rate too.

To help demonstrate a lack of bias in the data collected, the survey researcher should make every attempt to gain information about nonrespondents (Barriball & White, 1999). In some studies there may be little difference between respondents and nonrespondents; in others the difference may be large. A survey examining the attitudes of employees who refused to complete an employee survey found that noncompliants had a greater likelihood of quitting, less company loyalty, less satisfaction with supervisors, and more negative beliefs about how their employer handled the survey data (Rogelberg, Luong, Sederburg, & Cristol, 2000). While there are different strategies to address nonresponse (Barriball & White, 1999), Sully and Grant (1997) suggest using a "reasons for not responding" form. They found that this yielded responses that increased to the level obtained with traditional follow-up procedures and also collected demographic information on the nonrespondents.

In summary, the mail survey is a technique with much potential and several advantages. Nonetheless, drawbacks do exist, and many factors influence the rate of return and adequacy of response. The decision to use or not use a mail survey must be couched within the framework of the entire study and in particular the objectives of that study.

The Personal Interview as a Research Technique

Traditionally, interviews have dealt with an individual on a face-to-face basis. It may be the principal method of investigation in some studies, but in others it is more of an exploratory tool to acquire more information (e.g., a pilot study to develop a more extensive questionnaire). Less traditional is the group interview. While not appropriate for all occasions, it may be an excellent technique if the researcher is concerned with a behavior that takes place in a group interaction setting. The advantages of the group technique over the individual approach are (1) greater efficiency in time and money, (2) observation of group interaction patterns, (3) reflection of group behavior in results, and (4) productivity of others can be stimulated. On the other hand, the group approach may (1) intimidate and suppress responses, (2) promote conformity, (3) polarize opinions, and (4) be susceptible to manipulation by an influential group member (Isaac & Michael, 1981).

Advantages of Personal Interview Studies

Some of the major advantages of the individual interview study are (1) personalization of the study to the participant; (2) flexibility so that further probing may occur or questions can be repeated; (3) a response rate that is usually higher than with a comparable mail survey; (4) observation of both verbal and nonverbal behavior; (5) control over question order that cannot be accomplished by a mail questionnaire; (6) spontaneity and "no help from others," as contrasted with either the mail survey or the group interview technique; (8) recording of the time of the interview (this may be important if events affecting the object under study have occurred); and (9) ability to use more involved and complex questionnaires.

Disadvantages of Personal Interview Studies

As with all research methodologies, the interview study has some inherent disadvantages. Some of these are (1) cost in terms of money and time (including training period and travel allowance); (2) openness to manipulation or interviewer bias; (3) vulnerability to personality clashes; (4) lack of anonymity; (5) inconvenience to the respondent as well as lack of opportunity to consult records (e.g., medical records for immunization or booster shots); (6) lack of standardization in questions because probing or question repetition may bring about a rewording that produces different responses from different respondents; (7) lack of access to respondents because of distance or other factors that may make the mail survey appear more desirable; and (8) difficulty in summarizing the findings.

Factors Influencing Personal Interview Studies

As in the mail survey, several factors may influence the quality of the data received through the interview technique. The principal one, of course, is the effect of interviewer characteristics.

Berg (2001) noted that interviewee's perception of the interviewer plays a principal role not only in the decision to consent to interview but also in the presentation of biased information. Other researchers (Burns & Grove, 1993) have shown that, in addition to race and gender, style of dress, age, hairstyle, and speech mannerism all play a role.

Interview Structure

Several interview structures may be employed by the researcher, all of which may be placed into one (or more) of three categories. All three will be presented briefly. The researcher should note that reliability increases with objectivity.

Unstructured interviews offer broad freedom to the respondent in terms of both response and time. This type of interview is usually reserved for obtaining information that is very personal and/or potentially threatening. As to be expected, this format is the most susceptible to subjective bias or error.

The middle road is the *semistructured interview*, which contains a core of structured questions from which the interviewer may move in related directions for in-depth probing. This can produce accurate information on certain questions with a built-in opportunity for exploration. Training is important so that the interviewer knows when and how to probe as well as how to avoid the introduction of interviewer bias.

In the *structured interview*, a well-defined pattern is followed, similar to a questionnaire. The interviewer only strays from the pattern to clarify questions or allow for elaboration. The type of information sought through this technique must be factual and specific. The interview itself is usually brief.

Whatever structure is used, Berg (2001) has constructed commandments for interviewing; a synopsis is presented here. You should spend a few moments with small talk so that you never enter an interview cold. All interviewers should practice a lot to become proficient. You should always remember your purpose and be respectful to the interviewees. While you need to think about your appearance, you should act naturally allowing questions to "pop up" rather than appear overrehearsed. Being a good listener is extremely important, as is being cordial and appreciative at the end of the interview. Of course, you should not accept single-syllable answers.

Telephone Interviewing

The use of the telephone in interviewing has increased greatly over the past few years. Its chief advantage over face-to-face interviewing is cost savings. One study by Graves and Kahn (1979) estimates a savings of 50% by telephone, while others purport a reduction of 75 to 80% (Klecka & Tuchfarber, 1978; Taylor, Wilson, & Wakefield, 1998).

A second advantage is that telephone interviewing is much faster than either a mail survey or personal interview study. Third, the researcher can select subjects from a much broader area because travel is not involved. Fourth, the respondent remains more anonymous in a telephone interview. Fifth, monitoring and quality control are much easier in telephone interviews, because all calls can be made from a central location. Sixth, if no one is home, frequent callbacks can be made with little expense, as contrasted to an interviewer having to return to the household or business. Seventh, the researcher has access to secure buildings and dangerous neighborhoods with the telephone interview. Finally, the telephone interview may be better than the face-to-face interview for collecting sensitive data.

However, the telephone interview does have some drawbacks. Generally, respondents are less motivated and often may see the interview as a hoax or cover for some ulterior motive. Of course, the use of checklists and visual aids are eliminated, as compared with the interview study. Further, the telephone interviewer has very little control over the situation; all the respondent has to do is hang up the telephone. However, Graves and Kahn (1979) in their study found that, while a 74% response was obtained in personal interviews, a 70% response was received through the telephone interview. Because the same questionnaire was employed for each method, the results could be compared easily. It was discovered that the results were very similar over a wide range of topics.

Conklin (1997; 1999) has done extensive work on telephone survey use among colleges and universities, particularly as it relates to mail surveys and nonrespondents. She found little difference between the two approaches. Similarly, Fowler, Gallagher, and Nederend (1999), when comparing telephone and mail responses, found data collection method had little bearing on the key results.

The telephone is productive for qualitative interviews, especially if used as a follow-up to face-to-face interviews (Rubin & Rubin, 1997). To accomplish a qualitative telephone interview, Berg (2001) recommends following three steps. First, the interviewer must establish legitimacy; second, the interviewee must be convinced that it is important to participate in this research activity; and third, detailed information must be collected if it is to be of value to the investigation.

A potential problem with telephone interviews is that of unlisted numbers. Random digit dialing (RDD), however, has allowed the researcher to circumvent this dilemma. The researcher simply selects four-digit numbers from a table of random numbers and adjoins them to the prefix (first three numbers) and then dials that number. This makes unlisted numbers available.

Computer-assisted telephone interviewing (CATI) has been around for quite some time. This method allows the questionnaire to be displayed on a screen, and the interviewers simply ask the question and enter the answer via the keyboard or mouse. CATI can virtually eliminate the recording of data in the wrong place and the incorrect asking of questions. For example, if the question, "Do you smoke?" arises in a health interview and the answer is affirmative, the interviewer may be required to turn two pages to a set of questions about smoking (e.g., about inhaling or frequency). If the interviewer fails to do this, that data may be lost and/or the respondent may be asked other questions that could be embarrassing and shorten the interview. However, a personal computer can be programmed so that an answer automatically moves the interviewer to the next appropriate question. Response accuracy is increased, especially because the interviewer does not even see the questions that do not have to be asked. Other advantages are the detection of "wild" or meaningless codes, the production of error-free data ready for analysis, and the use of help menus. In order to achieve these advantages, the researcher needs to have a computer that will perform RDD, store and retrieve telephone lists, dial automatically, present questions, check codes, input to a data set, and perform interviewing management.

While CATI is a widely recognized approach, computer-assisted personal interviewing (CAPI) is new by comparison. Lightweight laptop computers with large memories have made this technique much more user-friendly. The interviewer brings the questionnaire to the screen and enters data for each answer, similar to the CATI approach. The U.S. Census Bureau has been experimenting with CAPI. The U.S. Department of Agriculture used laptop computers over a decade ago in their Nationwide Food Consumption Survey. The National Household Education Survey (National Center for Education Statistics, 1997) is a national study on educational issues that uses both RDD and CATI.

The use of a computerized self-administered questionnaire (CSAQ) requires the respondents to have access to a computer. Respondents are given instructions on how to access the questionnaire and steps involved in completing it. The World Wide Web now has several computerized self-administered questionnaires on many topics. As computers become more accessible and software more usable, it is likely that all forms of data collection will be computer-assisted or computer-driven.

The Computer Revolution: Web-Based Surveys, Including Electronic Mail

The Internet has dramatically changed how we communicate with one another. E-mail, websites, listserves, chatrooms, and newsgroups allow researchers almost instant communication.

Nesbary (2000) outlined three types of Internet surveys. The first is the e-mail survey, which is the oldest form of Internet survey and is very similar to regular mail surveys, since questionnaires are employed. The principal difference, of course, is the speed and nature of transmission. Another difference may be that e-mail is a better way to obtain reflective data. Heflich and Rice (1999) found that using a semistructured interview protocol via electronic mail produced reflective dialogues with deep, qualitative data. Furlong (1997) believes electronic mail, when compared to postal mail, is faster, increases the likelihood of the recipient getting the survey, and may encourage participants to respond more rapidly. Research by Meha and Sivadas (1995) supports this contention. However, Mavis (1998) found postal surveys to be superior to e-mail surveys with regard to response rate. The decision to use e-mail, at least in the next few years, must be situation-specific (Hughes & Pakieser, 1999). In other words, the researcher must consider survey cost, convenience, timelines, response rate, and most importantly, representative sampling.

The second form of Internet survey discussed by Nesbary is the disk-based survey. The questionnaire is placed on a diskette in either a word-processing format or an executable (.exe) format. A respondent simply opens the questionnaire in the appropriate format and fills in the blanks. A database format (Access, Paradox) can be used in the executable form, allowing the researcher great flexibility in developing and answering questions. Of course, both formats could be sent by e-mail as attachments instead of being sent as diskettes.

The third type of Internet survey is the forms-based survey. This survey instrument is located on the researcher's website. The researcher can contact respondents by e-mail to alert them to the website and ask them to respond. Of course, depending upon the nature of the research, only people who frequent the website can be asked to respond. For example, a cancer site may ask all people who visit to complete the questionnaire. This technique allows for the flexibility of a database format and the accuracy of a written survey. Needless to say, it can be a cost saving in terms of both time and money.

Response and Other Rates

When reading about response rates in survey research, it is important to identify how they were determined (Frey, 1989). The more common way is comparing the number of completions to the number of potential respondents who were eligible. This formula is as follows:

$$\text{response rate 1} = \frac{\text{number of completions}}{\text{number in sample}} \times 100$$

A second response rate that is sometimes used compares the number of completions to the completions plus partial completions and the number of refusals, less all uncompleted interviews. This formula is expressed as:

$$\text{response rate 2} = \frac{\text{number of completions}}{\text{number in sample} - (\text{noneligible and nonreachable})} \times 100$$

Response Rate 1 is the preferred method and should be used by Elizabeth in her survey research. It establishes a much more honest evaluation of returns. As a general rule, response rates for personal interviews are highest, followed by telephone and self-administered questionnaires, especially mail. This should not be too surprising since interviewers can be persuasive and respondents are much less likely to end a face-to-face interview.

Refusal rates are of importance in survey research because refusals are the most common reason for nonresponses. This rate is calculated as follows:

$$\text{refusal rate} = \frac{\text{number of respondents refused}}{\text{number of eligible respondents contacted}} \times 100$$

The noncontact rate is simply the ratio of nonresponse not attributed to direct refusals from the potential respondents. This rate is important since it lets the researcher know the degree to which respondents are accessible or can be located. The formula is:

$$\text{noncontact rate} = \frac{\text{total not contacted}}{\text{total known eligible}} \times 100$$

In reporting your research, you should show that the loss of data from nonrespondents is not detrimental to the findings. This might be done by showing that no obvious differences exist among respondents and nonrespondents in such factors as age, race, gender, socioeconomic status, education, and so forth.

Survey Sampling

The results of survey research, in fact perhaps the results of all research, rest heavily on the sampling foundation. That is, if our sampling is flawed, then our results will not be as useful. Ideally, the researcher would like to observe the entire population to add more weight to the findings. For example, in Elizabeth's situation she may wish to obtain answers from all residents in the two-county area. However, limitations of resources, time, and money frequently preclude a study of the entire population. This would be even more evident if the study were to survey her entire state. Subsequently, a subset of some predetermined size must be selected from the population of interest. The sample or subset should represent the total population so that the data collected from the sample will be as accurate as that from the entire population.

The logic involved is simple. Nonetheless, the importance of this step cannot be overemphasized. As stated by Leedy (1980), "The results of a survey are no more trustworthy than the quality of the population or the representatives of the sample" (p. 35). A knowledgeable researcher commences with a population and works down to the sample. In other words, the population of interest is designated and then a sample is derived. The neophyte, on the other hand, often works from the bottom up by attempting to ascertain the minimum number of respondents needed for a successful study. The inherent problem with this approach is that it is next to impossible to assess the representatives of the sample because the entire population has not been identified. In the case study, Elizabeth must determine her target population. Is it to be all residents? Or does she just wish to include taxpayers? Her population could be limited to all those who may potentially use the services of the hospital. Once this decision is made, she may then proceed to the selection of the sample.

The savings in both time and money are obvious reasons to deal with a sample of the population. There are additional advantages, too, as described by Bailey (1994). The sample may achieve a greater response rate owing to greater cooperation than might occur in the full population survey. This in itself would tend to make the results more accurate. In health surveys with sensitive items, this point is particularly important. Concomitantly, the researcher can keep a low profile by using a sample. That is, less people may be offended, thereby negating an opportunity for several people to organize a common resistance. In the case of interviewing, a sample reduces the number of interviews and interviewers. This is beneficial in that supervision of an enormous number of interviewers is difficult at best, and necessary attention to details such as follow-ups becomes very cumbersome as numbers increase.

There is little doubt that in many instances the use of a sample is much more advantageous than an entire population survey. Yet, the benefits only hold true if the sample is drawn with precision.

The National Health Interview Survey (1999) was redesigned to improve the reliability of the statistics for racial, ethnic, economic, and geographic domains. Patrick, Pruchno, and Rose (1998), in comparing five recruitment strategies, found that even nonprobability sampling can be very successful for recruiting large, diverse groups if very careful planning, implementation, and good funding exist. Wang and Fan (1997) discuss six criteria for survey sampling design evaluation. Four of the six involve sampling procedures. The four criteria are (1) clearly specifying the population, (2) explicitly stating the unit of analysis, (3) specifying a method to determine sample size, and (4) giving a detailed description of selection procedures. The next chapter addresses sampling techniques and sample size in detail.

Questionnaire Design and Construction

Questionnaire design and construction involve much more than drafting the questionnaire itself. The researcher needs to complete prequestionnaire planning, draft the questionnaire, prepare the final copy, and then pretest it. The following points illustrate the necessary components:

1. Prequestionnaire planning:
   a. Define the problem and hypothesize solutions.
   b. Determine the information needed to test the hypothesis.
   c. Review previous research and speak with resource personnel.
   d. Develop preliminary questions.

2. Drafting the questionnaire:
   a. Considerations for researcher, respondent, and interviewer
   b. Types of questionnaires
   c. Types of questions
   d. First draft of the questionnaire

3. Preparing the final questionnaire:
   a. Physical layout
   b. Reproduction and materials
   c. Identification of respondents in the questionnaire

4. Pretesting:
   a. Determining the value to questionnaire design.
   b. Evaluating the pretest.
   c. Revising the questionnaire, if necessary. (This may warrant another pretest.)

The emphasis in this section will be on drafting the questionnaire.

Researcher, Respondent, and Interviewer Considerations

Once the hypotheses have been carefully specified and the sample drawn, the next step in the research chain is development of the data collection instrument. Herein, the major consideration is questionnaire relevance to the researcher, the respondent, and the interviewer (when appropriate). The researcher must be certain that the questionnaire is relevant to the goals and objectives of the study as set. No matter how well worded or designed the questionnaire, if it fails to produce the data relevant to the objectives, it is worthless.

Overall, the study and subsequent questionnaire must be relevant to the respondent. This is not always self-evident because research objectives are frequently housed in scientific jargon; therefore, they must be clarified and justified in lay terms. This can be accomplished by means of a cover letter. There must be a connection between the respondent and all those questions that apply to the respondent. That is, can the respondents understand the questions? Are they likely to know the answers? Are they willing to respond to the questions? The answer to the last question could be "no" if the questions are not relevant and thereby offer no motivating force. To make the questions applicable, skips or contingency questions (e.g., "If you answered 'yes' to this question, skip to Question 22") can be used. With this method the respondent has to read and answer only items that are personally relevant.

In drafting the questionnaire that is to be used in an interview schedule, all elements that could lead to interviewer bias must be removed. Questions have to be phrased so as not to be misconstrued. Further, questions should follow a logical order, with a smooth transition from topic to topic. Needless to say, all directions to the interviewer and the respondent should be clear and concise.

Types of Questionnaires

Generally, questionnaire forms are closed, open, or a combination of the two. The *restricted*, or *closed*, form provides fixed-alternative questions that can be answered by a simple "yes" or "no" or by checking an appropriate box. Some of the advantages of this form are (1) ease of completion for the respondent; (2) simplification of coding and analysis, particularly because the questionnaire can be precoded; (3) greater chance that respondents will answer sensitive questions (e.g., about age or income) because they are usually categorized rather than demanding an exact number; and (4) a minimum of irrelevant responses.

On the other hand, some disadvantages of the closed form are (1) given a list of potential answers, the unknowledgeable respondent may guess or randomly select an answer; (2) variations in answers among respondents may be reduced since only certain categories are available; (3) there may be too many answer categories to be printed simplistically; (4) the respondent may become frustrated since there is no room for a separate, nonprovided opinion; and (5) the respondent may circle the wrong answer (e.g., circle a 3 instead of a 4).

It is suggested that the categories of "don't know" and "other" be included in a closed-form questionnaire. In this way, the respondent is not forced to work with just the alternatives provided. Further, it gives the researcher the opportunity to receive more relevant information.

In the *open*, or *unrestricted*, questionnaire form the response categories are not specified, and the respondent is allowed to answer in his or her own words. Some of the advantages of this type of questionnaire are that it is (1) usable when all the response categories are unknown, (2) preferable for controversial, sensitive, and complex issues, and (3) allows for respondent creativity, clarification, and detail. The disadvantages include (1) difficulty in coding and analysis; (2) greater demands on the respondent in terms of time, writing ability, and thought; (3) questions may be too general for the respondent to comprehend or answer; and (4) data collected may not be relevant to the objectives of the study.

Many questionnaires have *combined* forms, including both closed and open items. A questionnaire that is primarily closed should have at least one open-ended item to allow the respondent to express a personal opinion or thought. Each health science researcher must decide which type is more likely to supply the information desired.

Types of Questions

A variety of questions and response category formats are available to the questionnaire builder. In closed-form questionnaires the usual types are dichotomous, multiple choice, rating, and ranking. Open-form questionnaires generally consist of a blank space where the answer is to be written. On occasion, sentence-completion questions are incorporated into both forms.

To illustrate the different types, suppose that Elizabeth in our case study were to develop a questionnaire with primarily a closed format and a few open-ended items. The basic rule she would follow for writing questions would be to provide all possible answers in as clear a fashion as possible.

In *dichotomous* questions the answer comprises two parts, one of which is to be selected by the respondents. Examples of this type are:

> Circle the appropriate number:
> 1. Gender: Male 1   Female 2
> 2. Setting: Urban 1   Rural 2

With *multiple-choice* items, each potential answer is listed for the respondent such as:

> How far would you be willing to travel for a health program of interest to you? (Check One)
>
> 1 mile or less   [ ]
> 2 to 4 miles   [ ]
> 5 to 7 miles   [ ]
> 8 to 10 miles   [ ]
> 11 or more miles   [ ]

It can be readily noted that this format takes much more space than if answers are placed side by side; however, the answers are recognized quickly.

Many questionnaires include *rating* questions in which the respondent indicates a particular view about the psychological object. For example:

> Several educational services are listed below. Please indicate the importance of each to you:

	Very Important	Somewhat Important	Not Important
1. Diabetic training	_____	_____	_____
2. Smoking cessation	_____	_____	_____
3. Stress reduction	_____	_____	_____

This format allows several items to be categorized as a series with directions stated only once.

Another fixed-alternative approach is that of *ranking*. Here the respondent simply orders the given answers in rank. For example:

1. The following are some of the health problems faced by residents of our two counties. Please place them in order of greatest problem (rank it 1) to the smallest problem (rank it 5) within the counties, as you see them:

_____ Unintentional injury
_____ Alcoholism
_____ Drug addiction
_____ Teen pregnancy
_____ High blood pressure

For the *sentence-completion* format, an example item would be:

1. In regard to education, I feel the Community Hospital should

_____ .

Frequently, the *open-ended* questions are placed at or near the end of the questionnaire. For example, Elizabeth might ask the following question:

1. In the space below, please write out any particular interests or concerns that you have about attending programs at the Community Hospital:

_____

Branching questions need to be handled with care so that the correct target group responds to the questions. An example for Elizabeth could be as follows:

In the past month, have you or a member of your family been injured?

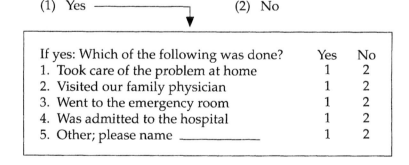

Or, this could be written in the following way.

In the past month, have you or a member of your family been injured?

1. Yes (complete section A)
2. No (go to section B)

It is important that the health science researcher consider the target population when deciding on the type of questionnaire and the types of questions. Further, when writing the questions, several pitfalls should be avoided. The following list can serve as a guide:

1. Phrase questions to be comprehended by all those in the target population.
2. Avoid double-barreled questions.
3. Be careful of double negatives.
4. Define terms that could be easily misinterpreted.
5. Underline or boldface a word if special emphasis is demanded.
6. Watch for inadequate alternatives to a question.
7. Do not use adjectives that fail to have an agreed-on meaning.
8. Be sure questions are not leading questions.
9. There should be no ambiguity in the questions.

On completion of the questions, it is necessary to combine them into the final questionnaire in an order that will bring about the greatest response. To assist in this task, some general rules should be followed:

1. Put sensitive questions as well as open-ended ones near the end of the questionnaire.
2. Place questions in a logical order when possible.
3. Simpler questions should be ahead of more difficult ones.
4. Avoid establishing a response set.
5. Request information needed for subsequent questions first.
6. Vary questions by length and type.
7. Separate reliability-check question pairs (i.e., pairs of questions in which one is stated positively and the other negatively). For example, if one of your questions is, "The Mental Health Center should offer educational classes (agree/disagree)," you should wait until later in the questionnaire to include the item, "the Mental Health Center should *not* offer educational classes (agree/disagree)."

Attitude Scale Construction

Likert Scaling

Scales may be included in a questionnaire to gather data in a different fashion. One type of scale was devised by Rensis Likert (1932), who employed ordinal scaling and summated rating techniques to develop an attitude scale. In *summated rating,* several items are used in an attitude scale, and, to ascertain an individual's score, the researcher adds (sums up) each item score circled. For example, if the attitude scale comprises 10 items and the person circles 1 for every item, the summated rating score would be 10, whereas the summated rating score of 50 would be obtained by the person who circles 5 for each of the 10 items.

One of the major problems of summated rating is that all the items may fail to measure the same concept. Perhaps some of the items in the 10-item scale just mentioned really do not measure what the others measure. Likert created a technique to eliminate such items and thereby improve internal consistency. This will be discussed in more detail later.

In constructing a Likert-type scale, the first step is to assemble a large number of items considered relevant to the attitude under investigation. These items or statements should fall in approximately equal numbers with respect to their relative favorableness or unfavorableness toward the object of interest.

Next, each statement must be weighted from 1 to 5, with 3 as the neutral position. It makes no difference whether a rank of 1 is the favorable or unfavorable end of the continuum, as long as the weighting is consistent. For purposes of illustration, however, let us allow the higher score to indicate a stronger agreement with the attitude being scaled. Therefore, a positive statement would be scored by the following key:

strongly agree	agree	undecided	disagree	strongly disagree
5	4	3	2	1

A negative statement would be scored as follows:

strongly agree	agree	undecided	disagree	strongly disagree
1	2	3	4	5

The reason for reversing the negative items or statements is to provide a total score that reflects positiveness toward the object in question. In a scale of attitudes toward sexuality, for example, the program participants with a positive sexual attitude would agree with positive statements and disagree with negative ones, while patients with an unfavorable (negative) sexual attitude would disagree with positive items and agree with negative ones. To obtain a total score, the relative weightings of each response are summed. Subsequently, in this example the higher total score represents a more positive sexual attitude than a lower total score.

Now, all of these items should be administered to a sample of the population for whom the scale is intended. As a general rule, the sample size should be at least twice the number of statements desired in the final scale, and most Likert-type scales have 20 to 22 items.

Selection of statements for the final scale is based on an objective check for internal consistency and statement differentiation between the highest and lowest scores. If selection is being done by hand, the scores can be separated into quartiles so the upper 25% can be compared with the lower 25%. The median score for each statement is calculated. If any statement has the same median score for both the high and low groups, it should be eliminated from the scale. For best differentiation, only those statements that have widely different median scores for the highest and lowest groups are retained. An easier way is to use a computer and check for internal consistency by an item-total correlation. Herein, the responses for *each* statement are correlated with the *total* scores obtained by the subjects on the whole test. This technique reveals the amount of agreement between each individual item and the total test—that is, the degree to which each item measures what the total test measures. Those statements receiving a low correlation should be eliminated.

As a final note, retain items with a high correlation and be certain to have approximately an equal number of positive and negative statements covering a range of topics within the attitude being measured.

Some of the advantages of Likert scaling are (1) it is simple to construct; (2) each item is of equal value so that respondents rather than the item are scored (unlike Thurstone scaling, discussed under *Interval-Ratio Scaling*); (3) it permits the use of latent attitudes in that items that are not manifestly related to the attitude being measured can be employed; and (4) it is likely to produce a highly reliable scale.

Van-Alphen, Halfens, Hasmans, and Imbos (1994) suggest that scoring can be improved by using the Rasch model. In that model both respondents and items are scaled on the same continuum, whereas in the Likert scaling all items have the same weight. The Rasch model is based on item response theory and the Likert model is from classical test theory. The Thurstone and Chave (1929) method (see below) is another way to weight the items.

Interval-Ratio Scaling

Another method of quantification is the interval scale. Based on equal units of measurement, the interval scale demonstrates how much of a given characteristic is present. Further, the difference in amount of the characteristic present in the persons with scores of 25 and 26, for example, is assumed to be equivalent to the difference in persons with scores of 75 and 76. In other words, interval scales indicate the relative amount of a trait, which is something that neither nominal nor ordinal scales permit. However, because a true zero fails to exist in ordinal scales, it is inappropriate to claim that a score of 75 is three times a score of 25.

In contrast, a ratio scale possesses not only the equal interval properties of an interval scale, but also a true zero. For example, a zero on a pharmacy weight scale shows the complete absence of ounces or grams. Moreover, a ratio scale has the properties of real numbers, which can be added, subtracted, multiplied, divided, and expressed in ratio relationships. Therefore, a pharmacy scale that measures 10 grams has twice as much weight on it as one that measures 5 grams.

The most precise ratio scales are common in the physical health sciences (e.g., those for measuring blood pressure). The behavioral health sciences, which measure characteristics such as attitudes, are limited to interval scales or even less precise types, such as ordinal or nominal scales.

Thurstone and Chave (1929) developed the Thurstone technique of scaled values, frequently referred to as the method of equal-appearing intervals. Herein, a large number of attitude statements are collected and entered on separate cards. The statements, via the cards, are then submitted to a panel of judges, who are required to rank the statements into 11 equidistant piles. The 11 piles represent a continuum from extremely favorable to extremely unfavorable, with the middle pile being neutral.

The scale value for any particular statement is the median of the frequency distribution by the judges. If more than one statement has the same scale value, then the statement with the smaller Q statistic or interquartile range is retained for the final scale. It is believed that the smaller the interquartile range, the greater the degree of agreement among the judges with respect to that particular statement's position along the continuum.

The general goal is to obtain 20 to 22 statements to form the final scale. The 20 or 22 statements are then randomly arranged and administered to a group of respondents, who can either agree or disagree with each item. To score, the mean or median value of those statements with which the respondent agreed is calculated. In other words, the respondent is asked to only check those items to which he or she agrees, and the mean or median value of the checked statements is the scale score for that respondent.

A partial Thurstone-type attitude scale may appear thus:

Sexual Attitude Statements for Program Participants

1. Sexual relations are simply sources of frustration. (10.0)*
2. Hoping for a sexual relationship is senseless. (8.2)
3. Sex may or may not be important in a relationship. (5.0)
4. Partners should try new and different sexual approaches. (2.5)
5. Sex is the most essential part of a relationship. (1.0)

Some of the statements are unfavorable toward sexuality (Statements 1 and 2), while others are favorable (Statements 4 and 5) and still others neutral (Statement 3).

One of the advantages of the Thurstone scale is that the statements are weighted or valued rather than the respondents. Nevertheless, the Thurstone scale is disadvantageous in that it is much more cumbersome to construct than the Likert scale. Further, there is the question about the dependence of the scale values upon the

---

*This is the scaled value for the statement. The participant checks the statements with which he or she agrees, and the scale values of the statements checked are used to ascertain a scale score by finding the average or median score.

opinions of the judges (Murphy & Likert, 1937). Moreover, it has been shown that this method is no more reliable than the Likert technique (Ferguson, 1941).

Some Thurstone-type scales have been produced for current use in the health science field. One such instrument is a scale to appraise the attitudes of college students toward euthanasia (Tordella & Neutens, 1979). Another scale measures information priorities among health consumers seeking cancer care (Degner, Davison, Sloan, & Mueller, 1998; Bilodeau & Degner, 1996). Degner et al. (1998) explored the use of both the Likert and Thurstone approaches.

Semantic Differential Scaling

The semantic differential scale was developed by Osgood, Suci, and Tannenbaum (1957) to measure attitudes. The semantic differential (SD) has three elements: (1) the attitudinal concept to be measured; (2) a pair of opposite adjectives; and (3) a series of undefined scale positions, usually seven in number, between each of the polar adjective pairs. For example, for the concept of research, the polar adjective pairs forming the opposite ends of the seven categories could be "good-bad" or "simple-complex." If this were the case, then the SD might look as follows:

Research

good ——|——|——|——|—— bad
simple ——|——|——|——|—— complex

The polar adjective pairs should be selected according to the objectives of the study. In addition to the polar adjective pairs developed by the originators of the SD, Jenkins, Russell, and Suci (1958) created an atlas of semantic profiles for 360 words. In both instances, Osgood et al. and Jenkins et al., the pairs of polar adjectives can be used to measure three dimensions—evaluative (e.g., good-bad), potency (e.g., hard-soft), and activity (e.g., fast-slow).

Heise (1970) has researched question format to find that it makes no difference whether one concept is followed by all adjective-pair scales, one concept is followed by one pair only, or all concepts are rated on one polar adjective pair. Further, if one concept is followed by all adjective pair scales, the ordering of concepts makes no difference. However, it is recommended that evaluative, potency, and activity scales be mixed or combined to prevent response sets. Concomitantly, the polar adjective pairs should be randomly arranged so that left and right positions on the total scale do not encourage a response set.

Sorokin (1976) has developed a semantic differential to measure attitudes toward aspects of sexuality. Two of the concepts in his scale are shown for illustration:

Sexuality Scales
Concept 9: Getting Married

pleasing ——|——|——|——|—— annoying
constructive ——|——|——|——|—— destructive
desirable ——|——|——|——|—— undesirable

Concept 10: Having Sexual Relations with the One You Love

pleasing ——|——|——|——|—— annoying
constructive ——|——|——|——|—— destructive
desirable ——|——|——|——|—— undesirable

Different polar adjective pairs could also have been selected, such as:

Concept 10: Having Sexual Relations with the One You Love

important ——|——|——|——|—— unimportant
constrained ——|——|——|——|—— free
active ——|——|——|——|—— passive
approach ——|——|——|——|—— avoid

Here three principal factors or dimensions as well as a fourth situational dimension are represented. "Important-unimportant" represents the evaluative factor, and "constrained-free" and "active-passive" reflect the potency and activity dimensions, respectively. The situational component is rendered by the adjective pair "approach-avoid."

In administering and scoring the SD, the patients or subjects should be instructed to put down their initial impression. The scale positions are converted to numerical values so that various statistical assessments can be completed:

important –7–|–6–|–5–|–4–|–3–|–2–|–1– unimportant

The scores can be analyzed for differences between concepts, between scales, between subjects, or any such combination. Subsequently, a semantic differential generates a large amount of data. For information on analysis techniques, consult Kerlinger (1964), Nunnally (1962), Snider and Osgood (1969), and Osgood et al. (1957).

Two advantages of the semantic differential are that it is simple to construct and easy for the respondent to complete. Further, it allows for several types of analyses to take place. However, that also serves as a disadvantage, because some analyses can be very complex. If the researcher employs this method of attitude scale construction, it is important to outline the scoring technique in detail for the practitioner.

Factor Scaling

Factor analysis is a procedure used to determine the number and nature of variables underlying given measures. For example, if a researcher had 45 statements planned for a scale to measure attitudes toward sexuality, it would be advantageous to know whether all the statements or items are measuring that particular concept or if underlying concepts exist. In other words, is the scale unidimensional? Through factor analysis, one might discover that a number of statements have some variance in common such that they correlate highly with some underlying dimension. If so, this dimension will appear as a factor or construct, which can be considered as a separate scale. In essence, factor analysis is a method for extracting common factor variances from sets of measures.

An instrument developed to measure attitudes about heterosexual relationships of teenagers with cognitive disabilities (Neutens, 1975) can be used as an example of factor analysis. Initially, 70 statements about dating and premarital and marital relations were obtained from a large population of educable mentally disabled students. After they were edited, these statements comprised a preliminary instrument, which was administered to 257 educable mentally disabled teenagers. All 70 statements were intercorrelated, yielding an R matrix. (Statement 1 correlated to Statements 1 through 70, Statement 2 correlated to Statements 1 through 70, and so on, until all statements were correlated with one another to form a matrix.) This matrix underwent factor analysis with the principal components solution and varimax orthogonal rotation to reveal three underlying concepts or dimensions within the 70 items. In other words, some of the 70 items correlated highly with one of the extracted factors or dimensions, others correlated highly with a second factor, and still others correlated highly with a third factor. Statements that failed to correlate at .300 were eliminated; this produced an instrument with 37 statements that measured three factors. Table 6.3 shows the three factors and the *factor loadings* (which can be considered the correlation between the statement and each of the three factors).

The factor structure is almost perfect. All I statements are loaded significantly on Factor I, all II statements on Factor II, and all III statements on Factor III. The only questionable statements are 31, 34, and 35, which have rather substantial negative loadings. Overall, the factor loadings are evidence for construct validity of the scale.

Unlike the Likert or Thurstone scaling techniques, the scales are not named until after factor analysis, rather than before construction. The factor scale name is usually derived from the content or theme of the statements contained within it.

In Neutens's heterosexual relations attitude scale, factor analysis was employed to validate attitude statements. If factor analysis is the only method employed in scale development, and if the scale is scored accordingly, the following rules apply. An individual's total score on a scale is calculated by taking the score on each statement in the scale (scored from 1 to 5 and corrected for negative items) and

TABLE 6.3 Rotated Factor Loadings of Heterosexual Relations Statements

Factor	Statement	Factor Loadings I	II	III
I	1.	.529	.122	−.184
	2.	.524	−.068	.002
	3.	.511	.101	.073
	4.	.473	−.012	.267
	5.	.456	.014	.117
	6.	.442	.098	.135
	7.	.438	.229	.038
	8.	.424	.055	−.026
	9.	.419	.142	.248
	10.	.417	.251	.086
	11.	.394	−.028	−.190
	12.	.390	.080	−.011
	13.	.369	.263	−.060
II	14.	.078	.582	.156
	15.	.068	.479	−.103
	16.	.023	.479	−.009
	17.	.249	.475	.105
	18.	.072	.458	.145
	19.	.228	.455	.007
	20.	.180	.432	.053
	21.	−.031	.431	.196
	22.	.191	.382	.089
	23.	.286	.312	−.026
	24.	.178	.301	−.105
	25.	.130	.300	.194
III	26.	.218	.059	.440
	27.	−.123	.136	.436
	28.	.030	.201	.434
	29.	−.083	−.182	.415
	30.	.064	−.043	.410
	31.	−.344	.184	.389
	32.	.151	−.121	.385
	33.	.052	.246	.375
	34.	.032	−.301	.373
	35.	−.314	−.023	.351
	36.	.297	.166	.331
	37.	−.236	−.023	.312

weighting it by the factor loading on that scale. For example, from Table 6.3, for Factor I, if a respondent scored 2 on Statement 1, 4 on Statement 5, and 3 on Statement 10, the total score for Scale I would be:

$$2(.529) + 4(.456) + 3(.417) = 1.06 + 1.83 + 1.26 = 4.15$$

Some of the advantages of factor scaling are (1) unidimensionality of each scale and (2) weighting of statements and continuous scores such that each statement is not of equal value (i.e., one statement may be weighted more according to its factor loading on the factor or dimension). The continuous score occurs when the discrete score (5, 4, 3, 2, or 1) is multiplied by the factor loading. Also, with the availability of computer programs to do the computations, construction is now easy. The disadvantages are the difficulty in hand computation and the necessity to name scales after their construction. A scale so developed may have descriptive value, but very little theoretical value. Other examples of factor analysis in scaling include those constructed by Kondo and Kamada (1998) to measure a sense of life worth living; by Santos, Reynaldo, and Clegg (1999) to use in extension surveys; and by Sanderson (2000) to develop dance attitude scales.

Cover Letter

When the questionnaire is complete, a cover letter should be developed. Though the instrument constructed is of prime importance, the beginning researcher should realize that an inappropriate cover letter or introductory statement may cause the respondent to discard the questionnaire without even looking at it, or to ask the interviewer to leave. As a matter of note, the letter should be on an organizational letterhead to indicate the legitimacy of the survey in the case of a mailed questionnaire. When an interview is conducted, the introductory statement serves as a public relations technique.

In regard to content, the cover letter or introductory statement should contain (1) identification of the person or organization conducting the study, (2) the reason the study is being conducted, (3) why it is important for the respondent to complete the survey, (4) assurance that there are no right or wrong answers, (5) assurance of confidentiality of information given, (6) assurance of anonymity of the respondent, when applicable, (7) length of time it will take to complete, (8) the date of return (for a mail survey), and (9) a notice of how to obtain results. Figure 6.2 shows the cover letter used by Elizabeth.

Scott (1961) reviewed several studies about cover letters and found that a "permissive" letter obtains a greater response than does a "firm" letter. Also, a "short, punchy letter" is better than a longer, logical appeal. Handwriting the address does not seem to increase the response rate. No difference in response rate was found whether a true signature or facsimile was used, or whether the letter was addressed as "Dear Mr. Smith," "Dear Friend," or "Dear Bulletin User." In short, he concluded that "the content of the letter is very much more important than its trappings" (p. 152). However, Wiersma (2000) has recommended that the letter be on official letterhead and be signed by a person in a professional position who is in some way associated with the respondents.

[Date]

Dear [Respondent Name]:

As you are aware, the Community Hospital is responsible for many health services in our bicounty area. We are conducting this survey to determine the need for selected health services and health education programs.

Enclosed is a questionnaire that we are asking you to complete as part of this survey. The questions are very easy to answer and should not take more than 20 minutes of your time. There are no right or wrong answers. You have our assurance that the information that you provide in this survey will be kept anonymous. Your answers will help us to plan health services and education throughout the bicounty region and to promote better health for all of our residents.

Since a limited number of these questionnaires are being sent out to select residents of the bicounty area, your individual opinion is highly important to the success of this undertaking. We, therefore, request that you please complete and return this questionnaire in the enclosed, self-addressed, stamped envelope *no later than [insert date]*. If you have any questions about this survey or want to have a copy of the results, please contact Elizabeth _____ at 555-9306.

Thank you for your cooperation.

Sincerely,

Jane Doe
Executive Director
Community Hospital

FIGURE 6.2 Cover Letter

Pretesting and Questionnaire Revision

The constructed questionnaire remains at rough draft stage until a pretest is done to identify flaws and to allow for corrections. Though the sample for the pretest is frequently fellow students, faculty, or co-workers, it is recommended that a subsample for the target population be employed for better results. Further, it should be administered in the same fashion as intended for the actual study (i.e., mail, telephone, or interview).

Those in the pretest sample should complete the questionnaire as directed and then do a critical analysis of all aspects of the instrument: sensitivity of issues, question wording and order, response categories, reliability checks, physical layout, length of time for answering, and instructions. Any comments given in the margins or elsewhere should receive special attention, particularly if several respondents hold the same view. In addition, the researcher should seek indicators of other problems by calculating the "no response" or "don't know" answers. Pattern of response should be observed for set responses.

Only when the corrections have been made should the questionnaire be used in the research project. If several alterations were required, another pretest should be conducted. All of this takes time and should be built into the time frame for the entire study. Omission of this step could prove to be a grievous error if the final data fail to correspond to the objectives.

Focus Groups

Focus groups, as an interview methodology, are becoming popular. This technique capitalizes on communication among the participants and the researcher. Rather than ask each person in the group to respond to the same question, although that could be done, the researcher encourages the participants to talk to each other—ask questions, give examples, provide comments. Focus groups arrive at opinions and can get to the reasons underlying those opinions. One of the highlights of the focus group technique is that it is culturally sensitive. It has been used extensively in cross-cultural research and in studying differential use of health services within a population (Kitzinger, 1995; Wilson, Pittman, & Wold, 2000). Critical comments can be generated with greater ease with this approach than with interviews (Watts & Ebbutt, 1987; Taylor et al., 1999). This is particularly important in evaluation studies and in marketing research.

The number of groups used in a singular study may range from 6 to 50, depending upon the nature of the research project and that old nemesis, available resources. Usually just a few groups are used. Sampling for focus groups can follow patterns similar to other types of research. That is, random sampling can be done. Depending upon the study objectives, imaginative sampling may be required. For example, Kitzinger (1990) found that it was important to include lesbians and women who were sexually abused in a study of women's experience with cervical smears. Focus groups can also be advantageous when sampling people who cannot read or write.

The number of participants per group should be between four and eight, and the sessions generally should last two hours, although they may be shorter or longer in duration. The sessions should be relaxed and the participants should be told that you are seeking interaction, not a question-answer format. Initially the researcher may sit back and observe but at some point will likely intervene to direct and guide the process. To stimulate discussion, you may want to have a series of large cards, each with a statement. The participants could place the cards in order of most important to least important, or they could separate the cards into "agree" and "disagree" piles. For example, Elizabeth could have cards dealing with quality of care at the hospital or the role of community health education carried out by the hospital.

Sim (1998) raises three issues in analyzing focus group data. First, it is difficult to infer attitudinal consensus. Second, measuring strength of opinion is very problematic. Third, attempts to generalize from focus group data can be met with methodological and epistemological objections. Therefore, analysis is generally qualitative in nature. Elizabeth, for example, could pull together and compare themes and how they relate to variables within the sample and population. Differentiation between group consensus and individual statements is important. Percentages and similar frequency data are not used. Deviant data (comments, themes) should be noted, since they can be valuable to the findings. Focus groups can be a stand-alone approach or can be combined with other survey techniques.

The Delphi Technique

The Delphi technique designed by Helmer (1967) is a method of reaching group consensus on any psychological object. It was originated to circumvent the traditional roundtable approach of group consensus with its inherent problems of the power of individuals to sway the group, the bandwagon effect of majority opinion, the manipulation of group dynamics, and the unwillingness of individuals to alter publicly stated positions.

While the Delphi technique is not new (Dalkey & Helmer, 1963), it is relatively recent to health science research. Two very different examples are those of Sowell (2000) and Annemans, Giaccone, and Vergnenegre (1999). The technique was used by Sowell to identify HIV/AIDS research priorities from the perspective of nurses in AIDS care. Annemans et al. employed a modified technique with clinicians to investigate the cost effectiveness of Taxol, an anticancer drug. Anderson, Goddard, Garcia, Guzman, and Vazquez (1998) used the Delphi technique to identify diabetes care and education issues for Latinos with diabetes. At the international level, WHO employed it to determine essential public health functions (Bettcher, Sapirie, & Goon, 1998). At the state level, Hahn, Toumey, Tayens, and McCoy (1999) used this approach to seek agreement among Kentucky legislators regarding tobacco control and tobacco farming policy. Elizabeth could use this technique as part of her overall data collection. For example, she could have a member of each hospital department involved in ambulatory care address the issue of necessary community health promotion programs in order to get consensus.

Generally, group members are identified who will generate the consensus position, and each member interacts individually to provide collective feedback. Individuals then reconsider their initial positions in light of group trends and can make adjustments accordingly. Eventually, this leads to an informed consensus isolated from the forces of the traditional approach.

Specifically, the sequence of events is as follows:

1. Identify the group members whose consensus opinions are sought. If they are representatives of a group (e.g., heads of departments of health sciences in universities), the sampling technique must be appropriate.
2. In the first questionnaire, each member of the group generates a list of concerns, goals, or issues toward which consensus opinions are desired (e.g., knowledge competencies for health educators or research issues confronting health education). The combined lists are edited, randomized, and placed in a format acceptable for a second questionnaire.
3. In the second questionnaire, each member rates or ranks the items derived from the initial questionnaire.
4. In the third questionnaire, the results of the second questionnaire are presented, revealing the preliminary level of group consensus to each item as well as repeating each member's previous response. The individual group member then rates or ranks each item a second time. If the member differs greatly from the group trend, a brief explanation should be given.
5. In the fourth questionnaire, the group trend becomes quite evident, as the results of the third questionnaire are presented for each item as well as the member's latest ranking or rating. Along with this is a listing by item of the major reasons for dissent from the group trend. In this questionnaire each member ranks or rates each item for a third and last time, keeping the group's emerging pattern in mind.
6. The results of the fourth questionnaire are calculated and presented as the final statement of group consensus.

If this technique is employed, it is necessary to have all the knowledge and skill required for survey design as well as questionnaire construction and design.

Case Discussion

As the newly hired Director for Outreach Education, Elizabeth definitely has her work cut out. The following steps would need to be taken or addressed if she were to carry out successful survey research:

1. She would need to identify her objectives and resources. One of her objectives is to demarcate the health needs of the people residing in the bicounty area. Another objective is to determine which health education/promotion programs are needed, while a third is to ascertain the best type of program delivery (when, where, size, and so forth).
2. Her overall design is likely to be descriptive—the "what" characteristics—with both cross-sectional and group-comparison items. Elizabeth may want to conduct a more detailed analytical design after she has analyzed information from her initial survey. The analytical approach might be best for a more focused survey effort.

3. It appears that her resources are limited, especially in regard to personnel. Nonetheless, it would be fruitful to recruit volunteers from the various departments to carry out a telephone survey. Assuming that the hospital has computer resources, she could seek assistance in designing her questionnaire so that it could be easily placed into an existing software package. Her volunteers would need to be trained to conduct computer-assisted telephone interviews. If the bicounty area had remote places with a poverty-struck population, then personal interviews would have to be arranged to collect those data.

4. Elizabeth's data analysis will be primarily descriptive in nature, with some cross-tabulations, such as gender and health needs, age, accessibility to programs, and the like.

5. In drawing a sample, her sampling frame would be all households residing in the bicounty area. For the CATI, she would use random sampling of households. She would need to ascertain the number of households and take a random sample. The remote households may require purposive sampling or convenience sampling (discussed in Chapter 7).

6. Her next step is to draft the questionnaire following the guidelines established in this chapter.

7. Using a subset of her intended population, Elizabeth should pretest the questionnaire and make revisions accordingly.

8. The next step is the actual administering of her precoded questionnaire.

9. The data collected should be cleaned or verified by both range and contingency checking.

10. The data will have been entered into the computer via CATI or CAPI, in the case of remote locations with no telephones.

11. Her data analysis will reflect percentages, means, and cross-tabulations, since the design is descriptive in nature.

12. Her final step will be to write the report and present it to the appropriate people at the hospital.

Summary

This chapter discussed survey research, commencing with the characteristics of such research. It was seen to be a more complicated matter than frequently perceived. The survey flow plan consists of 15 steps that outline the overall approach to doing a survey.

Overall design showed how both descriptive and analytical designs should relate to research questions. The descriptive designs included cross-sectional, longitudinal, and group comparison. Analytical designs addressed cross-sectional, case control, and prospective approaches.

The mail survey discussion included advantages, disadvantages, and many factors that influence the rate of return and the adequacy of data received. The latter included sponsorship, time and type of mailing, questionnaire length, color and format, ease of completion and return, incentives, nature of respondents, and follow-up procedures. There is little consensus as to what is an appropriate minimum number of returns. The chapter did discuss the issues of return rates and how they may be calculated.

The interview study was discussed, including the advantages and disadvantages of both the one-on-one interview and the group interview. The effects of interviewer characteristics—race, ethnicity, gender, social status and distance, age, clothing, and grooming—were presented and seen to have an effect on the interview process and results. Unstructured, semistructured, and structured interviews were presented according to reliability and ease of use.

The telephone interview was seen to have several advantages over the face-to-face interview methodology, despite some drawbacks. The increase in accessibility and the use of RRD combined with CATI has made the telephone interview more popular as a research technique. Computer-assisted surveys were addressed in regard to the telephone interview, personal interview, and self-administered questionnaires.

Four necessary components were presented for questionnaire design and construction: (1) planning the prequestionnaire, (2) drafting the questionnaire, (3) preparing the final questionnaire, and (4) pretesting. Emphasis was given to drafting the questionnaire with attention to researcher, respondent, and interviewer considerations; types of questionnaires (open or closed); and types of questions (dichotomous, multiple-choice, rating, ranking, sentence completion, and open-ended). A checklist of nine pitfalls in question writing was presented, as were seven general rules for arranging the final draft.

The importance of the cover letter accompanying the instrument, as well as its necessary content and trappings, was discussed. Pretesting was viewed as a critical analysis so that further modification may be made of the questionnaire.

Focus group interviews were addressed briefly. As a final note, the Delphi technique was reviewed in some detail, with reference given to various health science studies. This unique group consensus approach appears to be one that is of great benefit.

Suggested Activities

1. The State Department of Education has asked you to survey school administrators across the state regarding the use of tobacco funds awarded to the state by the courts for damages from smoking. Write out:
   a. The objective of the survey
   b. At least one research question
   c. The overall design of the survey
   d. A proposed method of data collection
   e. The size of the sample and how to obtain it

2. Go to the CDC website (www.cdc.gov) and click on *Visitor Survey*. After reviewing this forms-based survey, explain the value of the format and how you might improve the survey.

3. Go to the CDC website (www.cdc.gov) and click on *Data and Statistics*. Under the heading *Surveillance*, click on *Behavioral Risk Factor Surveillance System*. On that site, click on *Questionnaires* to review the most recent BRFSS Questionnaire. Evaluate at least one section on the questionnaire and be able to explain what you have learned about format, how to word questions, how to log answers, and how analysis could occur.

4. Design a ten-question survey to be administered to department chairs of university health education or health science programs. Which of the following methods would be your best option for delivery of the survey?

   a. Regular mail
   b. E-mail
   c. Disk-based survey
   d. Forms-based Web survey

   Justify your answer. Construct ten items in a fashion that fits your selected delivery option. In the case of a disk-based or forms-based survey, describe where drop-down boxes and the like would be used.

5. What are the differences between the Internet and the World Wide Web? What are the inherent methodological weaknesses of Web surveys? What role do you believe the World Wide Web will play in the future of health surveys?

References

Aday, L. A. (1989). *Designing and conducting health surveys: A comprehensive guide.* San Francisco: Jossey-Bass.

Anderson, R. M., Goddard, C. E., Garcia, R., Guzman, J. R., & Vazquez, F. (1998). Using focus groups to identify diabetes care and education issues for Latinos with diabetes. *Diabetes Educator, 24*(5), 618–625.

Annemans, L., Giaccone, G., & Vergnenegre, A. (1999). The cost effectiveness of paclitaxel (Taxol) + cisplatin is similar to that of teniposide + cisplatin in advanced non-small cell lung cancer. *Anti-Cancer Drugs, 10*(6), 605–615.

Bailey, K. (1994). *Methods of social research.* New York: Free Press.

Barriball, K. L., & White, A. E. (1999). Non-response in survey research: A methodological discus-sion and development of an explanatory model. *Journal of Advanced Nursing, 30*(3), 677–686.

Berg, B. L. (2001). *Qualitative research methods for the social sciences* (2d ed.). Boston: Allyn & Bacon.

Bettcher, D. W., Sapirie, S., & Goon, E. H. (1998). Essential public health functions: Results of the international Delphi study. *World Health Statistics Quarterly, 51*(1), 44–54.

Bilodeau, B. A., & Degner, L. F. (1996). Information needs, sources of information, and decisional roles in women with breast cancer. *Oncology Nursing Forum, 23*(4), 691–696.

Burns, N., & Grove, S. K. (1993). *The practice of nursing research* (2d ed.). Philadelphia: W. B. Saunders.

Centers for Disease Control. (2000). *School Health Policies and Programs Study (SHPPS)*. Atlanta: Division of Adolescent and School Health, CDC.

Conklin, K. A. (1997, May 18–21). *Telephone survey research*. Paper presented at the annual forum of the Association for Institutional Research, Orlando. (ERIC Document Reproduction Service No. ED 410886)

Conklin, K. A. (1999). Community college telephone survey research: An overview of methodology and utility. *Community College Journal of Research and Practice, 23*(4), 423–433.

Dalkey, N., & Helmer, O. (1963). An experimental application of the Delphi Method to the use of experts. *Management Science, 3,* 458.

Degner, L. F., Davison, B. J., Sloan, J. A., & Mueller, B. (1998). Development of a scale to measure information needs in cancer care. *Journal of Nursing Measurement, 6*(2), 137–153.

Ferguson, L. (1941). A study of the Likert technique of attitude scale construction. *Journal of Social Psychology, 13,* 51–57.

Fowler, F. J., Gallagher, P. M., & Nederend, S. (1999). Comparing telephone and mail responses to CAHPS survey instrument: Consumer assessment of health plans study. *Medical Care, 37*(Suppl. 3), MS41–49.

Frey, J. H. (1989). *Survey research by telephone* (2d ed.). Newberry Park, CA: Sage.

Furlong, D. K. (1997, May 18–21). *Between anecdote and science: Using e-mail to learn about student experiences*. Paper presented at the annual forum of the Association for Institutional Research, Orlando. (ERIC Document Reproduction Service No. ED 409320)

Graves, R. M., & Kahn, R. L. (1979). *Surveys by telephone: A national comparison with personal interviews*. New York: Academic Press.

Hahn, E. J., Toumey, C. P., Tayens, M. K., & McCoy, C. A. (1999). Kentucky legislators' views on tobacco policy. *American Journal of Preventive Medicine, 16*(2), 81–88.

Heflich, D., & Rice, M. (1999). *Online survey research: A venue for reflective conversation and professional development*. Paper presented at the international conference of the Society for Information Technology and Teacher Education, San Antonio, TX. (ERIC Document Reproduction Service No. ED 432283)

Heise, D. (1970). The semantic differential and attitude research. In G. F. Summers (Ed.), *Attitude measurement*. Chicago: Rand McNally.

Helmer, O. (1967). *Analysis of the future: The Delphi technique*. Santa Monica, CA: Rand.

Hughes, J., & Pakieser, R. (1999). Factors that impact nurses' use of electronic mail. *Computers in Nursing, 17*(6), 251–258.

Isaac, S., & Michael, W. (1981). *Handbook in research and evaluation* (2d ed.). San Diego, CA: Edits.

Jenkins, J., Russell, W., & Suci, G. (1958). An atlas of semantic profiles for 360 words. *American Journal of Psychology, 71,* 618–699.

Johanson, G., Green, S., & Williams, J. (1998, April 13–17). *Blunders and missed opportunities in survey research*. Paper presented at the annual meeting of the American Educational Research Association, San Diego. (ERIC Document Reproduction Service No. ED 420693)

Kerlinger, F. (1964). *Foundations of behavioral research*. New York: Holt, Rinehart, & Winston.

Kitzinger, J. (1990). Recalling the pain: Incest survivors' experiences of obstetrics and gynaecology. *Nursing Times, 86,* 38–40.

Kitzinger, J. (1995, July 29). Introducing focus groups. *British Medical Journal, 299.*

Klecka, W. R., & Tuchfarber, A. J. (1978). Random digit dialing: A comparison to personal surveys. *Public Opinion Quarterly, 42,* 105–114.

Kondo, T., & Kamada, J. (1998). The sense of a life worth living among contemporary college students and its scale. *Japanese Journal of Health Psychology, 11*(1), 73–82.

Leedy, P. (1980). *Practical research: Planning and design*. New York: Macmillan.

Likert, R. (1932). A technique for the measurement of attitudes. *Archives of Psychology, 21,* 140.

Mavis, B. E. (1998). Postal surveys versus electronic mail surveys: The tortoise and the hare revisted. *Evaluation Health Professions, 21*(3), 395–408.

Meha, R., & Sivadas, E. (1995). Comparing response rates and response content in mail versus electronic mail surveys. *Journal of the Market Research Society, 37,* 429–439.

Murphy, G., & Likert, R. (1937). *Public opinion and the individual.* New York: Harper.

National Center for Education Statistics. (1997). *National household education survey data files and electronic codebook.* Washington, DC: Office of Educational Research and Improvement, U.S. Department of Education.

National Health Interview Survey. (1999). National health interview survey: Research for the 1995–2004 redesign. *Vital and Health Statistics Series 2: Data Evaluation and Methods Research, 126,* 1–119.

Nesbary, D. K. (2000). *Survey research and the World Wide Web.* Boston: Allyn & Bacon.

Neutens, J. J. (1975). *Measuring attitudes about heterosexual relationships of educable mentally handicapped adolescents.* Paper presented at the National Council on Family Relations, Salt Lake City, UT.

Nunnally, J. (1962). The analysis of profile data. *Psychological Bulletin, 59,* 311–319.

O'Connor, K. G., Sharp, S., & Olson, L. (1999). The effect of monetary incentives on a survey of pediatricians. *Health Services Research, 16,* 42.

Osgood, C., Suci, G., & Tannenbaum, P. (1957). *The measurement of meaning.* Urbana: University of Illinois Press.

Patrick, J. H., Pruchno, R. A., & Rose, M. S. (1998). Recruiting research participants: A comparison of the costs and effectiveness of five recruitment strategies. *Gerontologist, 38*(3), 295–302.

Rogelberg, S. G., Luong, A., Sederburg, M. E., & Cristol, D. S. (2000). Employee attitude surveys: Examining the attitudes of noncompliant employees. *Journal of Applied Psychology, 85*(2), 284–293.

Rubin, H. J., & Rubin, I. S. (1997). *Qualitative interviewing: The art of hearing data* (2d ed.). Thousand Oaks, CA: Sage.

Sanderson, P. (2000). The development of dance attitude scales. *Educational Research, 42*(1), 91–99.

Santos, J., Reynaldo, A., & Clegg, D. (1999). Factor analysis adds new dimensions to extension surveys. *Journal of Extension, 37*(5), 21–27.

Scott, C. (1961). Research on mail surveys. *Journal of the Royal Statistical Society, 124*(A), 143–195.

Sellitz, C., Jahoda, M., Deutsch, M., & Cook, S. (1959). *Research methods in social relations.* New York: Holt, Rinehart, and Winston.

Sim, J. (1998). Collecting and analysing qualitative data: Issues raised by the focus group. *Journal of Advanced Nursing, 28*(2), 345–352.

Snider, J., & Osgood, C. (Eds.). (1969). *Semantic differential technique.* Chicago: Aldine.

Sorokin, W. (1976). *Personal health appraisal.* New York: John Wiley and Sons.

Sowell, R. L. (2000). Identifying HIV/AIDS research priorities for the next millenium: A Delphi study with nurses in AIDS care. *Journal of the Association of Nurses in AIDS Care, 11*(3), 42–52.

Sully, P., & Grant, P. (1997). Ethical and methodological improvements to mail survey research: An alternative follow-up method. *Canadian Journal of Program Evaluation, 12*(2), 81–104.

Taylor, A. W., Wilson, D. H., & Wakefield, M. (1998). Differences in health estimates using telephone and door-to-door survey methods. *Australian and New Zealand Journal of Public Health, 22*(2), 223–226.

Taylor, W. C., Yancey, A. K., Leslie, J., Murray, N. G., Cummings, S. S., Sharkey, S. A., James, J., Miles, O., & McCarthy, W. J. (1999). Physical activity among African American and Latino middle school girls: Consistent beliefs, expectations, and experiences across two sites. *Woman and Health, 30*(2), 67–82.

Thurstone, L., & Chave, E. (1929). *The measurement of attitudes.* Chicago: University of Chicago Press.

Tordella, M., & Neutens, J. (1979). An instrument to appraise attitudes of college students toward euthanasia. *Journal of School Health, 49*(6), 351–352.

Trow, M. (1967). Education and survey research. In C. Clock (Ed.), *Survey research in the social sciences.* New York: Russell Sage.

van-Alphen, A., Halfens, R., Hasman, A., & Imbos, T. (1994). Likert or Rasch? Nothing is more applicable than good theory. *Journal of Advanced Nursing, 20*(1), 196–201.

Wang, L., & Fan, X. (1997, March 24–28). *The effect of cluster sampling design in survey research on the standard error statistic.* Paper presented at the annual meeting of the American Educational Research Association, Chicago. (ERIC Document Reproduction Service No. ED 409320)

Watts, M., & Ebbutt, D. (1987). More than the sum of the parts: Research methods in group interviewing. *British Medical Journal, 13,* 25–34.

Wiersma, W. (2000). *Research methods in education* (7th ed.). Boston: Allyn & Bacon.

Wilson, A. H., Pittman, K., & Wold, J. L. (2000). Listening to the quiet voices of Hispanic migrant children about health. *Journal of Pediatric Nursing, 15*(3), 137–147.

Chapter *7*

Sampling Designs and Techniques

Case Study A

Moses, a health science researcher for ABC labs, was writing a proposal for a large study to test the effects of a new ABC pharmaceutical agent. The new agent, X, was developed to lower blood pressure. He had conducted a small pilot study with 20 patients (10 in the experimental group and 10 in the control group) and found no significant difference three weeks postinitial administration of pharmaceutical agent X. He believed that the new agent worked and that his pilot study was simply too small to detect any significant difference. He wondered how large a sample size would be needed if a significant difference were to be detectable.

Case Study B

Paige, like many other health care professionals, was alarmed at the rising incidence of communicable diseases in her immediate geographic area. She was fully aware that the medical profession was encouraging judicious use of antibiotics in order to reduce the rising resistance in the microorganisms. The chief public health officer for her two-county area requested that she do something to let the public know about childhood immunizations, flu shots, correct use of antibiotics, and the like. This was a high priority for the department. It was recommended that a survey be done to find out what the public knows about these items and to see what the best means of education would be—public health programs, mailers, TV ads, radio spots, school programs. She was given a two-year budget, which was to include both the survey and one year for education of the public. Since the survey was first on her agenda, she was concerned about how to select respondents and how many to select.

The Purpose of Sampling

Ideally, the researcher would like to observe the entire population to add more weight to the findings. For example, while it might be feasible for Paige to obtain answers from all residents in her bicounty area, this is not likely the situation for Moses. Limited resources, time, and money frequently preclude a study of the entire population. Subsequently, a subset of some predetermined size must be selected from the population of interest. The sample or subset should represent the total population so that the data collected from the sample will be as accurate as that from the entire population.

The logic involved is simple. Nonetheless, the importance of this step cannot be overemphasized. A knowledgeable researcher commences with a population and works down to the sample. In other words, the population of interest is designated and then a sample is derived. The neophyte, in contrast, often works from the bottom up by attempting to ascertain the minimum number of respondents needed for a successful study. The inherent problem with this approach is that it is next to impossible to assess the representativeness of the sample because the entire population has not been identified.

While savings in time and money are obvious reasons for sampling, there are additional advantages, too. The sample may achieve a greater response rate owing to greater cooperation than might occur in the full population survey. This, in itself, would tend to make the results more accurate. In health surveys with sensitive items, this point is particularly important. Concomitantly, the researcher can keep a low profile by using a sample. That is, less people may be offended, thereby negating an opportunity for several people to organize a common resistance. In the case of interviewing, a sample reduces the number of interviews and interviewees. This is beneficial in that supervision of an enormous number of interviewers is difficult at best and necessary attention to details such as follow-ups becomes cumbersome as numbers increase. There is little doubt that using sampling, in most instances, is more advantageous than using an entire population. However, the benefits are realized only if the sample is drawn with precision.

The Sampling Frame

The sampling frame is a list of all the persons (objects) from whom the sample is to be drawn. Understandably, the sample cannot be more accurate than the sampling frame from which it is selected. In constructing the sampling frame, the researcher lists every person in the population, but only once so as not to increase someone's likelihood of being chosen. If the study is small, it is recommended that the investigator construct the list personally to avoid omissions and repetitions that may be on existing lists. For example, Moses in Case Study A derived participants for his pilot study from those patients who frequented the Hypertension Center at a nearby university medical center. He listed all patients as his sampling frame, found out who was available, and of those, who would participate. In a larger study however, it is much more difficult and perhaps virtually impossible to procure an accurate and complete list. In Case Study B, it is probable that Paige would not be able to obtain a listing of all residents in the bicounty area. People are born daily, and others die, move, or give incorrect addresses so that they cannot be contacted. As the size of the study increases to include a city, county, state, or nation, the construction of the sampling frame becomes more formidable.

Employment of existing lists, such as telephone directories and county directories, is only a partial answer at best. Both poor people who may not own telephones and wealthy people who may have unlisted numbers will be excluded from the study. Those who have two telephones and multiple listings would have a greater opportunity for selection than those with a single listing. Unless the directory was recently compiled, address changes and people who have left the county would confound the list. If the researcher employs existing lists, an attempt should be made to ascertain the number of persons excluded and whether they differ in any systematic way from those on the list. If there is no common bond, that is, if people are excluded randomly from the total population, then little harm will be done.

A possible alternative to the time and monetary demands of listing individuals is to compile residence addresses of households. Residences are relatively stable, and a complete listing could serve as the sampling frame. Further, no groups should be excluded and the risk of bias should be decreased greatly. In attempting to survey the people in the bicounty area, Paige could use this approach and select a sample from the sampling frame of residential addresses.

In some situations, like that of Moses, a multicenter study is needed. However, without knowing approximately how many patients are needed, he is unable to determine the number of centers to involve. Once he has the sample size number, he can contact selected centers to find out if they wish to participate and how many patients are listed in each hypertension center. Since his unit of study is patients (not centers), he can then establish a sampling frame. Note that this is much different than Case Study B in which Paige knows the number of households.

Sampling Techniques

Once the population has been defined and the sampling frame established, the next step in arriving at a target group for research purposes is to select a method of sampling. Basically, there are two types of sampling techniques, which have several different procedures. *Probability samples* are those wherein the probability of selection of each respondent, address, or even object, is known. In contrast, *nonprobability samples* reflect an unknown probability of selection.

Probability Sampling

Probability sampling techniques include random sampling, systematic sampling, stratified random sampling, and cluster sampling.

Random Sampling. *Simple random sampling* is the basic building block of all probability sampling designs. In a random sample, each person (or address or object) in the population has an equal chance of being chosen for the sample. This is accomplished without bias for any personal characteristics. Of course, the underlying necessity is an adequate sampling frame with no one listed more than once and no one excluded. If either of these occurs, then by definition the sampling fails to be random.

An additional point about simple random sampling is that it is sampling without replacement. For example, if the sampling frame comprises 300 people, each person has a 1 in 300 chance of being selected. After 150 people have been chosen, the remainder will have only a 1 in 150 chance of being selected. This is considered adequate because the opportunity for selection is equal at any given stage of the sampling process.

While there are many methods for random selection, such as the flip of a coin, a lottery, or the spin of a roulette wheel, the usual one used by researchers is the table of random numbers. Each person in the sampling frame is assigned a number through identifiable characteristics (names, age, gender) to avoid bias. From the example above, each of the 300 people in the sampling frame would be given one number. The researcher would then employ the table of random numbers to commence selecting the sample.

Examination of a table of random numbers shows that there is no discernible pattern whether one moves up, down, or across the page. Initially, the researcher selects a predetermined pattern for moving through the table, that is, down columns or across rows. Next, a particular column and row are arbitrarily chosen from which to begin. If the names in the sampling frame are numbered in sequence, the researcher proceeds down the column (or across the row), pulling each name whose number corresponds to the number in the table. Because this is sampling without replacement, a number is simply ignored if encountered more than once. Similarly, if a number is found that is greater than that contained in the sampling frame, it is ignored. This procedure is continued until the desired sample size is obtained.

In Case Study B, Paige has a sampling frame of 50,000 addresses. Each would be numbered and she would then enter the table of random numbers. At this juncture, she decides to go down columns and arbitrarily choose column one, row three. Since her largest number is 50,000 (five digits), she needs to select five columns of numbers at a time. If the largest number had been 99 (two digits) or less in the sampling frame, she would only need to select two columns of random numbers. She would now proceed to pull out the required amount of numbers for her sample size. Each number extracted from the table of random numbers would be matched to the addresses in the sampling frame, and those addresses would be employed in her study.

It can be seen that Paige is just as likely to select a farmer as an industrialist. Moreover, it is highly unlikely that she would obtain all farmers or all industrialists by random sampling. However, it should be noted that her task would indeed be an arduous one unless it were computerized. This may be accomplished with software programs for most personal computers as well as with larger mainframes. If these routes are not feasible, alternative sampling techniques are available.

Systematic Sampling.   One alternative to the process of simple random sampling is *systematic sampling*. As the name implies, it is the selection of specific items in a series according to some predetermined sequence. The origin of the sequence must be controlled by chance. In other words, systematic sampling can be employed only when units in the sampling frame are random. In our case study, the residential addresses would have to be randomly ordered within the sampling frame. If they were not random, then Paige would be unable to use systematic sampling. However, if the items in the sampling frame were randomly listed, the health science investigator could choose $1/k$th of them, with k being any constant. If k were 2, then the sample would comprise one-half of the population. Similarly, if k were 5, the sample would be 20% of the entire population. Once again, in the case study, if Paige decided to survey 2% of the population, the k would be set at 50. The number of people in her survey would be 1,000.

Generally, the investigator randomly selects the first item from among the k items in the sampling frame. Next, by definition, a $1/k$th sample is established by choosing every kth item in the sampling frame. Subsequently, Paige would randomly select her first address for inclusion in the sample. Needless to say, like Paige, all health science investigators would need to determine sample size before beginning sample selection.

Although simple random sampling is more accurate and does not require the assumption of a randomized sampling frame, systematic sampling involves less work, thereby providing more information per dollar. Further, for the inexperienced survey researcher, it may reduce error because it is simpler to perform. In short, the greater the complexity of the method, the greater the opportunity for error. Nonetheless, it must be emphasized that systematic sampling is more dependent on the adequacy of the sampling frame than is simple random sampling. Because any ordering of the sampling frame is retained in systematic sampling, the results can be totally nonrepresentative. If evidence of biased ordering is found in the sampling frame, then steps must be taken to correct it. The most obvious step is to randomize the sampling frame (which is expensive and time-consuming), or if this is untenable, to return to simple random sampling or perhaps to draw a stratified random sample.

Stratified Random Sampling.   At times it is advisable to use *stratified random sampling*. This means to subdivide the population into smaller homogeneous groups in order to get a more accurate representation or to include parameters of special

TABLE 7.1 Stratified Random Sampling

Population Setting	County	
	County A	County B
Urban	Cell 1	Cell 2
Rural	Cell 3	Cell 4

interest. Herein, the population is broken down into nonoverlapping groups called *strata*, and then a simple random sample is extracted from each stratum.

The first step in stratified random sampling is to identify the strata (sometimes called *stratification parameters*). For example, Paige may wish to subdivide the population of the bicounty area into County A and County B. The residential addresses would be split exclusively into the appropriate county, and a simple random sample would be taken from each list. Although a simple random sample could have been employed for a listing of combined counties and still have excellent representation, the stratified design could save time and money by requiring a smaller sample size.

If so desired, more than one stratification variable or parameter could be used. That is, the health science researcher can stratify on two or more variables simultaneously. In addition to the county parameter, Paige could stratify on the urban-rural parameter. Now, instead of having two groups, she would have four. Table 7.1 illustrates the four groups or strata. Once the groups have been formed, a simple random sample is taken within each group or stratum.

In proportional stratified sampling, each sample drawn should represent the population in the proportion in which it exists within the total population. For example, imagine that in County A there were 14,000 addresses in an urban setting and 16,000 in a rural setting, for a total of 30,000. Similarly, there were 8,000 urban and 12,000 rural addresses in County B, for a total of 20,000. Combined there would be 50,000 addresses that were in the original sampling frame. For Paige to establish a sample size of 1,000, the sample should include approximately the same propor-

TABLE 7.2 Proportional Stratified Sampling

	County A	County B
Urban Addresses	14,000	8,000
Proportion	28%	16%
Sample Size	280	160
Rural Addresses	16,000	12,000
Proportion	32%	24%
Sample Size	320	240

tions as the entire population. Table 7.2 illustrates the proportional stratified sampling design.

Each subgroup or cell is drawn randomly in proportion to the total population. Cell 1, comprising 14,000 addresses, makes up 28% of the population and subsequently has a sample size of 280 (28% of 1,000). The remaining cells follow a similar pattern.

In other situations, the researcher may decide to stratify by gender, socioeconomic status, racial origin, education, or religious preference. Obviously, those in the health sciences may wish to stratify by health parameters such as smoking-nonsmoking, hypertensive patients–nonhypertensive patients, pregnancy-nonpregnancy, and many others. The characteristics of the entire population must be considered together with the objectives of the research before the stratified sample design is used. On occasion, stratified random sampling is disproportionate in that a larger proportion of the population is sampled in one stratum than in another. Two reasons for this design are (1) differences in population size; and (2) homogeneity among strata. When the population of a particular stratum is very small, proportionate sampling may leave the researcher with a sample size that is statistically unworkable. Similarly, a larger proportion of the population would have to be sampled in a very heterogeneous stratum. For example, if the health science investigator were to select a stratified sample of nonsmokers, cigarette smokers, and pipe smokers in a company that has 1,000 nonsmokers, 800 cigarette smokers, and 200 pipe smokers, a greater proportion of pipe smokers would have to be sampled than either nonsmokers or cigarette smokers to obtain a sufficient size for sampling adequacy. This dilemma of disproportionate sampling will be discussed further in the *Sample Size* section of this chapter.

Overall, stratified random sampling is a technique to maintain the same proportionality on stratification parameters in the sample as occurs in the population. The researcher may stratify by demographic characteristics or by health variables. In any case, the characteristics of the entire population must be considered together with the objectives of the research before the stratified sample design is used.

Cluster or Area Sampling. *Cluster or area sampling* is a variation of the simple random sample and is especially useful when (1) the population to be studied is infinite; (2) a list of members of the population is nonexistent; or (3) the geographic distribution of the population is widely scattered. For example, if an investigator proposed to survey all public school health educators in the United States, a simple random sample would be impractical.

In multistage cluster sampling, the investigator can first randomly sample 20 of the 50 states. In the second stage, from a sampling frame that lists all counties within the 20 states, a random sample of 100 counties could be selected. Then, in the third stage, a random sample of 50 school districts could be drawn from all the school districts within the 100 counties. The fourth stage could consist of random selection of 100 school health educators in the 50 school districts. The successive random sampling of states, counties, school districts, and finally health educators is relatively inexpensive and efficient.

Cluster sampling samples among clusters. While it has some advantages over simple random sampling, it does hold the possibility of more error. This is because it is not a single sample but rather two or more, each open to error. Further, there may be sample bias because of the unequal size of some of the subsets or clusters selected. The first stage of sampling may be representative, but the second stage may not be. The researcher must be concerned about the sample size and accuracy at every stage of the cluster sample.

In summation, all of the techniques we have discussed—simple random sampling, systematic sampling, stratified random sampling, and cluster sampling—may be combined into a single procedure to suit the needs of the researcher. In so doing, the investigator must be familiar with the idiosyncrasies of each method.

Nonprobability Sampling

In some instances, the researcher may decide to employ *nonprobability sampling*. In this method, the probability that a person will be chosen is not known, with the result that a claim for representativeness of the population cannot be made. Concomitantly, sampling error (the degree of departure from representation) is unknown. Subsequently, the researcher's ability to generalize findings beyond the actual sample is greatly limited. This may be a major disadvantage, depending upon the purpose of the study. Nevertheless, nonprobability sampling has an advantage over probability sampling in that it is less expensive, less complicated, and lends itself to spontaneity (spur-of-the-moment investigations). It is particularly useful in small studies or pilot investigations to perfect questionnaires. Nonprobability sampling includes convenience sampling, quota sampling, dimensional sampling, purposive sampling, and snowball sampling.

Convenience Sampling. A common example of *convenience sampling* is the captive-audience approach, such as using a classroom full of health science students. While the researcher forgoes representativeness in this case, time and money are saved. It is a simple matter of selecting the closest and most convenient persons.

Quota Sampling. *Quota sampling* is the nonprobability sampling equivalent of stratified sampling. Initially, the researcher determines which strata are relevant to the investigation and then proceeds to establish a quota for each stratum that is proportionate to its representation in the population. For example, in Paige's study it was found that in County A, 28% of the addresses were urban and 32% rural. In County B, 16% were urban and 24% rural. In selecting her sample Paige would not want all rural residences nor all urban ones. Preferably, the sample would be drawn proportionate to the urban-rural realities of the actual population. Once a quota is set, the sampling merely consists of finding addresses (persons) that fit into the stratum. In Paige's study, a total of 200 residents would mean 56 urban and 64 rural addresses in County A, and 32 urban and 48 rural addresses in County B. Although there is no random selection, at least the strata are in the same proportions as the entire population.

The researcher must make every effort to prevent bias. Bias is most likely to occur when the route of least resistance is chosen (e.g., avoiding houses in questionable neighborhoods or ones that contain unfriendly people). Confining the research to friends and acquaintances is not acceptable.

Dimensional Sampling. *Dimensional sampling* is principally a multidimensional form of quota sampling wherein the variables (dimensions) of interest in the population are delineated. Each variable and combination thereof must be represented by at least one case. It is a method in which only a small sample is required so that each case selected can be examined in more detail.

Purposive Sampling. This technique falls somewhere between quota sampling, in which various strata are to be filled, and convenience sampling, wherein the nearest and most available people are used. In *purposive sampling,* the researcher employs his or her own discretion to select the respondents who best meet the purposes of the study. This is a great advantage to the experienced researcher who can apply prior knowledge and skill.

Snowball Sampling. There is a multistage technique that literally "snowballs." In the first stage of *snowball sampling,* a person possessing the requisite characteristics is identified and interviewed. This person then identifies others who may be included in the sample. The next stage is to interview these persons, who in turn identify still more respondents who can be contacted and interviewed in following stages.

Mixed Sampling Designs. When a population or sample is very large, a mixed model of judgment and probability sampling is often used. Discretion procedures are frequently employed in the early stages and probability procedures in the later stages. This combined approach offers a savings in time, money, and effort as well as a sample that can be representative of the entire population.

Sample Size

The determination of sample size usually perplexes many researchers because they often have no conception of a minimally adequate sample size. They need to understand that correct sample size is dependent on both the nature of the population and the purpose of the study. Usually, a trade-off is discovered between the desire for a large sample and the feasibility of a small one. An ideal study would have a sample large enough to represent the population so generalization may occur, yet small enough to save time and money as well as to reduce the complexity of data analysis.

Considerations in Sample Size. It is a popular misconception that a sample is a small carbon copy of the original population, identical in every way. If this were the case, then the researcher would not have to worry about having a sample size that is representative of the population under study. Needless to say, one can never be certain of representativeness unless the entire population is used. An obvious deduction at this juncture is that the larger the sample, the greater the likelihood of representativeness. This is especially true if the population is quite heterogeneous on the given variable; the greater the heterogeneity, the greater the necessity for a larger sample. For populations in which there is no heterogeneity on a variable (complete homogeneity), a sample size of even one would suffice.

Sampling Error. Since use of an entire population rules out total homogeneity in most studies, the researcher must have representativeness as the primary consideration. Lack of representativeness is commonly referred to as sampling error. *Sampling error* is the degree to which the sample means of repeatedly drawn random samples differ from one another and from the population mean. Imagine, for example, that a large number of health science researchers each selected random samples of 50 hypertensive patients from the population of all hypertensive patients in Minnesota. The mean or average blood pressure of each of the random samples would not be identical. Although most of them would tend to cluster around the population mean, some would be relatively high by comparison, while others would be relatively low. This variation in sample mean is a result of sampling error. It is not a mistake in the sampling process but rather an inevitable variation when a number of randomly selected sample means (herein blood pressure) are compared.

Probability Level Alpha (α). Since means are not identical, it is logical to assume that any one of them differs from the population mean (average blood pressure of all hypertensive patients in Minnesota). Because a researcher deals with only one sample as a base for generalization about the population, it is necessary to determine whether the particular sample is representative. To make this determination the use of statistical techniques and probability theory is required. To put it briefly, the researcher attempts to establish that the sample is representative of the population on critical parameters at an acceptable level of probability. This *probability level*, also called a *confidence level,* is usually set at 95%, frequently referred to as the .05 level of significance. In lay terms, this means that there is a 95% chance that the sample is distributed in the same way as the population. If deemed appropriate, the researcher may decide to set the level more stringently—at the .01 level, in which there is a 99% chance. Of course, the restrictions could be eased by establishing the level at .10, thereby making it a 90% chance that the sample is distributed in the same way as the population. In the past, z critical values of the normal probability table for large samples have always been used; today, *t* critical values are employed for small sample sizes (fewer than 30 cases).

Probability Level Beta and Power Analysis. In hypothesis testing the *probability level* known as *alpha* refers to Type I errors (rejecting a null hypothesis when it is in fact true). Until the recent past, health science researchers have focused on this probability at the expense of Type II errors (incorrectly accepting a null hypothesis when in fact it is false), known as *beta* (β). A technique called *power analysis* uses 1 − β for the probability of procuring a significant result. This is referred to as the *power of a statistical test* (Polit & Hungler, 1995). The four factors involved in power analysis are: (1) level of significance (α, sometimes described as *p* level); (2) the probability of obtaining a significant result (power, or 1 − β); (3) the population effect size, which is a measure of the degree of effect of the independent variable on the dependent variable; and (4) the sample size. Knowing any three factors allows you to compute the fourth. In other words, power analysis can be used to estimate a sample size large enough to detect errors.

For example, in Case Study A, Moses needs to have some idea of an appropriate sample size before the study can actually begin. Following conventional research, he would set the risk of a Type I error at α =.05 and power 1 − β at .80. This is a general standard and means that he has a 20% risk of making a Type II error. The third factor he must know (to calculate the fourth factor, sample size) is the effect size or magnitude of the relationship between the independent and dependent variables. While the value of the effect size is determined by the nature of the study and the statistical tests to be used, the principles remain the same. To estimate effect size (for that matter any parameter necessary to compute sample size—means or standard deviations), the researcher should review previous work or conduct a pilot study. Fortunately, Moses did the latter.

Therefore, knowing all this information Moses can calculate the necessary sample size for each of his two groups. Rosner (1990, p. 273) provides the following formula for estimating sample size when comparing the means of two normally distributed samples of equal size using a two-sided test with an established significance level α and power 1 − β for each group:

$$n = \frac{(\sigma_1^2 + \sigma_2^2)(z_{1-\alpha/2} + z_{1-\beta})^2}{\Delta^2}$$

where $\Delta = \mu_2 - \mu_1$ (the respective means) and σ_1^2, σ_2^2 are the variances.
Moses had the following information from his pilot study.

Group 1 $M = 138.20$ Group 2 $M = 133.50$
Group 1 $s = 15.11$ Group 2 $s = 17.22$
Group 1 $n = 10$ Group 2 $n = 10$

where M = mean, s = standard deviation, and n = number in group.
He set α = .05 and power 1 − β = .80. Using all this information in the formula, he did the following calculations.

$$n = [(15.11)^2 + (17.22)^2][1.96 + 0.84]^2/(138.20 - 133.50)^2$$
$$n = [524][7.84]/22.09$$
$$n = 4114.75/22.09 = 186.27$$

This can be interpreted as Moses requiring a sample size of 186 hypertensive patients in each group, when significance level is set at 5% and 80% power is desired. It is no wonder that no significant differences were found in his pilot study of 10 patients per group.

Using this formula, an accurate sample size can be determined. However, Table 7.3 presents approximate sample size requirements for various powers, effects, and two values of α (for two-tailed tests) in a two-group mean difference situation (Polit & Hungler, 1995). To use the table, the researcher must know the effect size symbolized by γ. The formula for effect size is:

$$\gamma = \frac{\mu^1 - \mu^2}{\alpha}$$

TABLE 7-3 Approximate Sample Sizes[a] Necessary to Achieve Selected Levels of Power as a Function of Estimated Effect Size for Test of Difference of Two Means

Power	.10	.15	.20	.25	.30	.40	.50	.60	.70	.80
Part A: $\alpha = .05$										
.60	977	434	244	156	109	61	39	27	20	15
.70	1,230	547	308	197	137	77	49	34	25	19
.80	1,568	697	392	251	174	98	63	44	32	25
.90	2,100	933	525	336	233	131	84	58	43	33
.95	2,592	1,152	648	415	288	162	104	72	53	41
.99	3,680	1,636	920	589	409	230	147	102	75	58
Part B: $\alpha = .01$										
.60	1,602	712	400	256	178	100	64	44	33	25
.70	1,922	854	481	308	214	120	77	53	39	30
.80	2,339	1,040	585	374	260	146	94	65	48	37
.90	2,957	1,324	745	477	331	186	119	83	61	47
.95	3,562	1,583	890	570	396	223	142	99	73	56
.99	4,802	2,137	1,201	769	534	300	192	133	98	

Estimated Effect[b]

Note. Reprinted with permission from Polit, D. F., & Hungler, B. P. (1995). *Nursing Research: Principles and Methods* (p. 455). Philadelphia: J. B. Lippincott.
[a]Sample size requirements for each group; total sample size would be twice the number shown.
[b]Estimated effect (γ) is the estimated population mean group difference, divided by the estimated population standard deviation, or:
$$\gamma = \frac{\mu^1 - \mu^2}{\sigma}$$

In this formula, γ is the difference between the population means divided by the standard deviation of the population. Using the results of his pilot study, Moses would determine the pooled standard deviation. This would give him the following:

$$M_1 \text{ (mean of Group 1)} \qquad = 138.20$$
$$M_2 \text{ (mean of Group 2)} \qquad = 133.50$$
$$\alpha \text{ (pooled standard deviation)} = \ 16.20$$

The value of γ would be:

$$\gamma = \frac{138.20 - 133.50}{16.20} = .29$$

Using this information, he would estimate his needed sample size to be 174 for each group, assuming $\alpha = .05$ and a power of .80. This means he would need a total sample size of 348. This approximates the earlier formula, which showed he needed 186 per group for a total sample size of 372. Cohen (1988) explained that effect size for this type of investigation (two-group test of mean differences) is estimated at .20 for small effects, at .50 for medium effects, and at .80 for large effects. In health education research, it is likely that most effect sizes will range from .20 to .40.

The formula is modified (see Rosner, 1990, p. 275) when the test of significance is one-sided. Using the same parameters for *alpha* and power, Moses would use the formula below for each group with an equal n:

$$n = \frac{(\sigma_1^2 + \sigma_2^2)(z_{1-\alpha} + z_{1-\beta})^2}{\Delta^2}$$

where $\Delta = \mu_2 - \mu_1$ (the respective means) and σ_1^2, σ_2^2 are the variances:

$$n = [(15.11)^2 + (17.22)^2][1.645 = 0.84]^2/(138.20 - 133.50)^2$$
$$n = [524.84][6.18]/22.09$$
$$n = 3243.51/22.09 = 146.83$$

Knowing that the pharmacologic agent would make a difference allows for a one-sided test and a decrease in the number of patients needed. Herein, Moses would need 147 patients per group rather than the 186 necessary for the two-sided test of significance for means. Rosner (1990) provides formulas for samples with unequal means, too.

Suppose that Moses could not find two groups to compare. In this situation, he would have to use one group, administer the new pharmacologic agent X, and watch for a change in blood pressure. From a design standpoint he would lack a control group; nonetheless, pragmatically, health researchers are sometimes forced into less than desirable research designs. If this were the case, he would need to use a formula for one sample inference. Rosner (1990) provides formulas to determine sample size for both one-sided and two-sided tests of significance for means.

The one-sample inference formula to conduct a two-sided test for means with a designated significance level (α) and power $1 - \beta$ (Rosner, 1990, p. 218) is:

$$n = \frac{\sigma^2 (z_{1-\beta} + z_{1-\alpha/2})^2}{(\mu_0 - \mu_1)^2}$$

The one-sample inference formula to conduct a one-sided test for means with a designated significance level (α) and power $1 - \beta$ (Rosner, 1990, p. 219) is:

$$n = \frac{\sigma^2 (z_{1-\beta} + z_{1-\alpha})^2}{(\mu_0 - \mu_1)^2}$$

In our calculation with a control group, we used a two-sided formula, assuming we did not know the effects of the new agent. However, let's assume that Moses is quite certain that the new agent will lower high blood pressure, thereby allowing him to use a one-sided test of significance. Suppose he wants to have at least 80% power for detecting a significant difference if the pharmacologic agent is to change blood pressure by 10 mmHg. Using the sample size estimation formula and information from his pilot study, he would calculate the following:

$$n = (15.11)^2(0.84 + 1.645)^2/10^2$$
$$n = (228.31)(6.18)/100$$
$$n = 1410.96/100 = 14.11$$

He would only need 14 patients for a one-sided test, with one sample.

Imagine that the standard deviation was 20.11 mmHg (this makes the variance greater than in the pilot study). If you use this in the same formula, you would find that Moses would need 25 patients rather than 14. The point herein is that the greater the variance, the greater the number of subjects required.

There are books of tables (Cohen, 1988) and computer programs (Borenstein & Cohen, 1988) available to estimate sample size using power analysis. As in the examples with Moses, you need to be armed with some information—alpha, power, and effect size. In addition to testing the difference between two group means (*t*-test), the tables and computer programs can be used when comparing the means of more than two samples (ANOVA situation); when testing the significance of a bivariate linear relationship such as the Pearson *r*; and when comparing the differences in proportions between two groups (chi-square test).

To assist you with any of these calculations, computer-based programs such as Statistical Packages for the Social Sciences (SPSS), Statistical Analysis System (SAS), Biomedical Programs (BMDP), Minitab, and Statistica can be used on your personal computer. On the other hand, there are websites in which you can enter your information. For example, the University of California at Los Angeles posts a power calculator to determine sample size (http://ebook.stat.ucla.edu/calculators/powercalc/). A website at York University in Toronto provides links to many statistical packages that you can purchase or find on other websites (http://www.math.york.ca), including the UCLA site. Once you locate the York site, go to *Resources* and then to *Statistical Consulting Services*. World Wide Web resources, including statistics departments, are listed therein.

Special Considerations for Health Surveys. Conducting health surveys may require special considerations for both sampling design as well as sample size. Insofar as sample size, Aday (1989) notes that several criteria should be employed. This section addresses some of those considerations briefly. For a more extensive discussion, other resources should be used (Aday, 1989).

Step 1: Identification of Major Study Variables. As noted in Chapter 6, one of the principal steps of survey research is to delineate the variables under study. In Paige's study, her major area of interest is the use of antibiotics during the preceding year.

Step 2: Types of Estimates of Study Variables. Paige has a choice of several different ways to summarize the study variable—percentages, ratios, means, and so on. She should pay heed to the level of measurement that will be used in her analysis. In this example, she chooses to use percentages—the percent who used antibiotics correctly (i.e., those who complied with physician directions).

Step 3: Population or Subgroup Selection. The design of the study dictates the population or subgroup in question. For example, is the survey descriptive or analytical in nature? Is it a group comparison, cross-sectional, or longitudinal approach? Paige plans to use the whole sample to represent the bicounty population.

Step 4: Relevant Standard Error Formula. There are several ways to calculate sampling (standard) error when determining sample size. The method chosen should correspond with the analysis and study design for the variables—percentages, means, ratios, differences. Procedures for calculating standard errors of selected types of estimates can be found in several texts (Kalton, 1983; Lee, Forthofer, & Lorimor, 1989; Levy & Lemeshow, 1991). Listed below are formulas for the standard error of the mean and the standard error of percentage (Aday, 1989).

The standard error of the mean (SE_M) for a simple random sample is calculated by dividing the standard deviation for the sample by the square root of the sample size:

$$SE_M = \frac{s}{\sqrt{n}}$$

The standard error of percentage (SE_M), or proportion for a simple random sample, is:

$$SE_p = \frac{\sqrt{p \times 100 - p}}{n}$$

As you recall, Paige chose to use percentage or proportion to summarize her variables. Consequently, the standard error of a percentage estimate of 50% for a sample of 100 cases would be:

$$SE_p = \frac{\sqrt{.50 \times (1.00 - .50)}}{100}$$

$$SE_p = \frac{\sqrt{.50 \times .50}}{100}$$

$$SE_p = \sqrt{.0025}$$

$$SE_p = .05$$

This means that for a sample of 100 cases, the standard error of the estimate of 50% $(p = .50)$ is 5% (.05). She can be confident that 95% of the time the true value of the population was between 40 and 60% (almost two standard errors above and below). Remember that 68% of the time, the true value would lie between 45 and 55% (one standard error, and in this study that is 5% above and 5% below).

Step 5: Expected Estimate. Health survey researchers should use other studies or theories to arrive at an expected value of the estimate. In our study, Paige used data to expect that 50% $(p = .50)$ of the sample will have been on antibiotics in the past year.

Step 6: Tolerable Range of Error in the Estimate. Needless to say, the figure derived in Step 5 is an estimate and subject to error. All investigators must decide what would be a reasonable range of error. The range varies with the precision needed in reporting survey results (for example, ± 10% versus ± 5%). Keep in mind the more precise the estimates, the greater the need for a larger sample size.

Step 7: Level of Confidence. Herein the researcher establishes the level of statistical confidence—99%, 95%, or 90%. The confidence level chosen is used with the formula for the relevant standard of error estimate to obtain the minimal sample size to have that level of statistical confidence. In our case example, Paige selected the typical 95% level of confidence with a ± 1.96 standard error around the estimated population value. Her calculations would be:

95% confidence interval = 1.96 × standard error

$$= 1.96 \times \frac{\sqrt{p \times (1.00 - p)}}{n} = .05$$

where, therefore,

$$n = (1.96)^2 \, [p \times (1.00 - p)]/(.05)^2$$
$$n = 3.84 \, (.50 \times .50)/.0025 = 384$$

The size of her sample, thus far, is 384. However, as the following steps show, this can be modified for several reasons.

Step 8: Estimated Sample Design Effect. The sample size, n, derived from the formula in Step 7 pertains to a simple or systematic random sample design. More complex designs generally require larger sample designs. Kalton (1983) discusses the effects of various sample designs on the variances (standard error squared). For example, in cluster sampling the design effect is 1.3, which means that the standard error for any estimate based on the sample is 30% higher than that derived from a simple random sample. Consequently, if Paige were to use a cluster sampling she would need to increase her sample size to 499 (384 × 1.3). In contrast to cluster sampling, stratified designs usually require less subjects than a simple random sampling. This is because the strata are less diverse (i.e., more homogeneous). "The net result of taking the weighted average of the standard errors of these relatively homogeneous strata is that the standard errors for a stratified design will be less than those that result from a simple random sample of the same population" (Aday, 1989, p. 116).

In our example, Paige plans to conduct a simple random sample so her estimate of 384 respondents remains.

Step 9: Response Rate Adjustment. Unfortunately, almost any health survey will have less than a 100% response rate. This step allows the researcher to adjust the size of the sample to accommodate the response rate. For example, Paige feels that she will have a 65% response rate. The adjustment is determined as follows:

$$n = 384/65 = 591$$

Step 10: Adjustment for Expected Proportion of Eligibles. At this step, the number of respondents determined from Step 9 are divided by the expected portion of respondents who will actually be found eligible, once they are contacted. Paige estimated that 95% will be eligible with the revised sample size being:

$$n = 591/.95 = 622$$

Step 11: Cost Computation. The researcher should repeat these steps for each of the major estimates to be analyzed. The resulting range of sample sizes can be reviewed, as can the cost for each sample size. The final size selected can be based on the number of ideal respondents, the budget, and what compromises can be made. Costs are determined by multiplying the dollar amount per respondent by the total number of respondents. Herein, Paige estimated her cost at $55 per respondent (if she uses the telephone), with a total cost of $34,210.

In summary, Paige found that she needs approximately 622 respondents to have 95% confidence that the hypothesis that about 50% of the people in the bicounty area have used antibiotics in the past year is true, should the value for the sample drawn from the area fall between 45 and 55%.

Additional Sample Size Considerations. Two key elements that play a role in sample size are design, specifically stratified random sampling, and weighting where necessary.

Stratified Random Sampling. Stratified random sampling presents several issues in regard to sample size. As noted in the discussion of sampling types, the sample within each stratum is drawn randomly and as such can be considered an independent sample of the population stratum. Stratified random sampling is such that a very heterogeneous population can be subdivided into several relatively homogeneous strata, each demanding a fairly small sample.

Investigative studies involving a single dichotomous stratification parameter (urban-rural, smokers-nonsmokers, private hospitals–public hospitals) with random sampling in each stratum may employ a formula to determine sampling size. The formula considers confidence level and sampling error in calculating a representative sample size:

$$N = (z/e)^2(p)(1 - p)$$

where N = sample size
  z = the standard score corresponding to a given confidence level
  e = the proportion of sampling error in a given situation
  p = the estimated proportion or incidence of cases in the population

Confidence level indicates the probability that the sample proportion will reflect the population proportion with a specific degree of accuracy (sampling error is designated as e in the formula). With a 95% confidence level, z = 1.96; whereas with a 99% confidence level, z = 2.58, and with a 90% confidence level, z = 1.65.

Suppose that a health researcher decided to investigate patient education programs in public and private hospitals in West Virginia. In ascertaining the sampling frame, it was found that private hospitals accounted for 25% of all hospitals in the state. The proportion of private hospitals in the population of all hospitals would be .25 (p = .25). Employing the usual standard of a 95% (z = 1.96) confidence level and a sampling error of .10, the following calculations apply:

$$N = (1.96/.10)^2(.25)(.75)$$
$$N = (19.6)^2(.25)(.75)$$
$$N \doteq (384.16)(.1875)$$
$$N = 72$$

As a point of interpretation, a sample size of 72 private hospitals would give representativeness with no more than a plus or minus .10 sampling error with a confidence limit of 95%.

However, a stratified random sampling is often disproportionate in that a greater proportion is sampled in one stratum than another. The two major reasons for this are (1) differences in population size and (2) differences in homogeneity among strata. As an illustration, an investigation was conducted in West Central Illinois to ascertain the relationship of religion and health habits. The population comprised 1,000 Protestants, 800 Roman Catholics, and 200 Mormons. It is evident that a proportionate sample would leave the Mormons misrepresented or at least without a statistically functioning sample. Further, the decision to work with a sample of 100 from each of the religious strata revealed that the odds of being randomly selected varied tremendously. The Protestants had a 1 in 10 chance of being chosen, Catholics had a 1 in 8 chance, and Mormons had a 1 in 2 chance.

One way around this dilemma is to use weighted sampling. With this procedure the additional problem of combining subsamples (strata) into one overall sample for the purpose of data analysis can be overcome. Weights are assigned to each of the strata. Mormons are given a weight of 2 because they have a 1 in 2 chance of selection. Catholics have a weight of 8 because they have a 1 in 8 chance of selection, and similarly Protestants have a weight of 10. To make calculations more workable, each weight is divided by 2 to arrive at smaller numbers. This provides weights of 1, 4, and 5 for Mormons, Catholics, and Protestants, respectively.

The researcher can weight the data during analysis using the appropriate weight for each stratum. For example, suppose the following unweighted data shown in Table 7.4 were obtained. To obtain proportional data, each stratum would be weighted by the appropriate amount. The result would be as seen in Table 7.5.

TABLE 7.4 Distribution of Smokers by Religion

Smoking	Religion		
	Mormon	Catholic	Protestant
Cigarette	2	25	26
Pipe	10	21	34
Nonsmoker	88	54	40
Total	100	100	100

TABLE 7.5 Weighted Distribution of Smokers by Religion

| | Religion | | |
Smoking	Mormon	Catholic	Protestant
Cigarette	2	100	130
Pipe	10	84	170
Nonsmoker	88	216	200
Total	100	400	500

The figures are changed, but the relative values of the data are not altered. Thus, weighting provides adequate and equal representation of all strata. Aday (1989) provides a more detailed discussion of weighting.

In conclusion, there are several considerations in determining sample size, which are listed below:

1. Select as large a sample size as possible, because the larger the sample, the smaller the sampling error.
2. Cost, in terms of money and time, and subject availability are legitimate concerns in ascertaining sample size.
3. Surveys require a greater sample size than experimental studies because of response failure, item omission, poor interviewing, and so on.
4. When a sample is to be subdivided into smaller groups for data analysis, a large enough sample is required to allow for statistical treatment within each subgroup.
5. Stratification allows for greater homogeneity, thereby requiring a smaller sample size than a simple overall random sampling.
6. Assigning weights is a technique applicable to disproportionate sampling.

Case Discussion

Moses had conducted a pilot study to provide some background information for his larger proposal. Using that information in conjunction with related information about the new pharmacologic agent, he elected to use two groups, equal numbers, a 95% percent confidence level and power at 80%, and a one-sided test of means. Applying the sample size formula, he arrived at 147 patients per group, for a total of 294 patients. He would now need to contact other hypertension centers with similar patients to see if they would be interested in participating. He could randomly select some sites, and if they agree to be in the study, then have the patients randomly assigned to each of the two groups.

In regard to Paige's survey, she explored the possibility of using a telephone survey of households in her two-county area. They would be randomly selected. (Chapter 6, on survey research, discusses this in greater detail.) The method Paige used to arrive at the size of a sample was much different than the method used by Moses. She had several steps involved beyond his taking into account design effect, response rate, and eligibles. This brought her to a total of 622 respondents. Given this information, Paige can decide whether a telephone survey is too costly. However, if she believes that mailing would be less expensive, she would need to recalculate her steps, especially in light of response rate and eligibles.

Summary

Limited time, money, and resources frequently preclude a study of the entire population. Therefore, a sample of the population is required. The sample, however, must be of a size that represents the population and provides opportunity to detect significant differences when appropriate. The sampling frame is a list of all the persons from whom the sample is to be drawn. This can be difficult to obtain in some instances.

Sampling techniques can be subdivided into two broad categories: probability and nonprobability sampling. Probability sampling means that the likelihood of selecting each respondent is known; examples are random sampling, systematic sampling, stratified random sampling, and cluster sampling. In contrast, nonprobability sampling reflects an unknown probability of selection. Types of nonprobability sampling techniques include convenience, quota, dimensional, purposive, and snowball sampling. Depending on the nature of the research objectives, mixed sampling designs may be used.

Sample size was discussed from two broad perspectives: the first was based on power analysis while the second was seen from a health survey perspective. Considerations in determining sample size include sampling error, alpha probability level, and, for power analysis, probability level beta. The standard alpha level of significance is .05, while power is generally established at $1 - \beta = .80$. Formulas were given for two sample inferences for both two-sided and one-sided tests for means. Similarly, formulas were given for one sample inferences for both two-sided and one-side tests for means. It was noted that similar tests are available for (1) comparing the means of more than two samples, (2) comparing proportions between two groups, and (3) testing the significance of bivariate linear relationships.

In regard to health surveys, 11 steps were outlined as considerations for sample size. These steps included:

- Identification of major study variables
- Estimates of study variables
- Subgroup selection
- Relevant standard error formula
- Expected estimate
- Tolerable range of error in the estimate
- Level of confidence

- Sample design effect
- Response rate adjustment
- Adjustment for expected proportion of eligibles
- Cost computation

The steps are like building blocks in that each step depends on the preceding steps for appropriate calculation. Additional considerations were stratified random sampling and weighting. A brief summary list of considerations was presented.

Suggested Activities

1. Imagine that you had a population of 931 people, and that a simple random sample size of 75 is to be selected. How would you use a table of random numbers to select the first 10 people?

2. A population is divided into four strata (urban-rural, male-female) with the population sizes being 15,000, 8,000, 17,000, and 9,000, respectively. A sample of 500 is to be selected using proportional stratified random sampling. What is the sampling fraction, and what would be the number selected from each stratum?

3. Go to the website http://ebook.stat.ucla.edu/calculators/powercalc/ to select a power calculator for sample size. Choose normal distribution for two-sample, unequal variances. Enter the data from Moses's study using $\alpha = .05$, a power of .80, and $M_1 = 138.20$ and $M_2 = 133.50$. What do you obtain for a sample size for each group? How does this answer compare to the formula and to the table?

4. Visit the website http://ebook.stat.ucla.edu/textbook/calculators/sampsize.phtml for a different sample size calculator. This site allows you to compute sample size needed for a given confidence and a given maximum allowable deviation. It is currently used for means, proportions, and totals. Assume you are trying to estimate the mean. In the calculator, make the population size 3,000, with a maximum allowable difference of 0.1, confidence interval of 0.95, and variance estimate of 1.0. Submit this information to find out the required sample size using a random sample.

5. You wish to conduct a survey on health education in your school district. You have a list of 6,125 households, and this is to be your sampling frame. The sample size is limited to 600. What is the sampling fraction? How would you go about selecting the sample? If you were encouraged to do a systematic sampling, how would it be conducted? Why might it be better than a simple random sampling?

6. Go to the website http://www.math.york.ca. From there click on *Resources* and then click on *Statistical Consulting Service*. At that site, go to *WWW Resources* and

search various links. Become familiar with sites that provide services to calculate sample size for various studies.

References

Aday, L. A. (1989). *Designing and conducting health surveys.* San Francisco: Jossey-Bass.

Bailey, K. (1982). *Methods of social research.* New York: Macmillan.

Borenstein, M., & Cohen, J. (1988). *Statistical power analysis: A computer program.* Hillsdale, NJ: Erlbaum Associates.

Cohen, J. (1988). *Statistical power analysis for the behavioral sciences.* New York: Academic Press.

Kalton, G. (1983). *Introduction to survey sampling.* New York: Sage.

Lee, E. S., Forthofer, W., & Lorimor, R. J. (1989). *Analyzing complex survey data.* New York: Sage.

Levy, P. S., & Lemeshow, S. (1991). *Sampling of populations: Methods and applications.* New York: Wiley.

Polit, D. F., & Hungler, B. P. (1995). *Nursing research: Principles and methods.* Philadelphia: J. B. Lippincott.

Rosner, B. (1990). *Fundamentals of biostatistics.* Boston: PWS-Kent.

Chapter *8*

Qualitative Research

Case Study

Health Data Analysts, a research consortium, has been awarded a contract to examine the efficacy of a hospital's Wellness Center. Steven has been named the project director of this study, and he will head a team comprised of several staff people who are all trained and educated to gather and interpret data for the layperson. The consortium devised a methodology to use qualitative research in order to best reach the goals and objectives of the project.

Some of the previous chapters of this textbook have dealt with collecting and reporting data in a quantifiable manner. This chapter discusses another method of gathering data that is different from experimental and survey research in that it is *qualitative*. As an introduction to this chapter, Table 8.1 compares the two approaches of qualitative and quantitative research. After you review the table, you will be able to see that the need, setting, and type of problem to be studied will eventually determine the research approach you will use.

Characteristics of Qualitative Research

What is different about qualitative research? The following characteristics, adapted from Bodgan and Biklin (1998), help to describe some traits about this methodology:

1. *Qualitative data has the natural setting as the direct source of data, and the research is the key instrument.* The data are collected at the location of the study. Steven, in our case study, will go directly to the Wellness Center to study the actual goings-on first-hand. The researcher is really the instrument most readily used. Even if tape recorders or other equipment is employed, the researcher has the insight into where he or she should be and exactly how to collect the necessary

163

TABLE 8.1 Comparisons Between Qualitative and Quantitative

Qualitative		Quantitative
Phrases Associated with the Methodology		
Case study	Naturalistic	Empirical
Documentary	Observation	Experimental
Ecological	Participant	Hard data
Ethnographic	Phenomenological	Positivist
Field work	Soft data	Social facts
Life history	Symbolic interaction	Statistical
Key Concepts Associated with the Methodology		
Common sense	Negotiated orders	Hypothesis
Definition of situation	Process	Operationalize
Everyday life	Social construction	Reliability
Practical purposes	Understanding	Replication
Meaning		Statistically significant
		Validity
		Variable
Academic Affiliation (beginnings)		
Anthropology		Economics
History		Political science
Sociology		Psychology
		Sociology
Goals		
Describe multiple realities		Establish the facts
Develop sensitizing concepts		Predict
Develop understanding		Provide statistical description
Test grounded theory		Show relationships between variables
		Test theory
Relationship with Subjects		
Empathy		Circumscribed
Emphasis entrust		Detached
Equalitorian		Distant
Intense contact		Short-term
Instruments and Tools		
Tape recorder		Computers
Transcriber		Indexes
		Inventories
		Questionnaires
		Scales
		Test scores

TABLE 8.1 *Continued*

Qualitative	Quantitative
Data Analysis	
Analytical induction Constant comparative method Induction Models, themes, concepts Ongoing	At end of data collection Deductive Statistical
Problems in Using the Approach	
Data reduction difficult Difficult to study large populations Procedures not standardized Reliability Time-consuming	Controlling extraneous variables Obtrusiveness Validity
Design	
Design is a hunch as to how to proceed Flexible, evolving General	Design is a detailed plan of operation Specific Structured
Data	
Descriptive Fieldnotes Official statistics Personal documents Photographs Subjects' own words	Counts, measures Operationalized values Quantifiable coding Quantitative data Statistical data
Sample	
Nonrepresentative Small Theoretical	Control for extraneous variables Control groups Large Precise Random selection Stratified
Methods	
Observation Open-ended interviewing Participant observation Reviewing of documents	Data sets Experiments Quasi-experiments Structural interviewing Structured observation Survey research

Note. Adapted from Bogdan, R., and Biklin, S. *Qualitative Research in Education.* Boston: Allyn & Bacon, 1998, pp. 45–48.

data. The reason that qualitative researchers go to the location under study is that they are concerned with context and feel that situations can best be understood when they are directly observed. The setting has to be understood in the history context of the institution of which it is a part. When the data with which qualitative researchers are concerned are produced by subjects, as in the case of official records, the researchers want to know where, how, and under what circumstances the data came into being. Of what historical circumstances and movements are the records a part? Qualitative researchers believe that behavior is influenced by the setting and therefore always go to that location to collect the necessary data.

2. *Qualitative research is descriptive.* Numbers are not used to collect data, but rather words and pictures form the basic methods of data collection. The data include transcripts of in-depth interviews, field notes, photographs, tapes, memos, personal documents, and other official records. In our case study, Steven might ask the director of the Wellness Center for files pertaining to the goals and objectives stated when the center first opened.

Quotations are very often used in collecting qualitative data. In addition, a record is made of everything that occurs in certain situations. For example, when observing a conversation between two people, the researcher would probably describe the initiator (i.e., the person who did most of the talking and listening), the immediate surroundings (e.g., near a drinking fountain), and so on. The researcher is attempting to get a very comprehensive and deep understanding of the situation being studied. Therefore every detail must be described, and this is a very laborious task.

3. *Qualitative researchers are concerned with process rather than with outcomes or products.* The researcher is concerned with the natural history of the situation being studied. Questions related to how decisions are made in the context under study and to what becomes "common sense" are areas of concern. Qualitative studies tend to decipher exactly what goes on in an institution so that the expected outcomes are fulfilled. That is the *process* leading to the outcomes. In quantitative research, subjects are given tests (pretest and posttest) to determine the effectiveness of a program. The qualitative process discerns activities that would occur between the pretest and posttest and analyzes those events, with no concern for the outcome.

4. *Qualitative researchers tend to analyze their data inductively.* Qualitative investigators do not collect data to prove or disprove a prior hypothesis, but rather they collect the data first and then group them together. Glaser and Strauss (1967) describe a type of theory that builds from the bottom up as *grounded theory.* The qualitative investigator puts together a theory after the data have been collected and after much time has been spent at the location with the subjects. Part of this process is to find out what the concerns are, as opposed to quantitative research in which investigators come into a situation with predetermined questions.

5. *Meaning is of essential concern to the qualitative approach.* Qualitative researchers are concerned with how different people live their lives and make sense of them; this is called *participant perspective.* For example, investigators might ask what

people in a certain situation take for granted. In our case study, Steven may ask Wellness Center personnel for their perspectives on the efficacy of the center. He would ask other personnel in the hospital the same question. In other words, he would attempt to get the participants' perceptions about the Wellness Center and relate them to the perspectives of other people, looking for common ground.

Many situations in which qualitative research is conducted will not include all of the characteristics we have discussed, but they should include a majority. Investigators using this research method must have time and patience, as the study will undoubtedly demand much painstaking effort.

Theoretical Foundations

For any researcher to adequately collect and analyze data, he or she should be aware of and have an understanding of the theoretical foundation on which the research is based. The theoretical foundations of qualitative research are similar to those in anthropology and sociology, in which paradigms are used to guide research. A *paradigm* is a research perspective that holds views about how research is to be conducted and that has its own assumptions about how the world works and about what is important in that world. Most qualitative researchers use a phenomenological perspective, which is the basis for most research in this area.

Phenomenological Perspective

Max Weber was the leading proponent of the phenomenological approach to research. The phenomenologist is concerned with attempting to understand human behavior through the eyes of the subjects in the study. This has been called *verstehen*, which is the interpretive understanding of human interaction. The phenomenological approach is used throughout most qualitative studies because of the importance of interviewing the subjects in a program or institution. Here the investigator has not made any presumptions about how the subjects view something, and goes about conducting an informal interview without any structure. This perspective is ever present as a theoretical framework for qualitative researchers.

Symbolic Interaction

Symbolic interaction originated with George Herbert Mead in his book *Mind, Self and Society* (1934). He viewed communication as the key to understanding the connection between intelligence (mind), self-consciousness (self), and the community (society). Gestures (verbal or not) made by people are symbols, taken to mean acts that stand for something else. Another aspect of Mead's work dealt with the fact that humans have a self-conscious awareness of themselves. Interaction between people depends on the degree to which it possesses a self-conscious quality.

How others interpret the interactions depends on experience and history. In other words, symbolic interaction theory asserts that people's self-concepts are influenced by the way others respond to them.

People act not according to predetermined responses but as interpreting, defining, symbolic animals whose behavior the researcher can only understand by entering the defining process (Bogdan & Biklin, 1998). This is accomplished with a type of qualitative research called *participant observation*, which will be discussed later in this chapter. Defining is a shared event, and the people involved have usually developed congruent definitions of interpretations. As people see a need, they may change their definition of an interpretation, and this is where the qualitative investigator steps in to determine how definitions develop.

Culture

Cultural anthropologists study other cultures, sometimes from a phenomenological perspective. *Ethnography* is the term used for the description of a particular culture. All anthropologists use the theoretical framework of culture in their research studies, and this organizes the ethnographic work. The ethnographer has few if any hypotheses, and there is no structured instrument with which to collect the data. The goal of the ethnographer is to describe in as much detail as possible the customs, religious ceremonies, mores, language, and other pertinent variables of a subculture or group. The best way to do this is for the investigator to become a participant observer and in so doing attempt to put aside his or her own culture.

Ethnomethodology

Harold Garfinkel (1967) coined the term *ethnomethodology* to refer to the study of how individuals create and understand life. It is the study of everyday, commonplace, routine social activity. Ethnomethodologists attempt to understand how people make order out of the complex world in which they live. A more complete discussion of ethnomethodology will appear later in this chapter, because it is a type of qualitative research that has taken on importance in the last 35 years.

Methods of Qualitative Research

Qualitative methodologies are research procedures that enable the investigator to produce data. The methods that will be discussed include observation, participant observation, ethnomethodology, and document study. Although in-depth interviewing is also a qualitative research method, we chose to discuss it in Chapter 6, on survey research.

Observation

One of the primary methods of qualitative research is *observation*. It is a scientific technique if conducted under the proper circumstances. Observation must (1) serve a research purpose; (2) be planned systematically; (3) be recorded systematically; and (4) be subjected to checks and controls on validity and reliability (Bickman, 1981). The following section will describe the value and purposes of observation, methods of observation, what to observe, and observer training.

Value and Purposes of Observation. Observational data are collected in a natu-ralistic setting in that the researcher does not manipulate or control people or other significant things related to the study. It is a discovery-oriented approach carried out in the field. Because the investigator is in the field, he or she can become very close to the situation and better understand the context within the program and its various complexities. Therefore, the value of observational data is that it enables those who asked for the information (the users) to understand the entire program through detailed and very descriptive information that is provided through the collection of observational data.

The collection of observational data may have three purposes: (1) to provide descriptions of behavior; (2) to record situational behavior; and (3) to study a topic that lends itself to this method. First, providing detailed descriptions of the behavior patterns of people is one of the purposes of health science research. The observa-tional method of data collection enables researchers to accomplish this task. When observational data are recorded, it is done at the same time a behavior pattern is occurring. This allows investigators to get a true sense of individual and group behavior under real and accurate circumstances.

A second purpose for using observational data is that behavior can be recorded as it actually occurs. In our case study, Steven will use observation so that he and his staff can directly observe behaviors as they happen. In this manner they will be able to observe how Wellness Center personnel interact with each other under varied circumstances and in several situations.

The remaining purpose of observational methods is that there are certain circumstances under which they are the *only* feasible method to collect the appro-priate data. Infants and toddlers, for example, cannot be interviewed or given a survey to complete; hence, observation becomes the method used to collect data concerning these types of subjects. Another example would be a study of people with severe diseases (terminal cancer, schizophrenia), which is not possible except through observation.

There are several values or advantages of direct observation. Patton (1990) has best described the advantages of direct, personal observations:

1. By directly observing program observations and activities, the investigator is able to understand the *context* within which the program operates.
2. The first-hand experience with a program enables the experimenter to use the inductive approach.
3. The study personnel can observe things that are routine to those in the program.
4. The investigator can learn things about the program that cannot or will not be revealed in an interview or questionnaire.

5. The observers are able to present a comprehensive view of the program because they can move beyond the perception of the participants.
6. The investigator uses his or her knowledge and experience in terms of feelings, reflection, and introspection about a program.

Methods of Observation.   There are two major types of methods of observation: relatively unstructured and structured. In the former method, the investigator attempts to get directly involved in the situation and to describe it as nonselectively as possible. In structured methodologies, the investigator codes or categorizes the observed behaviors of the program participants.

Unstructured methods may involve being involved as a participant observer, filming and videotaping an occurrence, using specimen records, and recording anecdotes. Because participant observer methods will be discussed later in this chapter, we will focus here on the other unstructured methods.

By using *film or videotape,* one could ideally get a complete and accurate view of a program. However, is this really the goal of observation? Or is it to summarize, systematize, and simplify the event, rather than depict an exact replication (Bickman, 1981)? Even if one does use film to record the program, the film really is not an exact reproduction because of biases caused by the presence of the camera and microphone.

Specimen records are descriptions of behavior over a brief continuous time period. They allow for extrapolations of one event to several or a series of events. Behaviors are noted with painstaking care, and the interventions of those observed are recorded so as to define a standing pattern of behavior. If these patterns of behavior can be observed under various environmental settings, a behavioral consistency can be determined. This is the major advantage of using specimen records.

Anecdotes are used widely by many people attempting to observe behavior. The observer selects places and particular events to observe before actually recording the anecdote. This is not true of specimen records or films. Anecdotal records are objective and usually written after the incident has occurred. This type of record can test hypotheses if proper sampling is used. In the previously mentioned methods, hypotheses are generated *after* the observations are made. Anecdotal records should not be interpretive, but merely descriptive and accurate.

Generally, unstructured methods lead to problems of reliability, observer bias, and memory distortion. Because these problems can damage any study, we suggest that unstructured methods be used to generate rather than to test hypotheses.

Structured methods are more formal methods used to observe behavior and to set up or test hypotheses. The investigator is able to select activities to observe before they occur and can plan a systematic recording of observations. There are several ways to record this type of information: duration, continuous, frequency-count, and interval.

Duration recording is used when the observer wishes to record the elapsed time during which the behavior occurs. In our case study, if Steven wanted to find out how long the coordinator of the Wellness Center talked during a staff meeting, he could use a stopwatch to accomplish this task.

Continuous recording occurs when the observer records all the behaviors of the subjects and thereby creates a *protocol*. A protocol is a narrative in chronological order of everything that occurred in a given setting, such as the Wellness Center staff meeting. This is a very comprehensive method in that the observer must use a content analysis system to classify the observed behavior.*

When using *frequency-count recording,* an observer simply counts the number of times a particular behavior occurs. This is especially useful when behaviors occur at low frequency and observers can count several different behaviors at the same time.

Interval recording is used to study the sequence of behaviors of subjects. The observer records a specific behavior at specific intervals (e.g., every ten seconds). If Steven were to record, at intervals, when the coordinator of the Wellness Center asked a rhetorical question, he could get an idea of the sequence of that behavior. In addition, if Steven had a frequency count of rhetorical questions and multiplied it by the interval, he could get the duration of that behavior, which could prove to be very important in diagnosing possible personnel problems.

What to observe. Many program aspects should be observed to get a comprehensive view of that program. We will discuss (1) program setting; (2) program activities and participant behaviors; (3) informal interactions and unplanned activities; (4) nonverbal communication; and (5) unobtrusive measures. Much of the following has been abstracted from Patton's *Qualitative Evaluative and Research Methods* (1990). These occasions can help an observer organize a methodology that will emphasize certain kinds of observations. These are called *sensitizing concepts,* and they provide a framework to enhance the importance of behaviors and events.

The *program setting* is the physical environment in which the research takes place. When the reader can visualize the setting through a complete and detailed description provided by the investigator, then the program setting is helpful. The researcher should avoid using interpretive words such as "very," "wonderful," and "lovely." Rather, words that actually describe the setting—colors, dimensions of space, or quotations of participants—should be used.

Program activities and participant behaviors are observed by asking questions such as: What do the participants do? What is it like to be a participant? What do the observers see while the program is in progress? Units of activity are generally regarded as organizers for the researcher. These units may include staff meetings, formal sessions, patient-client sessions, and the like. The investigator must focus the sequence of events in a chronological order: When did the activity begin, who introduced it, and who is in charge?

Gradually, the researcher attempts to observe each activity by asking questions that deal with statements made by staff and participants during the event, such as: How did behaviors change over the duration of the activity? How did it feel to be engaged in that activity? At the end of the activity, the observer asks: What signals that the event has ended, what is said by whom, and what is the relationship of this particular activity to the other parts of the program?

---

*For a more complete discussion of content analysis see Bergs (2001).

Observation of *informal interactions and unplanned activities* is just as valuable as viewing formal activities in a program. Investigators should ensure that time is allotted for this activity. It can occur during breaks or meals, before and after formal working hours, and during the workday. The researcher will probably overhear conversations or conduct face-to-face or small-group interviews. The way people interact or do not interact after a meeting or part of a program should also be observed. The fact that people do not interact is a part of the data and should be noted.

Nonverbal communication has received much attention by behavioral scientists, who of course include health scientists. When observing groups, noticing how people sit, what they do in their seats, how they dress, and how they space themselves in discussion groups (e.g., who sits next to whom and how often) enriches description of the process of a program. Investigators should describe the nonverbal cues of others, as well as their own reactions to those cues. And by watching for behavior patterns, they can learn about significant nonverbal behaviors.

Unobtrusive measures are helpful in obtaining data without the participants realizing that they are part of the study. Examples of this type of data collection include analyzing contents of wastepaper baskets, counting cigarette butts before and after meetings, and noting what is written on a blackboard or memo pad. These unobtrusive measures are very helpful, because once people know that they are in a study, their reactions may become self-conscious and inhibited. Unobtrusive measures should not contaminate the way people respond. Additional ways to collect unobtrusive data include looking through directories, calendar diaries, and other such documents.

In our case study, Steven could observe reactions of people leaving a conference room, witness daily calendars to see the meetings scheduled, and look at internal memos. These would be unobtrusive measures and could possibly reinforce the results of other reactive data-gathering methodologies, such as surveys and interviews. The more varied the data-gathering techniques, the more congruence should appear among the results. This provides a more true and accurate picture of the program being observed.

The Observation Form.   There are so many types of observations and situations in which they take place that we encourage all investigators to prepare their own forms. Each time an observation takes place, a new form is required. Researchers should attempt to plan their observations so they can devise appropriate forms. Table 8.2 is an example of a form that Steven might utilize when observing a staff meeting of the Wellness Center.

As is evident in the table, observation forms can be easily devised, and, when utilized properly, can provide necessary and valuable information for the study.

Observer Training.   Many reviews on observer training (Hartman & Wood, 1990; Berg, 2001; Thomas, 1993) provide helpful information on the training of observers. You should refer to these references for a more complete review. We will discuss the

TABLE 8.2 Observation Form

1. Every time the Wellness Center coordinator asks a question, place a check next to one of the following general categories that best describes the question:

		Frequency	Total
a.	Asks personnel for direct input	×××	3
b.	Asks personnel to answer specific questions	××××	4
c.	Asks for general questions	×××××	5
d.	Other	×××××××	7
	Total		19

Note. Adapted from Gall, M., Borg, W., & Gall, J. (1996). *Educational Research.* New York: Longman.

observation manual, observer orientation, training for the observational setting, and training in the observational setting.

The *observational manual* becomes the bible for all observers. The manual should discuss and explain ethical issues, dress codes, courtesy protocols, and all other matters that pertain to the collection of data by the observational method. The manual should clearly define all code categories, and positive and negative examples should be included to more explicitly depict the coding techniques. Health Data Analysts, the research consortium that Steven is employed by, would have a well-developed manual for use in most of the research projects the consortium conducts. Steven will have worked on this manual before contacting his staff.

In cases in which the observational method fits into the specific research project, *observer orientation* occurs when observers have been selected by the project director to be oriented to the purpose of the study. All observers must be encouraged to follow the coding system exactly and not allow other information to interfere with completion of the forms. The observers should not be told about any hypotheses, if any exist, because this knowledge might bias them when they are completing the necessary observation forms.

During orientation the observers must be informed about subjects' rights and the confidentiality of the study. Observers should not discuss their reactions with each other until the observations are complete.

Training for the observational setting includes having observers memorize the manual, especially the coding rules and definitions. This will eliminate confusion and disorganization when the actual observations occur. It might be worthwhile for Steven to ensure his staff's knowledge of the manual by having them practice and then demonstrate mastery on a test regarding the manual. Observers should be exposed to and trained in using the actual forms and any other equipment (videotape or audiotape recorders, etc.).

One way for training to occur is to place the trainees in settings that require them to use the materials that will be used in the actual study. This can be accomplished by having trainees watch videotapes and listen to tape recordings, called *analogue tapes.* These are made by experienced observers. They enable the trainees to proceed from the simple to complex tasks, approximating an actual situation.

While the trainees are using the analogue tapes, they should receive constant, consistent, and constructive feedback as to the accuracy of their responses. This can be done by comparing trainees' responses to experienced observers' responses and discussing the discrepancies. In addition, this method can be useful in reconstructing forms and/or categories of behavior on the forms.

After the analogue tape training is completed and the trainees have demonstrated almost perfect accuracy in their response to the tapes, they should begin *training in the observational setting.* This is the final phase of the training and is conducted under supervision. Steven would take one of his staff to a very straightforward observational setting (behind a one-way mirror in a person's office) and encourage the staff member to begin making observational recordings. Afterward, Steven would review the staff member's forms to check for accuracy. Each staff member would go through the same type of procedure before attending larger, more complicated observational situations.

Participant Observation

Participant observation involves the collection of data in the field that combines document analysis; interviewing of respondents and informants; and direct participation, observation, and introspection (Denzin, 1989). The field of anthropology is best known for using participant observation, but more recently, sociology, education, and health science researchers have used this method of qualitative data collection. The aforementioned disciplines have used participant observation in natural settings such as schools, hospitals, and clinics. Our case study would lend itself to participant observation as a methodology.

The participant observer becomes part of the setting and "goes native." The observation may take several forms and may vary as to the degree of the researcher's participation, how much is disclosed to the subjects in the study, and the degree to which the activities and subjects are directly observed by the investigators (Glesne & Peshkin, 1999). Researchers can become totally involved in the setting (e.g., become a staff member of the Wellness Center in our case study), or be a partial participant in a tribe or religious group without becoming an actual member of that group. When an observer "goes native," he or she wants to understand the values and experiences of that group. The participant observer must disregard her or his own values, because they might cause the participant observer to become emotionally involved with the group. This becomes a difficult dilemma for the participant observer. He or she must share experiences of the group but cannot become totally involved, because some sort of detachment must be retained to accurately report the observations.

How much is told to the subjects can vary from everything to nothing at all. At times it is necessary to conceal the fact that there is a study being conducted. This may result in some ethical problems. However, compromises are usually achieved by using partial disclosure. Here, only a few select people are informed about the

participant observer. Junker (1960, pp. 35–38) has described four types of partici-
pant-observation situations:

1. *Complete participant:* In this role, the observer's activities are entirely concealed. The observer is a complete member of an in-group, thus sharing secret information guarded from outsiders. The observer's freedom to observe outside the in-group system of relationships is severely limited. Such a role tends to block perception of the workings of the reciprocal relations between the in-group and the larger social system, and makes it difficult to switch from this to another role to observe the details of the larger group.
2. *Participant as observer:* Here, the observer's activities are *not* entirely concealed, but are "kept under wraps," or subordinated to activities as participant. This role may limit access to some kinds of information, perhaps especially at the secret level.
3. *Observer as participant:* This is the situation in which the observer's activities as such are made publicly known at the outset, are more or less publicly sponsored by people in the situation studied, and are not kept under wraps. This role may provide access to a wide range of information, and even secrets may be given to the participant observer.
4. *Complete observer:* This describes a range of roles where, at one extreme, the observer is behind a one-way mirror, and at the other extreme, the observer's activities are completely public.

Participant observation must involve direct observation and is usually supplemented by other data collection methodologies. One of the most common complementary sources of data collection is the use of informants. *Informants* are a group of members who are in a position to reveal worthwhile information or who are wholly representative of the group under study.

Advantages and Disadvantages of Participant Observation.   The first advantage of participant observation is the ability of the process to *explore* a theory or a type of measurement. In addition, it allows for hypothesis formation where it is impossible to do so before the beginning of the study. A further point of exploration lies in the investigator being able to research a new area as a participant observer.

A second advantage to participant observation is that it allows investigators to gain *access* to subjects or data where it might not otherwise be feasible. Organizations that might feel threatened, such as in our case study, would be prime candidates for participant observation. This methodology would enable a researcher to gain valuable data as an insider of the organization. A further consideration is that in some instances subjects are unable to recall events or may not view events as important, thereby not giving the investigator accurate, reportable information. Additionally, participant observation becomes advantageous when subjects cannot self-report data, as in the case of very young children, impaired persons in hospitals, or those who are afraid to self-report data (prisoners, gang members, etc.).

The third major advantage to participant observation is that it offers the possibility of obtaining a *richness* of data. While other methods provide hard data in terms of numbers and statistics, participant observation enables the researcher to see variables within the context of the natural setting. Because subjects are off-guard, the descriptions garnered are accurate as to what exactly occurred.

As with any methodology there are both pros and cons; there are several disadvantages with participant observation. The most serious of these is the ethical element, especially when no one under study is apprised of the investigation. The problem then is one of deception and of the reactions of subjects who were, in effect, duped. Another disadvantage of participant observation is the possibility that the participant observer will become too emotionally involved, lose objectivity in reporting, and then later provide personal interpretation to the data. A third disadvantage lies in the reliance on the participant observer's memory to recall all aspects of the events that occurred. This can be a slow and arduous process, because the observer must covertly write or dictate notes whenever feasible.

Being a Participant Observer. Many of the considerations previously discussed concerning validity, reliability, sampling, and subject selection must be adhered to in participant observation. However, as Walizer and Wienir (1978) discuss, some special concerns pertain to participant observation.

Selecting the problem is a consideration for participant observation. Investigators may have relied on previous research to pose the problem or even have used participant observation to find the problem. There are some major things to look for when observing a particular group that guide the problem selection. The following has been adapted from Walizer and Wienir (1978, p. 338):

1. How is the institution or program organized?
2. What is the nature of the social relationships that exist within the program?
3. What types of technology are utilized to make the work environment plausible?
4. What are the relationships between management and staff?
5. What activities do employees do together? Apart?

These questions are just a few examples of how participant observers begin to construct a framework for their study. These questions naturally lead to others and thus can readily focus the problem to be studied. There are times when participant observers are given the problem before embarking upon the research.

A second consideration is *choosing the setting* for participant observation. If the problem has previously been delineated, then the participant observer must choose an appropriate site that would contain that problem. For example, if one wanted to study the relationship between secretaries and middle managers, the chosen site must include both these characters, and both must have expressed the desire to participate in the study. Another aspect to consider in choosing the setting is to ensure that the participant observer will be comfortable in the setting. If you were asked to be a participant observer in a nuclear power plant and did not feel at ease in the situation, the study would not benefit from your participation.

Another consideration is *establishing social relationships* with the subjects. This is the most important part of the design, because the entire concept of participant observation relies on acceptance of the observer by group subjects. Before the study commences, it would be wise to obtain the necessary approval from high-level employers, presidents of corporations, chieftains of tribes, and so on. In our case study, Steven would get permission from the hospital director and clinic president if he wanted to conduct part of the research by using participant observation.

Once the study is in progress and the necessary permissions have been granted, the participant observer should begin to become associated and acclimated to the program. In this regard, the observer should attempt to remain in the background and not attract attention. This prohibits people from being too curious about the "new person on the block."

A fourth consideration in attempting to become a participant observer is *finding informants*. These persons are used to observe for the participant observer, and to suggest to and inform the participant observer about the program and its problem or problems to be studied. The observer must make sure that the informant is reliable and relaying truths about what he or she sees and hears. The informant should be tested by the participant observer to verify his or her comments and perceptions.

A further consideration for the participant observer is *establishing rapport* with the subjects. The goal of the investigator is to blend in with the program and act as natural as possible. Bogdewic (1999) has delineated ways in which a participant observer may establish rapport:

- *Be unobtrusive:* You should be more observer than participant. Your behavior and attire should not draw attention, as your goal is to learn what it takes to fit in.
- *Be honest:* People in the setting you are studying will have a limited understanding of why you are there. Questions about your interests and what you hope to find should be dealt with in an open and direct manner. You should assure people that their participation is voluntary and that their identities will remain anonymous.
- *Be unassuming:* Try not to threaten the subjects by your expertise in technical and professional matters. You can play down your expertise.
- *Be a reflective listener:* This communication skill helps build rapport and is an excellent way to learn the language of the participants. Particular words in a social situation have significance and meaning to the subjects.
- *Be self-revealing:* Participants will have some degree of curiosity about you, and your willingness to discuss common interests and life experiences can open the door to a more trusting relationship.

Participant observation is absolutely demanding and can take a great deal of time, patience, and effort. While the observer is spending the day with the subjects in a group, the other waking hours are spent recording, collating, and analyzing data. Hence, participant observation can be a very time-consuming activity, especially if it persists for a long period of time. However, the rewards are great in that participant observation, as a qualitative research method, gives the richness and completeness needed for obtaining information and drawing conclusions concerning some research problems.

Ethnomethodology

Ethnomethodology is the study of methods used in everyday, commonplace, and routine social activities. Garfinkel (1967) defines ethnomethodology as an organizational study of a person's knowledge of his or her ordinary affairs, or of his or her own organized enterprises, where that knowledge is treated by investigators as part of the same setting that it also makes orderable. It should be made clear here that ethnomethodology is not an alternative methodology aimed at a more effective solution of traditionally formulated problems. Focusing upon the complicated character of action scenes, ethnomethodology necessarily develops a style of research responsive to its subject matter. In other words, ethnomethodology is *not* a research method per se, but rather it is a method to attempt to find out how people make sense out of ordinary situations in which they live. Ethnomethodologists, then, examine common sense in an attempt to understand how people see, describe, and explain order in the world in which they live.

As an example, Wieder (1974) explored how narcotic addicts in a halfway house used a "convict code" (e.g., "do not snitch," "help other residents") to explain and account for their behavior. He illustrated the way in which residents "tell the code" by applying maxims to specific situations when they are called upon to account for their behavior. He wrote: "The code, then, is much more a method of moral persuasion and justification than it is a substantive account of an organized way of life. It is a way, or set of ways, of causing activities to be seen as morally, repetitively, and constrainedly organized" (p. 158). This is an example of how ethnomethodologists suspend their own commonsense assumptions to study how common sense is used in everyday life.

Advantages and Disadvantages of Ethnomethodology. The *advantages* of ethnomethodology are many. The first is that it studies nonverbal as well as verbal behavior. Second, it is longitudinal because it is ongoing, and changes in behavior can be viewed over a long period of time. Third, this type of study can provide insight into what and why people think about commonplace activities and behaviors, thus enabling health scientists to make better order of why people behave the way they do in areas of health.

One of the *disadvantages* of ethnomethodology in relation to the health sciences is that this type of study involves investigating the *process* of how something occurs, rather than the *product* of that occurrence. As an example, in our case study Steven would not use ethnomethodology to ascertain the attitudes of Wellness Center personnel toward centralized management, but would use ethnomethodology to study the process of how those attitudes were formed. Another disadvantage is that ethnomethodology does not lend itself to large-scale studies, but is better for process-oriented, smaller investigations.

An interesting point to include here is that ethnomethodology actually studies all the previously discussed methods as a means to garner knowledge about the process of how people make sense of their commonplace lives. In this manner, researchers can gain valuable insights into questionnaire construction and coding of other survey materials.

Indexical Expressions. Indexical expressions are situation-specific words and/or phrases whose meanings change from situation to situation and may depend upon who is uttering the word or to whom the remarks are directed. Garfinkel and Sacks (1970) listed the following indexical words: *she, we, he, you, here, there, no, this, that, it, I, then, soon, today,* and *tomorrow.* These words have varying meanings, dependent upon the context. The indexicals have to be interpreted by an individual who is participating in the interaction before the meanings of the words are clear. The ethnomethodologist does not want to convert these indexical expressions into objective, nonindexical expressions, as a traditional researcher might approach this situation. Instead, the ethnomethodologist wants to study the rules people set to make sense of these indexicals in everyday conversation. This can be a very important aspect of a research project: the interpretation of important words.

Another aspect of ethnomethodology is that conversation and interaction are regulated by rules or norms. Ethnomethodologists discover how sense is made out of the structuring and ordering of indexicals. They can put meaning to indexicals that are made clear through a situationally specific process in which the context may be problematic and differ from place to place or time to time. However, the rules by which meanings are explicated remain objective, constant, and nonproblematic (Bailey, 1994). Topics that are usually studied by ethnomethodologists are:

1. Formulating, or the process by which one conversationalist interprets or explains a part of a conversation
2. Sequencing of a conversation
3. Terminating of a conversation

All of these and many other topics provide invaluable information to the health scientist, especially when conducting a qualitative research study. Experimental and survey research results may tell us what the subject knows or thinks, but ethnomethodology takes it one step further in an attempt to find out why the respondent answers in particular ways. Ethnomethodologists are indeed interested in human behavior in that they seek to find the rules that govern behavior.

Document Study

We shall discuss the study of documents with specific reference to nonpersonal documents. Personal documents will be discussed in a later section of this chapter, under *Techniques of Collecting Qualitative Data.* A very valuable source of information is retained in a program's or institution's records and documents. The investigator will have a better understanding and increased knowledge about a program once he or she reads its documents. At the outset of the project in our case study, Steven should negotiate receiving at least the following types of documents: routine client records, correspondence from and to staff, financial charts, and official or unofficial documents generated by or for the program (Patton, 1990). These documents can avail the investigator of basic sources of information regarding the activities and processes of the organization, and they can enable the researcher to view other questions not previously considered to follow up on observations, participant observation, or ethnomethodological research.

Types of Documents. There are many official documents that the researcher should attempt to obtain: minutes of meetings, memos, newsletters, policy documents, code of ethics, philosophy statements, and the like. The qualitative researcher is looking for how the organization or program is defined by those who are involved in that program. Therefore, a review of these documents will prove beneficial.

Internal documents include memos and other communications that abound in any organization. In a hospital, such as our Wellness Center, the amount of paper that flows from the top to the bottom is immense. Of course, some flows in the opposite direction as well. These documents can reveal the true chain of command, the interoffice fighting and subsequent negotiation, and the rules and regulations. In addition, leadership styles might emerge from these documents. It is advised, as we stated in the beginning of this section, that the researcher ensure that he or she will have access to this information before the project actually commences.

External communication includes those materials that are circulated outside the organization. This would include newsletters, public philosophic statements, news releases, marketing advertisements, and public access programs (e.g., health fairs, open houses). These documents can provide official points of view and insight into administrative hierarchy. Many organizations, especially hospitals, have hired public relations firms. This makes it a little difficult to ascertain who wrote what. In any case, the researcher should obtain the necessary information regarding the public relations organization, such as whether all external documents get reviewed in-house previous to publication. These documents are readily accessible because they are produced for outside consumption. In many instances, files will be kept of these types of documents, so they will be very easy for the researcher to obtain.

Personnel records can provide valuable information about hiring and firing practices, promotion and reward systems, and administrative policies regarding personnel. In addition, these files also can provide information about the people (e.g., personnel managers, supervisors) who add paper to the file. Access to these files may be granted if researchers agree not to identify people but instead use a coding system to describe the content of the files.

Document study can provide a well-rounded view of the organization or program that the researcher is studying. The aforementioned methods of qualitative research—observation, participant observation, ethnomethodology, and document study—all enhance the researcher's ability to gain an understanding of the events and activities of a particular program or an organization. A good qualitative study would most likely put to use most of these methods, because they will prove to be beneficial. The next part of this chapter will discuss how, using various techniques, Steven may actually collect the necessary data concerning the efficacy of the hospital's Wellness Center.

Techniques of Collecting Qualitative Data

There are several techniques to use when you are collecting qualitative data. These include field notes, subjects' written words, photography, and official statistics. The following sections briefly describe these techniques.

Field Notes

Field notes are the most important part of collecting data in qualitative research. They are used in *all* methodologies: observation, participant observation, ethnomethodology, and document study. Field notes contain everything and anything that the observer feels is worth noting. Any information that will enable the observer to gain a better understanding of the program must be written down immediately. If one leaves observation to memory, one is leaving much to chance.

Descriptions are the basics of field notes. Basic information as to who was there, what was happening, and where the observation took place should be included in the notes. In addition, a description of the event, what took place, and the interactions between people should be recorded. Field notes also should contain quotations of what people said. In addition, the notes should reflect the observer's feelings and reactions to the experience, as well as the meaning and significance of the event. Furthermore, the notes should contain the observer's insights, interpretations, beginning analyses, and working hypotheses regarding the situation (Patton, 1990). These comments are noted by using observer's comments (OC).

Lofland (1995) has some suggestions for those writing field notes:

1. Record the notes as quickly as possible after the observation.
2. Discipline yourself to write notes quickly and reconcile yourself to the fact that the recording of the notes can be expected to take as long as the actual observation.
3. Dictating rather than writing is acceptable, but writing may have the advantage of stimulating thought.
4. Typing field notes is preferable to handwriting because it is faster and easier to read.
5. Make at least two copies of the field notes. One original copy is retained for reference, and other copies can be used as rough drafts to be cut up, rewrittten, and reorganized.

Content of Field Notes. Two types of materials are included in the field notes: descriptive and reflective (of the observer's ideas and concerns). The *descriptive* part of the field notes includes the following (Bogdan & Biklin, 1998):

1. *Portrait of the subjects:* Include their physical appearance, dress, style of talking, and mannerisms.
2. *Reconstruction of dialogue:* The conversations between subjects, as well as what subjects might say to the observer, are recorded. Use direct quotations, especially when they are unique to the setting.
3. *Description of the physical setting:* The observer should draw a diagram of the furniture arrangements, and where people are sitting. Note also any blackboard writing and what may be on bulletin boards.
4. *Accounts of particular events:* Note who was involved in the event, in what manner, and the nature of the action.
5. *Depiction of activities:* Include detailed descriptions of behaviors.

As we discussed previously, the *reflective* part of the field notes should be recorded as well as descriptions of events, activities, and behaviors. These notes should be designated by "OC." Bogdan and Biklin (1998) offer the following comments on what should be included in the reflective part of the field notes:

1. *Reflections on analysis:* Speculate about what the observer is learning, emerging themes, patterns, and additional ideas.
2. *Reflections on method:* Include comments on the study design, accomplishments, and plans for what to do next.
3. *Reflection on observer's frame of mind:* Observers may have preconceived notions about the subjects. When these are changed or reinforced, they should be noted.
4. *Points of clarification:* Make additional notes to add or clarify a previous notation.

Field Note Form. Observers should adopt a standard form for their field notes. They should include at least the following:

1. *Title page:* This should include the date, time, and place of observation, as well as when the notes were recorded. The title of the event may also be included here.
2. *Diagram of setting:* As mentioned previously, a diagram of the activity or event should be included at the beginning of the notes.
3. *Wide margins:* They are necessary because the observer or someone else might want to make appropriate comments.
4. *Paragraphs:* New paragraphs should be formed very frequently to correspond with each new person speaking or with every change in the setting.
5. *Quotation marks:* They should be used as often as possible. Even though the observer may not quote exactly, if the notation is very close to an exact replica, enter the quotation marks.

Field Note Techniques. There are various ways to record field notes, but the observer must find the technique that is most comfortable for herself or himself. Most people use pen and paper on site and then use a typewriter, dictating machine, or word processor to rewrite and embellish the notes later on. Another on-site method used is a tape recorder. If an observer wishes to use a tape recorder or other equipment (silent typewriter, portable word processor, etc.), then the observer must make sure that the equipment does not interfere with the natural workings of the subjects within the group. In other words, the equipment must be unobtrusive.

Another mechanism available for recording field notes is called the Stenomask. It is a sound-shielded microphone attached to a portable tape recorder that is worn on a shoulder strap (Patton, 1990). The handle contains the microphone switch and allows the observer to talk into the recorder during an activity without the subjects being able to hear the dictation. Of course, this can be distracting to the group, and therefore should be used with caution.

Field notes provide the basis from which qualitative data is recorded and then analyzed. Recording field notes is a tedious task that requires patience and long hours after the observations have been completed. It is necessary that notes be organized and clear so that all involved in the project may benefit from the effort.

Personal Documents

Much information can be obtained from studying people's personal effects. This may include their clothing and the furnishings in their home or office. What may be of greater significance to qualitative researchers is examination of documents that indicate how people lead their everyday lives. These include calendars, diaries, letters (personal and business), autobiographies, scrapbooks, books read, and poetry written. Thomas (1923) was an early proponent of utilizing personal documents to make inferences about people's lives. He believed that autobiographies, letters, and the like, were an important source of data because they were capable of presenting life as a connected whole and of showing the interplay of influences on individuals. Thomas's research focused upon immigrants at the beginning and later analyzed their diaries, letters, and other personal documents. From these analyses he was able to depict some central themes of these people: individualization, demoralization, and deregulation.

The use of personal documents usually does not allow for a large sample size, although the Thomas study, as just described, must be considered an exception. Using personal documents enables the qualitative researcher to make a generalization about a subject and then use excerpts from the documents to illustrate them. In our case study, if Steven believed that the coordinator of the Wellness Center was autocratic, he would search the personal documents of that coordinator to look for a sense of autocratic personality.

How to Obtain Personal Documents. Obtaining personal documents such as diaries, autobiographies, and letters is not an easy task. One way that was used by

Thomas and Znaniecki (1927) was to advertise in a newspaper to find the appropriate materials. Some people might be willing to share diaries and letters. In our case study, organizational files would be very helpful. These personnel files should contain references to people in the organization, indicating how people define themselves in their respective positions.

The written words of subjects can be of invaluable assistance to the qualitative researcher who is attempting to gain an understanding of how and why a system works. Although obtaining these personnel documents may be difficult, it allows the investigator to exercise her or his imagination.

Photography

Qualitative research can be greatly enhanced by photography. The following section is taken from Bogdan and Biklin's (1998) excellent work on the benefits of photography in collecting qualitative data.

Social scientists have used photography since the nineteenth century to depict social documentaries on how people live (Thomson & Smith, 1877; Riis, 1980; Stott, 1973). The adage "a picture is worth a thousand words" has been adhered to by recent social scientists utilizing photography (Becker, 1978; Wagner, 1979). The advent of photography has enabled researchers to study aspects of life that cannot be researched through other approaches: images are more telling than words. There are two categories of photographs that qualitative researchers may use: found photographs (pictures others have taken) and those that the researcher has produced.

Found Photographs. Many organizations have archives of photographs depicting groundbreaking ceremonies, outings, and other events germane to an organization. Newspapers usually have photo libraries as well as book libraries. In addition, county offices will have aerial photographs of land.

Photographs can reveal factual information that may shed light onto organizational structure. Parties may have been photographed, thus depicting who was there, seating arrangement, mistress or master of ceremonies, and general ambiance.

A photograph is like all other forms of qualitative data: to use it, the investigator should place it within the proper context and understand what it is capable of telling. Photographs can represent the photographer's point of view, a superior's orders, or even the subject's demands. This can present valuable information in that when photographs are studied, clues are ascertained as to what people value by the images they prefer. These add to the evidence that the other qualitative techniques have enabled the investigator to gather.

Photographs may present anomalies: images that do not fit the theoretical constructs that the investigator has been forming. This can enhance the researcher's analysis and insights and even alter preconceived notions about the subject. Researchers may utilize photographs to discern how people define their world: what people take for granted, what they assume is unquestionable, and what organizational assumptions exist.

Researcher-Produced Photographs. Investigators can collect factual information by using photographs to depict utilization of facilities. The technique requires the use of hidden cameras, but it is a technique that is acceptable. Participant observers take photographs in the course of the study so they can more accurately recall events, activities, people, what they were wearing, seating arrangements, and so on.

There are the usual advantages, disadvantages, and cautions when researchers are about to use photography as a data-collection technique. In certain instances picture-taking may inhibit the establishment of rapport (the researcher appears to be an outsider), and there are other occasions when it is advantageous to developing rapport (other cultures may feel a sense of pride at being asked to pose—this serves as a discussion tool). We recommend that you do not take pictures at the very beginning of a project but wait until you have established rapport; you might even wait until subjects themselves start snapping—thus giving you a chance to join in the photography session.

Photographs, whether found or taken by the investigator, can serve as a tool for enabling the researcher to better understand the values and inner workings of the organization or program being studied. Photography can be a researcher's tool as well as a cultural product.

Official Statistics

Quantitative data that have already been collected can serve to help qualitative researchers in that the data may suggest trends (e.g., the Wellness Center has had five coordinators in four years) and also provide descriptive statistics (e.g., age, sex, race, and socioeconomic status of Wellness Center staff). In addition, hypotheses may be broadened and/or delineated dependent upon what the official statistics delineate.

Qualitative researchers tend to be critical of quantitative statistics because they are asking questions that cannot easily be answered with numbers: "Rather than relying upon quantitative data as an avenue to accurately describe reality, qualitative researchers are concerned with how enumeration is used by subjects in constructing reality. They are interested in how statistics reveal subjects' common-sense understanding" (Bogdan & Biklin, 1998, p. 118).

Types of Official Statistics. There are several different kinds of official documents that provide statistics for researchers. They include census documents; health statistics provided by insurance companies; statistics provided by voluntary health organizations; and personality inventories provided by hospitals, schools, clinics, personnel departments, and social service agencies. For the purpose of brevity, we will discuss census documents and other directories that can provide data for the qualitative research.

Census surveys are conducted every 10 years in the United States. They supposedly enumerate every person living in the country. (The first modern U.S. census was taken in 1790.) These massive undertakings are computed to make sure that apportionment of government representatives remains accurate and truly representative, and to provide data for a wide variety of research interests. The census asks general questions regarding age, sex, socioeconomic standing, number of people living in a household, and the like. It should be noted here that not all households are asked the same questions, because the census, at times, uses sampling to gather some of its information.

Directories are another source of vital statistics that can be valuable to the investigator. Telephone directories and city directories usually have information that is needed and useful when conducting a study. City directories usually list the name, address, and occupation of a person, but these are not representative of the population because people have to agree to be listed in the directory. There are also professional directories, such as the *American Association of Sex Educators, Counselors, and Therapists Directory*. These are compendiums that may include brief biographies, which will be helpful to the researcher.

Occupational directories, such as the *Dental Association Directory*, can provide information that allows construction of indexes to compare cities. This has been especially useful in depicting utilization and placement of physicians. There are also a vast array of *Who's Who* directories, many with regional and professional classifications. In addition, county and state governments keep records that provide information concerning financial transactions. These include automobile registration, pet ownership, collected fines, and residential taxes.

Problems in Using Statistical Records. There are several problems inherent in amassing voluminous amounts of data, which the qualitative researcher should take into account.

1. *Data collection methods:* For example, the reporting of deaths in a region is created locally and may not mean the same thing to the entire universe. Undercounting is another problem inherent in data collection.
2. *Ambiguous terms:* Categorical definitions that are used by governmental agencies are not always used in the same way by nongovernmental agencies. Boundaries of districts and regions may change as the population changes. In addition, technical definitions (for example, the U.S. census defines an urban area as a town of at least 2,500 people) do not always coincide with common usage of these terms.
3. *Bias:* Lists for directories are not assembled for research purposes, and are not usually completed with the care of accuracy necessary for a research project. Professional directories might be incomplete because a fee was charged for inclusion, which causes a bias in the reporting.

Official records and statistics can be an invaluable aid for the qualitative researcher. Easy access to a great deal of information may enable an investigator to get a good picture or sense of an organization or of the place where that organization exists. As with any compilation of large amounts of data, cautions must be observed in the use of these compendiums. While we have reported on only a few types of census-like compilations, the U.S. government garners many special subtopic reports from the census and other mass surveys.

Analyzing Qualitative Data

After collecting reams of data, most of it containing voluminous words, the researcher asks, "How can I make sense of this mess?" What needs to be done then is to make coherent sense out of these many pages of words. The qualitative investigator will look in the data for themes and patterns that might help construct and/or support hypotheses.

Recognizing Themes and Constructing Hypotheses

Taylor and Bogdan (1998) offer the following suggestions for constructing hypotheses and recognizing themes:

1. *Read the notes carefully:* Read everything, even notes of minor incidents, very carefully. Write margin notes recording possible patterns and trends leading to themes and hypotheses.
2. *Construct typologies:* These are classification schemes that can be useful when formulating hypotheses. They are formed by denoting how your subjects classify people and behavior and the differences between and among subjects that allow them to be classified.
3. *Read the relevant literature:* Consult the professional literature to compare the literature findings with what is beginning to appear in your data. In addition, utilize the concepts, models, and paradigms of others.
4. *Code important conversation topics:* Code those conversation topics that keep recurring. (Coding will be discussed below.)

It is very important that the researcher be able to determine common threads and themes through analysis of the data. This process then leads to hypotheses formulation and support for those hypotheses. To accomplish what at times seems like an insurmountable task, the investigator must develop a coding mechanism by which to organize and assemble the data.

Coding the Data. Once the notes have been reread, typologies constructed, and literature reviewed, an elaborate coding system must be devised. This system will serve to organize and assemble the mounds of data that have been collected. When

TABLE 8.3 **Section of a Coding Sheet**

Administrative Hierarchy (AH)	AH (DUR) (END)	2.1
Style = ST	AH–ST	2.1.2
Role = RO	AH–RO	2.1.3
Demeanor = DR	AH–DR	2.1.4
Subject use = SU	AH–SU	2.1.5

the review of the notes commences, the investigator makes notes and begins to code as described in the previous section. There are several types of codes, including (1) descriptive; and (2) explanatory. *Descriptive* codes do not require interpretation but indicate a class of phenomenon in the notes. As an example, in our case study, Steven would note "PERS" in the margin to denote "personality" wherever appropriate. This will enable him to quickly note where all relevant personality notes appear in the text.

Explanatory codes indicate where patterns or themes have emerged. Steven could use "PAT" (pattern) or "TH" (theme) to indicate an administrative style that he has seen as evident in the data. Codes, no matter which kind, tend to pull the data together and make sense of the field notes.

Creating the Code.   There are several methods to help the investigator create the code. Miles and Huberman (1994) suggest devising a *start list* previous to doing fieldwork. The list develops from the conceptual framework—the list of research questions, problem areas, and key variables that were determined at the beginning of the study. Usually, a master code is developed. For example, in our case study, "ADM ST" might mean "administrative style," and "AUT" (for "autocratic") might be a subcode under ADM ST. This list may have as many as 90 codes and should be kept on one piece of paper for easy reference. Table 8.3 is an example of a section of a code sheet. The first column denotes a descriptive level for the general categories, the second column indicates the code, and the third column keys the code to the research question from which it derives.

Bogdan and Biklin (1998) suggest other items to be considered when determining coding subsections:

1. *Setting/context:* information on surroundings
2. *Definition of the situation:* how people define the setting
3. *Perspectives of subjects:* ways of thinking, orientation
4. *Ways of thinking about people and objects:* subjects' understanding of each other, of outsiders, and objects that are included in their world
5. *Process:* categorizing events, changes over time, and flow
6. *Activities:* regularly occurring kinds of behavior
7. *Events:* specific activities
8. *Strategies:* tactics, methods, techniques, plays, and other conscious ways subjects accomplish things
9. *Relationship and social structure:* behaviors not officially defined by the organization
10. *Methods:* material pertinent to research-related issues

These coding patterns can enable the investigator to think about the categories for which codes are to be developed. This method has its advantages and disadvantages over the start list. However, it is recommended that the researcher find the coding method that is easiest to work with and that will provide the most complete listing of codes to organize the data.

Data Organization. Now that the investigator has developed a coding system, the mechanics of actually going through the data and organizing them becomes the main task. The first step is to number all the pages of data so that the location of sources is easily accessible. Numbering the data in chronological order of their occurrence is a good way to sequence the data.

A second step is to begin coding the data using any of the methods previously discussed, or even one that the investigator may construct on his or her own. After the coding categories have been designed, the third step is to go through the data and mark each paragraph (or sentence) using the appropriate coding category. The fourth step is to sort the data.

Sorting the Data. Bogdan and Biklin (1998, p. 171) have several recommendations for sorting data and encourage researchers to utilize the method that is best suited to them and the data:

1. *Cut up and put in folders:* After creating a manila folder for each coding category, cut the field notes apart and file them in the appropriate folder. Go through all the notes, placing a number next to each coded unit of data that corresponds to the number of the page it is on. It is less confusing if you circle that number or in some way mark it so you do not confuse the coding numbers with the page numbers. The page numbers enable you to refer back to the master copy if confusion arises concerning the original context.
2. *File cards:* To utilize this method, each line on the pages on which the original field notes were written must be numbered consecutively. In addition, a stack of notecards with the code number and corresponding phrase and word written on the top is needed. Record on each card on what page and on what lines on that page the data relevant to the category can be found.
3. *Information retrieval cards:* These cards are available at most college book stores; two brands are McBee and Indecks. Each card contains a large space where data is typed according to each paragraph or sentence. Each card comes with the same numbered holes around the rim. After each paragraph or sentence is typed on the card, cut off all holes except those that correspond to the number of the coding categories to which the sentence or paragraph pertains. After all data have been transferred to the cards, place them in the box that originally held them. The box has the same dimensions as the face of the card, and thus the holes with the numbers line up perfectly. A long, needle-like instrument, which comes with the cards and box, is used to pull cards out of the box. Line up the cards and pass the needle through the hole that corresponds to the category and pull on the handle. The cards not wanted fall off, and the others are available for study.

Each method of sorting the data has advantages and disadvantages that should be obvious. A researcher may try all three of the methods discussed, at different times, to find out which is most appropriate.

The analysis of qualitative data can be a taxing and tedious task, and at the same time the most rewarding. Hypothesis construction and the recognition of themes are the primary reasons for analyzing the data. Coding of the data enables the researcher to organize the substantial amount of data collected. Once the data have been coded, they then have to be sorted so that themes, patterns, categories, and trends can become evident.

Using Computers in Data Analysis

With the advent of computer programs to assist in analyzing qualitatively collected data, such tasks as those listed below can be made easier (Miles & Huberman, 1994, p. 44):

- Making notes in the field
- Writing up or transcribing field notes
- Editing: correcting, extending, or revising field notes
- Coding: attaching key words or tags to segments of text to permit later retrieval
- Storage: keeping text in an organized database
- Search and retrieval: locating relevant segments of text and making them available for inspection
- Data "linking": connecting relevant data segments to each other, forming categories, clusters, or networks of information
- Memoing: writing reflective commentaries on some aspect of the data as a basis for deeper analysis
- Content analysis: counting frequencies, sequences, or locations of words and phrases
- Data display: placing selected or reduced data in a condensed, organized format, such as a matrix or network, for inspection
- Conclusion drawing and verification: aiding the analyst in interpreting displayed data and in testing or confirming findings
- Theory-building: developing systematic, conceptually coherent explanations of findings; testing hypotheses.
- Graphic mapping: creating diagrams that depict findings or theories
- Preparing interim and final reports

The programs used in data analysis can be categorized into five major types (Weitzman & Miles, 1995):

1. Text retrievers (examples: Metamorph, Orbis, Sonar Professional, The Text Collector, Word Cruncher, ZyINDEX)
2. Textbase managers (examples: ask Sam, Folio VIEWS, MAX, Tabletop)

3. Code-and-retrieve programs (examples: HyperQual2, Kwalitan, Martin, QUALPRO, The Ethnograph)
4. Code-based theory-builders (examples: AQUAD, ATLAS/ti, HyperRE-SEARCH, NUD.IST, QCA)
5. Conceptual network-builders (examples: Inspiration, MECA, Meta Design, SemNet)

Choosing the appropriate computer program is an important part of the data analysis. You should consult with professionals who have utilized these types of programs to determine which program or programs will best suit your research needs.

Case Discussion

Steven, the project director of the study to determine the efficacy of a hospital's Wellness Center, has a highly skilled team of professionals who are familiar with qualitative methodologies. They decided to utilize computer programs to assist them in coding and retrieving their data. The program they chose was Ethnograph, as they believed this program was most appropriate for their project. The project team utilized a variety of mechanisms for collecting the data as discussed throughout the chapter.

Summary

Qualitative research is an approach utilized to collect data and report the findings. It differs from quantifiable methods by having as its main goals the description of multiple realities; development of sensitizing concepts; and understanding of a particular program, organization, or setting. The designs used are generally flexible, and they evolve as the study progresses. Data come in different forms: field notes, official statistics, personal documents, photographs, and subjects' written words. Methodologies used are observation, participant observation, ethnomethodology, and document study. The samples utilized are usually nonrepresentative and small. Analysis of the data is very time-consuming because it is done by hand, without the aid of mechanical devices (computers).

There are several problems in using qualitative research methodologies. These include the fact that (1) the data reduction is difficult; (2) large populations are not easily studied using this approach; (3) the procedures are not stabilized; (4) reliability is subjective; and (5) the method is very time-consuming. However, qualitative approaches are very useful when a researcher wants to study naturalistic settings such as schools, hospitals, organizations, and the like. In our case study, the consortium Health Data Analysts decided quite appropriately to utilize qualitative methods to study the efficacy of the hospital's Wellness Center.

Suggested Activities

1. Devise a list of topics that could be studied utilizing the qualitative approach.

2. Conduct a literature search on one of the topics in your answer to Activity 1 and attempt to set up a coding system for those citations.

3. Describe, in detail, a situation wherein you could be a participant observer. What are the steps you would take, from the conception of the idea to the completion of the data analysis?

4. One of your assignments in your health evaluation class is to collect qualitative data about pharmaceuticals related to the relief of pain from arthritis. You are to use only the Web. Detail how you would go about collecting the appropriate data, and list the websites that were most beneficial.

5. Utilizing your library's on-line capabilities, create an annotated bibliography of the most recent (1998–present) sources concerning qualitative data collection for the health sciences. Which sources would you recommend? Why?

References

Bailey, K. (1994). *Methods of social research* (2d ed.). New York: Free Press.

Becker, H. (1978). Do photographs tell the truth? *After Image, 5,* 9–13.

Berg, B. (2001). *Qualitative research methods for the social sciences.* Boston: Allyn & Bacon.

Bickman, L. (1981). Observational methods. In C. Selitz, L. Wrightsman, & S. Cook (Eds.), *Research methods in social relations.* New York: Holt, Rinehart and Winston.

Bogdan, R., & Biklin, S. (1998). *Qualitative research in education* (3d ed.). Boston: Allyn & Bacon.

Bogdewic, S. (1999). Participant observation. In B. Crabtree & M. Miller (Eds.), *Doing qualitative research* (2d ed.). Newbury Park, CA: Sage.

Denzin, N. (1989). *The research act: A theoretical introduction to sociological methods.* Englewood Cliffs, NJ: Prentice-Hall.

Gall, M., Borg, W., & Gall, J. (1996). *Educational research* (6th ed.). New York: Longman.

Garfinkel, H. (1967). *Studies in ethnomethodology.* Englewood Cliffs, NJ: Prentice-Hall.

Garfinkel, H., & Sacks, H. (1970). On formal structure of practical action. In J. McKinney & E. Teryakian (Eds.), *Theoretical sociology* (pp. 338–366). New York: Appleton-Century-Crofts.

Glaser, B., & Strauss, A. (1967). *The discovery of grounded theory: Strategies for qualitative research.* Chicago: Aldine.

Glesne, C., & Peshkin, A. (1998). *Becoming qualitative researchers.* New York: Longman.

Hartman, D., & Wood, D. (1990). Observational methods. In A. Bellack, M. Harsen, & A. Kazdin (Eds.), *International handbook of behavior modification and therapy.* New York: Plenum.

Junker, B. (1960). *Field work: An introduction to the social sciences.* Chicago: University of Chicago Press.

Lofland, J. (1995). *Analyzing social settings.* Belmont, CA: Wadsworth.

Mead, G. H. (1934). *Mind, self, and society.* Chicago: University of Chicago Press.

Miles, M., & Huberman, A. (1994). *Qualitative data analysis: An expanded sourcebook.* Thousand Oaks, CA: Sage.

Patton, M. (1990). *Qualitative evaluation and research methods.* Newbury Park, CA: Sage.

Riis, J. (1980). *How the other half lives.* New York: C. Scribner's Sons.

Stott, W. (1973). *Documentary expression and thirties America.* New York: Oxford University Press.

Taylor, S., & Bogdan, R. (1998). *Introduction to qualitative research methods.* New York: Wiley.

Thomas, J. (1993). *Doing critical ethnography.* Newbury Park, CA: Sage.

Thomas, W. (1923). *The unadjusted girl.* New York: Harper & Row.

Thomas, W., & Znaniecki, F. (1927). *The Polish peasant in Europe and America.* New York: Alfred A. Knopf.

Thomson, J., & Smith, A. (1877). *Street life in London.* London: Sampson Low, Murston, Searle and Rurington.

Wagner, J. (Ed.). (1979). *Image of information.* Beverly Hills: Sage.

Walizer, M., & Wienir, P. (1978). *Research methods and analysis.* New York: Harper & Row.

Weitzman, E., & Miles, M. (1995). *Computer programs for qualitative data analysis.* Thousand Oaks, CA: Sage.

Wieder, D. (1974). Telling the code. In R. Turner (Ed.), *Ethnomethodology.* Baltimore: Penguin.

Chapter 9

Evaluation Research

Case Study

Rosewood Hospital has had a cardiac rehabilitation program for two years. A new chief of staff is searching for cost-cutting measures and has asked for an evaluation of the cardiac rehabilitation program. The chief of staff sought proposals from agencies, universities, and other groups to evaluate the program. The evaluation contract was eventually awarded to the Department of Community Health at the University of Dover. The department's evaluation team was headed by Sarah, a professor with experience in hospital-based evaluations.

Introduction

Evaluation research is yet another type of research that health scientists utilize for a myriad of reasons. Usually in evaluation research, scientists seek to determine if a program's goals and objectives have been achieved. Evaluation research has been defined as:

1. The application of scientific principles, methods, and theories to identify, describe, conceptualize, measure, predict, change, and control those factors or variables important to the development of effective human service delivery systems (Streuning & Brewer, 1983, p. 211)
2. The systematic application of social research procedures in assessing the conceptualization, design, implementation, and utility of social intervention programs (Rossi, Freeman, & Lipsey, 1999, p. 20)
3. An evaluation using an experimental or quasi-experimental design conducted to establish the efficacy or effectiveness—internal and/or external validity—and cost effectiveness or cost benefit of an intervention among a defined

population at risk for a specific impact or outcome rate during a defined period of time (Windsor, Baranowski, Clark, & Cutter, 1994)

These definitions give us a sense of what evaluation research is about: *a process of determining the effectiveness of a program.* We emphasize *process* as opposed to product. Once the process is completed, decisions are then made about the program being evaluated. For instance, in our case study Sarah may provide information about the cardiac rehabilitation program concerning its length, duration, and cost benefits, which can provide valuable information to the chief of staff. The chief of staff may decide to improve the program's weaknesses, terminate the program, or add more funds to the program.

Purposes of Evaluation Research

As we have stated, there may be many and varied reasons for a research evaluation project to be undertaken. We can look at the purposes for evaluation research from different vantage points: (1) the program evaluator; (2) the administrator; (3) the consumer or public; and (4) the organization, or in our case study, the hospital.

Sarah's team of evaluators from the University of Dover may wish to contribute to the knowledge and the discipline of evaluation research. In addition, the team may view this as a means for advancement in their area of expertise. An altruistic purpose for Sarah's group may be a belief that they can help the discipline of health science by conducting this evaluation.

The chief of staff of Rosewood Hospital may have other purposes for the evaluation, including (1) gaining control over the program, (2) bringing attention to the cardiac rehabilitation program, or (3) bringing the program to the attention of the hospital (Shortell & Richardson, 1978).

The Rosewood Hospital administration may want to be able to justify the money it spends on the program. Additionally, they may want to determine whether the program is indeed worth the expenditures and plan for its expansion. The government that helps fund the hospital may want the evaluation to ensure that its dollars are well spent. Furthermore, special interest groups, such as cardiac rehabilitation specialists, may have gotten community support for the program and therefore need to prove its worthiness.

Chelimsky (1978) describes the following purposes for evaluation research: management and administrative reasons, assessment of the appropriateness of program changes, identification of ways to improve the delivery of interventions, or accountability to funding agencies. In addition, evaluations may be completed to fulfill planning and policy purposes, to test innovative ideas, to decide if programs should be curtailed or expanded, or to support one program in lieu of another.

Whatever the purpose that underlies evaluation research, those involved in the process must be sure to accomplish the task by using appropriate methodologies, processes, and analyses. In other words, the research project must be able to be replicated by other evaluation groups.

What Can Be Evaluated?

Almost anything can be evaluated, and this usually is done in some manner or form. Listed here are some examples of things that have been or could be evaluated:

- Programs
- Drugs
- Health
- Databases (for computers)
- Lifestyles (single, married, etc.)
- Software programs
- Teaching styles
- Workshops
- Staff and personnel
- Management systems
- Organizations
- Needs-assessment strategies

Even evaluation models and schemes can be evaluated, and some have been so scrutinized. The next section will discuss some evaluation models and attempt to critique them.

Steps in Conducting Evaluation

Once Sarah was appointed to conduct an evaluation of the cardiac rehabilitation program, she had to determine a plan of action. We will use this portion of the chapter to describe the step-by-step process of setting up an evaluation of a program. Two major sources were utilized in the writing of this chapter: Rutman's *Evaluation Research Methods* (1984) and Shortell and Richardson's *Health Program Evaluation* (1978). Figure 9.1 depicts the process of evaluation. From the inception of the project to the final report, there must be interaction between the evaluator(s) and the person or group for whom the evaluation will affect: the decision-makers.

Who is the client?
What are the purposes of the evaluation?
What is the methodology to be utilized?
What is included in the contract?
How is the evaluation to be conducted?
Who will use the results of the evaluation?

FIGURE 9.1 The Evaluation Process

Although we have depicted the steps as separate entities, in reality some may be working at the same time. In other words, they are interactive.

Who Is the Client?

In our case study, Sarah has been hired by the chief of staff. Is the chief of staff the primary client, or is the hospital board the primary client? Sarah must determine the power structure of the hospital board and those persons who will be instrumental in making decisions with the added information provided by her evaluation group. She might interview the board members, or ask the chief of staff or informed health care workers to ascertain who the decision-makers are in Rosewood Hospital. This can become a cumbersome and complicated process, but one that is very worthwhile. If it does appear that the entire hospital board is the actual client, then the evaluation group must take this into consideration at every phase of the evaluation process.

What Are the Purposes of the Evaluation?

Sarah should determine the exact purposes for which the evaluation is to be undertaken. If possible, she should ascertain the covert as well as the overt reasons for conducting the study. Earlier in this chapter we discussed the major purposes of conducting an evaluation and refer you to that section for a brief review. In our case study, let us assume that the members of the hospital board and the chief of staff disagree about their evaluation goals. The board wants to know if the cardiac rehabilitation program is cost-effective and if they should keep it in lieu of other programs. Knowing the main purpose of the evaluation, the team will have the necessary insight as to what specific methodologies and techniques should be utilized to conduct the study.

What Is the Methodology to Be Utilized?

When determining the methodology to be used, the evaluator must be familiar with the purposes of the evaluation as we have discussed. We will discuss the various methods to use later on in this chapter. However, briefly, they are as follows: experimental and quasi-experimental designs, correlation, surveys, personnel assessment, expert judgment, and case study. Once the methodology is determined, it is then necessary to consider the feasibility of implementing that method. The following characteristics must be considered when determining the feasibility of the method: available funds; time schedule; availability of data; and the legal, political, ethical and administrative constraints that usually occur when conducting an evaluation.

What Is Included in the Contract?

When Rosewood Hospital sent its request for proposals (RFPs) across the nation, it specified funding levels, time frames, purpose of the study, and other information.

Once the hospital contracted with the University of Dover to perform the evaluation, Sarah had to develop a more inclusive contract between Rosewood Hospital and the evaluation team. The contract that they will develop should determine responsibilities of the evaluation team and should include:

1. A line-item budget
2. The entire scope of the evaluation
3. Details concerning the research design and data collection procedures
4. Levels of cooperation of the Rosewood Hospital board
5. Controls to ensure adherence to the evaluation plan
6. Determinations as to the publicity of the final report

How Is the Evaluation to Be Conducted?

As Rutman (1984) has so adequately explained, conducting a program evaluation entails three tasks: (1) measurement, (2) use of a particular research design, and (3) analysis of the data. Each of these areas must receive the necessary attention so that the evaluation process will produce usable results.

Measurement. The evaluation team decides on the type and amount of information that are necessary to answer the questions posed at the beginning of the study. Evaluations may obtain four categories of information: (1) program, (2) objectives and effects, (3) antecedent conditions, and (4) intervening conditions.

Program information is collected on how the program is run. Information on the process of the program can determine how the program was implemented: if it was implemented as designed; how the implementation process affected the results of the program; and whether the program was cost-effective.

Objectives and effects are the central point of evaluating programs. The extent to which a program reaches its goals and objectives can be measured in addition to the effects it has produced.

Antecedent conditions refer to the context within which the program operates, the characteristics of the client, and the background of program personnel. Antecedent information helps to interpret the findings, which enables the evaluator to determine what is most beneficial to the client; what type of personnel benefit the program best; and whether the context in which the program operates is best for meeting the program's objectives.

Intervening conditions are unplanned occurrences during the program's activities. For example, in our case study, the head teacher of the gifted health science program may leave that program, thus causing a disruption to the organization. Measurement of the impact of these intervening conditions can enable the evaluators to determine which factors help the program reach its objectives.

Another consideration is determining the methods by which the information will be collected. Data may be collected through questionnaires, interviews, observations, program documents, and official statistics. These methodologies have been discussed in detail elsewhere in this text; therefore we will not discuss them here.

Validity and reliability of instruments become important considerations. *Validity* refers to the extent to which a procedure measures what it is supposed to measure. There are several types of validity:

1. *Face validity:* On the face of it, it is obvious that the instrument measures what it purports to measure.
2. *Content validity:* The instrument will produce a reasonable sample of all possible responses, attitudes, and behaviors.
3. *Construct validity:* The extent to which scores on a proposed instrument permit inferences about underlying traits, attitudes, and behaviors.
4. *Predictive validity:* The instrument can accurately predict a future occurrence.

Reliability refers to the stability of the instrument. In other words, the same results will be consistently reproduced in subsequent administrations of the instrument. To avoid unreliability, evaluators must ensure that instruments are properly worded and administered in a consistent manner.

Research Design. Evaluation research treats research design as other types of research do—very importantly. A good research design enables researchers to ask the pertinent questions and determine the answers to those questions. In this regard Cook and Campbell (1994) state the importance of *attribution* and *generalizability* in the choice of a research design. Designs concerned about attribution (the fact that the program has produced the measured results) use several measurements, pretests and posttests, control groups, and random assignment to groups.

To ensure generalizability, the sample must comprise people who are representative of the population. In addition, the experiment should be replicable by other investigators.

Data Analysis. The final task in conducting a program evaluation is concerned with analyzing the data. For inferences to be made about the program, the correct statistical techniques need to be employed. Statistical methodologies are usually determined by the hypotheses (questions asked) and the research design. Conclusions and recommendations about the program are based on the data analysis; therefore, inappropriate techniques can lead to false or erroneous statements concerning the program.

Who Will Use the Results of the Evaluation?

At the beginning of this section we described the importance of determining who the decision-maker(s) will be or who the client is. The decision-makers will utilize the study's findings for a multiplicity of reasons. Therefore, it is imperative that the decision-makers are involved in the evaluation so they will feel a commitment to use the findings of the project. It is anticipated that if the many groups that have a stake in the program (in our case study, members of the hospital board, chief of staff, health care workers, patients, and administrators) receive information about the process and outcome of the program, then more appropriate decisions can be made concerning the program.

The steps in conducting an evaluation have been discussed with the idea that they are interactive with each other. The evaluation team should determine, in advance, a well-conceived plan of action to carry out the evaluation. Communication with pertinent personnel is of utmost importance when these procedures are drawn up. Planning is imperative, no matter the type of evaluation research.

Evaluation Models

Evaluation research dates as far back as 2200 B.C., when the Chinese emperor insisted that all of his public officials pass proficiency tests. Would that be possible today? Testing seems to have stimulated the evaluation movement when Alfred Binet was asked by France's public instruction minister to devise a test to screen for mentally disabled children in the classrooms. This test became the basis for the IQ tests currently in use in the United States. With time, evaluation and measurement took a firm foothold in science. Individual differences were characterized by evaluation studies, and toward the middle of the twentieth century evaluation strategies began to concentrate on groups, organizations, and curricula. The following discussion depicts several evaluation models and explains advantages and disadvantages of each model.

The Behavioral Objectives Model

The behavioral objectives model, advanced by Tyler (1949), Mager (1962), Bloom (1984), Suchman (1976), and Popham (1993), starts with a program's goals and collects data to determine if these goals were met. The program's success is measured by the outcomes of the program in relationship to the stated goals. The field of education has had much to do with this model, because Tyler (1949) defined educational goals in terms of student behaviors. These student behaviors were then assessed to determine if modifications or refinements in the curriculum were needed. The behavioral objective approach, as proposed by Tyler, included the following steps:

1. Derive a pool of candidates by examining learner studies and by soliciting suggestions from content specialists.
2. Pass the pool of candidates through a series of three screens: philosophical, psychological, and experimental.
3. Put the candidates who survive the screening process into a matrix whose rows depict the content areas and whose columns depict the student behaviors expected in relation to the content areas. The individual matrix cells represent individual objectives.

4. Identify situations in which students can express the behaviors mentioned in the objectives.
5. Develop instruments that can test each objective.
6. Apply the instrument, in pretest and posttest paradigms, so that behavioral changes assigned to the curriculum can be measured.
7. Examine the results to determine the strengths and weaknesses of the curriculum.
8. Develop the hypotheses that account for the pattern of the strengths and weaknesses.
9. Modify the curriculum and begin the process once more.

Tyler's approach led the way for program and organizational evaluations, in addition to the individual evaluations that were being conducted before Tyler came upon the evaluation research scene. In the health sciences, this model has been used in the area of dental health by the American Dental Association. More recently, his model has taken on additional refinements in the form of criterion-referenced tests, in which objectives are first set, and then the tests are based on that set of objectives. In addition, competency testing has become popular in many states. Here, objectives that are the basis for a test serve as the minimal objectives for a particular grade level. In other words, students must pass the competency test to go on to the next level or grade.

Education is not the only field in which the behavioral objective model has been used. Businesses and other organizations have utilized the *management-by-objectives* (MBO) approach, whereby personnel determine their own objectives and then are evaluated on the basis of how well they met those predetermined objectives. In the public health arena, Suchman (1976) wrote a book using a goal-based approach in which he identified goal activity and put it into operation. The reader was to assess the effect of the goal operation, form a value about that goal, set the goals and objectives, and finally measure those goals. Suchman (1976) said, "The most identifying feature of evaluative research is the presence of some goal or objective whose measure of attainment constitutes the main focus of the research problem" (p. 37).

This model has its *weaknesses* in that questions usually arise concerning who sets the goals and objectives, whose interests they represent, whether the goals really are a complete set of the desired behaviors, how these goals can be measured, and whether important outcomes are reflected by the respecification of objectives (House, 1999). These questions or inherent problems of this approach must be carefully thought out before one embarks upon a behavioral objectives model toward evaluation.

A *strength* of the behavioral objectives approach is that it provides validity. As we discussed in Chapter 5, *validity* means that the program, or instrument, does what it claims to do. By applying this model, the objectives should be directly linked to the measured outcomes of the program. A second advantage is that this model enables the evaluator to have a set plan of action by establishing predetermined steps to be taken.

The Systems Analysis Model

In the systems analysis model, a few output measures are determined, and then the differences in programs or their policies are measured as they vary against the predetermined indicators. This model had its roots in the Department of Defense and in what was once called the Department of Health, Education, and Welfare, and is now called the Department of Health and Human Services.

When the U.S. government began utilizing this model, it was to evaluate Title I, a program that provides funds for disadvantaged youth. There were 30,000 projects to be evaluated by using test scores as the measure of success. The results were to be reported in a normal curve and aggregated at the state and national levels. These evaluations led the government to act concerning certain programs. What developed was a systems approach to a cost-benefit analysis that would compare programs.

Cost-benefit analysis is a distinct and difficult methodology to undertake, even for a governmental organization. The goals are predetermined, and then the outcomes of the program are measured. Once the outcomes have been measured, the programs then must be compared on a cost level, which should determine the best outcome for the least amount of money.

Systems analysis can be used for evaluating management and planning procedures, policy structure, and budget procedures. Rossi et al. (1999) ask the following questions when preparing an evaluation:

1. Does the intervention reach the target population?
2. Is the intervention implemented in the manner specified?
3. Is the intervention effective?
4. How much does the intervention cost?
5. What are the intervention's costs relative to its effectiveness?

These types of evaluations must be very objective and leave no room for the commonsense type of qualitative research discussed previously. It is obvious that the social scientist's method of conducting this type of evaluation is relied upon very heavily. These evaluations usually can produce realistic evidence, which should be able to be duplicated by other researchers. A comprehensive evaluation can illuminate facts about program planning, program monitoring, impact assessment, and economic efficiency (House, 1999).

This model has been used with great success by many economists, especially within the governmental sector of our nation. Evaluators utilizing the systems-analysis model have a preconceived notion as to the function of the program under scrutiny. The role and function of that program have been well delineated by the government, thus enabling the evaluative researcher to answer concrete questions relative to that program. This model has recently begun to be used in the health science area. Investigators attempt to determine the cost-effectiveness of a program, such as a hospital's patient-education program. In our case study,

Sarah would most certainly choose this method as one of many to evaluate the program.

The major *disadvantage* of this model is that, because it is utilized so often by governmental agencies, it excludes the interest and concerns of the program participants. In an excellent critique of this model, House (1999) claims:

> At its worst, the systems analysis approach leads to scientism—the view that the only way to the truth is through certain methodologies. Objectivity is equated with reliability, with producing information from only certain types of instruments. Impartiality and validity are sacrificed. In reducing everything to a few indicators so that one can demonstrate reliability, do cost-benefit analysis, and discover the most efficient programs (thus maximize utilities), the outcomes of complex social programs are narrowed to a few quantitative measures. (pp. 226–227)

At times, the systems-analysis model takes an almost hard, cold approach to evaluation, and seems to not consider the human, social context of the program or organization.

There are *advantages* to this model, especially when the evaluator is looking for simple cause-and-effect relationships. In this case, a few indicators may indeed be enough to determine those relationships. For example, the systems-analysis approach may be used to determine physician shortages in certain areas of the country. A simple count would suffice, here using one indicator. However, the evaluators must ensure not to extrapolate a possible shortage of physicians to indicate insufficient health care delivery.

The Decision-Making Model

Evaluation research made perhaps one of its largest contributions in the field of decision-making. Evaluators believed that they could enable decision-makers (e.g., program leaders, administrators) to make more informed decisions based on the data they collected. Stufflebeam (1971) developed the CIPP model to enable evaluation to contribute to the decision-making process in program development. (CIPP is an acronym for the four types of educational evaluation processes in the model: context, input, process, and product.) The model also includes three settings in which decisions are made: homeostasis, incrementalism, and neomobolism. There are additionally four types of decisions that can be made: planning, structuring, implementing, and recycling. Stufflebeam also delineated three steps in the process of evaluation: delineating, obtaining, and providing. We have chosen to discuss the types of evaluation Stufflebeam described, because they have wide implications for health science evaluation research.

Context evaluation involves analyzing a program's problems and needs (a discrepancy between a desired condition and an existing one). In our case study, Sarah might find there are 200 cardiac rehabilitation patients in the program, but has determined that there is a need, by consensus, to reduce that number to 150. Hence a *need* has emerged. Once the needs have been determined, program objectives that will alleviate that need are proposed or determined.

Input evaluation considers the resources and strategies of the program. The data that are collected during this stage of the research project enable the evaluator to make decisions regarding (1) whether equipment or resources might be too expensive; (2) whether a particular strategy could be effective in achieving the program's goals; (3) whether strategies are legally or morally acceptable; and (4) how to best utilize staff as resources.

Process evaluation begins once the program is underway. For example, Sarah will begin to observe and collect data relative to the cardiac rehabilitation program. If she were to find that program patients did not attend the sessions and had higher absentee rates than other patients, the program decision-makers may take some action based upon this information. They might encourage patients to attend cardiac rehabilitation programs in other hospitals. In addition, process evaluation methods serve to keep records of the events that occur during the program. These records should be kept over a relatively long time period so that peaks and valleys can be ascertained.

Product evaluation determines the extent to which the program's goals and objectives have been achieved. The evaluators develop measures of the goals and then administer them to the proper audiences. The results enable program administrators to make decisions concerning modifying or ending the program. There is another approach to the decision-making model, as suggested by Patton (1990). He suggests that for evaluations to be successful and relevant, the decision-makers must be identified so that the gathered information gets to the people who can implement change. A second step in conducting this type of evaluation is to identify and focus the relevant questions. The program administrators also may specify how they would use the answers to questions, and thus provide much needed input into the research study.

Decision-making approaches primarily use survey methods such as questionnaires, face-to-face interviews, and small-group discussions. The evaluator goes to the setting (for example, Sarah would go to Rosewood Hospital), but does not necessarily set up an experiment. The program administrator, or decision-maker, plays a very important role in this type of evaluation model.

The major *advantage* of this model is that the methodology selects the information that would be most useful to the evaluator. Criterion measures are predetermined, so that the evaluation is actually focused for the evaluation team. In our case study, Sarah would meet with the administrator of the cardiac rehabilitation program to help determine the questions to be asked during the evaluation process. At this point, some might believe that the decision-maker (the administrator) may have too much to say concerning the evaluation, and thus not be objective in the approach.

This leads to some *disadvantages* of the decision-making model: the administrator is preferentially treated, the evaluator becomes very close to the managers of the program, and the evaluation can become undemocratic and unfair. In addition, the identification and specification of important decisions are difficult tasks for the evaluator. Who should be included in this process? How should these people be utilized before, during, and after the evaluation?

The Goal-Free Model

The goal-free model was developed by Scriven (1973) when he was employed as one of a group of advisors to the Educational Testing Service to screen candidates for a list of innovations and developments that had been funded by the federal government, and whose evaluations proved that they were worth giving to schools. During this experience he delineated intended and unintended effects, or side effects, of a particular program. If one knew the goals of a program, this might serve as a contaminating effect. Therefore, Scriven decided that evaluations should be goal-free, and that the organizational framework of the process becomes the effects of the program, rather than the goals.

Goal-free evaluation is not widely utilized because of two factors: (1) Scriven has not given much guidance as to the procedures of the model; and (2) evaluators cannot easily find criteria to judge the program if they are not to use the administrators' or the developers' goals and objectives. It is apparent that social science areas may find it difficult to utilize this model, but one good example of its use is offered by Consumers' Union. This group typically evaluates all sorts of products using what the members believe are criteria that consumers would prefer. Goal-free evaluation uses the reference group of the consumers of programs, rather than the producers or administrators.

Scriven has developed the concept of consumers' need to be analyzed and does so through needs assessments of a particular group of people. He has insisted upon a bias-free approach when conducting the research, so the evaluator can remain as objective as possible. The techniques that are utilized include double-blind experiments, in which neither the subject nor the evaluator knows which is the treatment and which is not. Scriven describes goal-free evaluation as a triple-blind experiment in which neither of the treatments is known.

The goal-free model, though not utilized very frequently, does serve to point evaluators to the important aspect of the unintended or side effects a program may offer. Evaluators have become sensitized to the not-so-evident effects and therefore have added a richness to the field of evaluation research.

Scriven's goal-free model is implicit in reducing bias in the evaluation. Because the evaluator has no contact with program personnel and does not have an inkling as to the goals of the program, a supposedly unbiased evaluation can occur. Unfortunately, there have not been many goal-free evaluations, assumedly because of the unwillingness of administrators to allow strangers to act as investigators, or "hunters." The major *disadvantages* of the goal-free model include (1) the lack of a clear methodology as to how to approach this model; and (2) the lack of social interaction between normally social people: evaluators and administrators of human service programs.

The *advantages* of the goal-free model lie in its ability to be completely bias-free from stated or predetermined goals. Consumers' Union does evaluate products in this manner. However, we must remember that products are not processes, and it is process that concerns most evaluations in the health sciences. It appears that goal-free evaluations, in combination with other models, make a contribution to program or organizational evaluations.

The Connoisseurship Model

Connoisseurship is the art of perception that makes the appreciation of complex educational practices possible (Eisner, 1994). In this model, a judge is used to determine the effects of a program, curriculum, or educational system. Just as an art critic might write about a painting, so will the connoisseur write of program evaluations. Connoisseurship consists of recognizing and appreciating the qualities of a program, and the connoisseur writes about that program, or, in other words, renders a critique or criticism of that particular program. Sarah, in our case study, would be the connoisseur.

The connoisseur, or critic, must be an experienced evaluator who will point out the significant aspects of a program through writing about his or her feelings about the program. With such an approach there are many methodological considerations to take into account: How can one know whether a critic is to be trusted? How can one be sure that the critic is not imagining the events? How can one know what confidence to place in the critic's description, interpretation, and evaluation of a program?

Eisner (1994) does suggest that to obtain validity for this model, one should look for instances of structural corroboration, where separate pieces of evidence validate each other if they fit together to form a coherent, persuasive whole. Another way to validate the critic's findings is to ensure that the language used is referentially adequate. This can be accomplished by having other critics view the program through analysis of videotapes and audiotapes to assess if the first critic's interpretation of the material was valid.

The critic must be experienced and trained in utilizing the connoisseurship model. The evaluator becomes totally involved in the program and becomes as familiar with it as is possible. The criticism that comes about through this model will usually lead the program to improve its standards and probably perform better. Although this model is not in the traditional mode of collecting and analyzing data, it does serve to supplement other approaches and to provide additional insight to what is being evaluated.

This model, because it is very closely aligned with art criticism, provides a very impressive and expressive idea for completing an evaluation. Because this type of method has worked very well in the arts (drama, music, painting, etc.), it should prove valuable to the science of evaluation. Connoisseurship has the *advantage* of adding another way to accomplish and augment an evaluation. It provides an expert review that, although biased, can detect weaknesses, flaws, and strengths of programs and/or organizations.

However, as with all of our evaluation models, there are *disadvantages* in utilizing the model. One is that the connoisseur, who is really an expert, must decide on criteria in making judgments about programs. But how does the evaluator decide on these criteria, and how are these criteria justified to the administrator of the program? A second disadvantage is that Eisner (1994), the creator of the connoisseurship model, maintains that the evidence for the criticisms is the behavior of the teachers of programs being evaluated. If this is so, can or will teachers readily accept the criticisms? Have they?

The Case Study Model

In this model, the *process* of a program or an organization is the focus of the study. The evaluator attempts to depict the program to those involved in the program by presenting a case study. This is usually accomplished through interviews that serve the same purpose as those that ethnomethodologists conduct. You will often hear the term *naturalistic* applied to these methodologies. The major proponent of the case study model has been Stake (1991), who stated that

> case studies will often be the preferred method of research because they may be epistemologically in harmony with the reader's experience and thus to that person a natural basis for generalization. . . . If the readers of our reports are the persons who populate our houses, schools, governments, and industries; and if we are to help them understand social problems and social programs, we must perceive and communicate in a way that accommodates their present understandings. Those people have arrived at their understandings mostly through direct and vicarious experience. (p. 5)

It is evident that the case study model enables people to gain an understanding of their world through complex descriptions of that world. The methodologies utilized to collect the data are interviews, as we stated previously. However, the writing becomes very informal, with illustrations and allusions. This evaluation model has led Stake (1991) to develop and implement responsive evaluation, which will be discussed later in this chapter.

The case study model comes from the qualitative research methodologies in which participant observation, interviews, document study, field notes, and subjects' own words are used to collect and record the data. Although the case study model is similar to the connoisseurship model, there is a difference: The case study evaluator determines the perceptions of other people, whereas the connoisseur relies on only his or her own experience and values. Sarah would utilize these methodologies and act as the sole case study evaluator.

The case study model is a subjective approach to evaluation and has met with criticism as compared to the more scientific methods of evaluation. Because of the nature of the methodology of the case study, different observers will emphasize different parts of a program. This leads to the *disadvantage* of inconsistency. Another disadvantage is the interpretation made by the evaluator. The evaluator must observe all parts of a program and then draw conclusions. Whose values are the basis of these conclusions?

There are many *advantages* to the case study model. As House (1999) has stated, these include (1) obtaining rich and persuasive information from program participants and other people removed from the program; (2) representing diverse points of view and different interests; and (3) potentially being persuasive, accurate, and coherent.

Accurately depicting a case study and trying to avoid becoming personally involved can be a difficult task for any evaluator. Although this model has many advantages, it suffers from the same weakness that other models do: not having written methods and procedures.

The Accreditation Model

Many professional associations conduct evaluations of their respective professional training programs. In the area of health sciences, one of these accrediting bodies is the Council for Education in Public Health (CEPH), which accredits schools of public health and community health programs outside schools of public health. Other examples of professional reviews involve lawyers, physicians, educators, social workers, and speech and hearing therapists.

The CEPH accrediting process is similar to that of many professional organizations, so we have chosen to use it as an example. Typically, the accrediting body sets up criteria that are organized into several sections concerned with the professional training program. The approach that CEPH utilizes involves a self-study evaluation of the program. The program personnel have several months to prepare an in-depth analysis of the program and submit it to the CEPH staff.

A subcommittee of CEPH is appointed as the visiting on-site group, and they review the self-study report previous to the on-campus visit. Once on the site, the committee interviews staff, faculty, and students associated with the program being evaluated. The committee prepares a brief report and gives its findings, informally, to the program director. Typically, a few months later, a formal report is forwarded to the director with comments regarding the strengths and weaknesses of the program. The program director is then given an opportunity to correct any perceived weaknesses or devise a plan to do so. Program representatives are then invited to a meeting of the full council for a final disposition. The results of this process are then communicated to the appropriate program personnel.

Accreditations are useful in that they provide a mechanism for self-evaluation as well as simultaneous peer evaluation. Programs that have been accredited are believed to have met criteria and standards set by the profession. The accreditation model has grown as professional groups come under increased pressure to evaluate their own programs. The *advantages* of this model include (1) the self-evaluation mechanism; (2) setting of criteria and standards for a profession; (3) a continual effort at evaluation; and (4) accountability to the public. Although these advantages place a great burden on the profession in question, it seems apparent that a review of methods and procedures of professions can only help to improve that profession.

TABLE 9.1 Evaluation Models

Model	Audience or Reference Group	Methodology
Behavioral objectives	Managers, social scientists	Behavioral objectives, achievement tests
Systems analysis	Economists, managers	Cost-benefit analysis, planned variation
Decision-making	Administrators	Surveys, interviews
Goal-free	Consumers	Bias control
Connoisseurship	Consumers, connoisseurs	Critical review
Case study	Client, practitioners	Case studies, interviews, observations
Accreditation	Professionals, public	Self-study review by panel

Note. From *Evaluating with Validity* by E. House, 1999, Beverly Hills: Sage. Copyright 1980 by Sage. Adapted by permission.

The accreditation model also has its *disadvantages* in that the public has challenged the model and the process, which can bring about disharmony within the profession itself. A second limitation is the procedure that professional organizations utilize in their evaluations. The accrediting teams may not always have fair and competent people, and each team may vary when conducting a site visit. This can lead to uneven evaluations among member programs and create a system of review that does not promote equality.

Table 9.1 summarizes the evaluation models we have discussed. These models can be utilized alone or in any combination. We have attempted to give a clear description of each model with a sense of its advantages and disadvantages so that evaluators may be able to decide which model is best suited for each evaluation situation. In our case study, Sarah might appropriately choose a combination of the decision-making and case study models. Can you suggest another model that Sarah could utilize to evaluate the cardiac rehabilitation program?

Types of Evaluation Research

There are several types of evaluation research, some of which have developed from or have been precursors to the models previously discussed. We have chosen to discuss four types of evaluation research: (1) needs assessment; (2) formative;

Outcome	Typical Questions
Productivity, accountability	Is the program achieving the objectives? Is the program producing?
Efficiency	Are the expected effects being achieved? Can the effects be achieved more economically? What are the *most* efficient programs?
Effectiveness, quality control	Is the program effective? What parts of the program are effective?
Consumer choice, social utility	What are *all* the effects?
Improved standards, heightened awareness	Would a critic approve this program? Is the audience's appreciation increased?
Understanding, diversity	What does the program look like to different people?
Professional acceptance	How would professionals rate this program?

(3) summative; and (4) responsive. These types of evaluation research can be utilized in the health sciences because they have broad application in the social sciences.

Needs Assessment

Usually, a needs assessment occurs when someone at the decision-making level feels there is a discrepancy between an acceptable condition and the existent condition. In our case study, the needs assessment would have been conducted *previous* to the implementation of the cardiac rehabilitation program. Often, needs assessments are conducted at the community level: Hospitals begin wellness centers, voluntary associations set up screening programs, and public health departments determine the *need* for free services.

Public support of a program should be demonstrated before that program becomes an actuality. Recently we have seen strong support for child and partner abuse education programs, both in hospitals and other community groups. This has resulted because of the exposure of several child abuse cases involving adults who were in charge of preschools and parents who were abusing their own children, as well as attention given to partner abuse through the media. Even though there appears to be widespread support for child and partner abuse education programs, it is best to carry out a needs assessment to determine if a *specific group* would support such a program.

Needs assessment has been called front-end analysis (Harless, 1973), which means that the assessment of the needs of a program, evaluation of the program's conception, a cost estimate, determination of feasibility, and projections of demand and support are researched before the program commences. Two factors that might determine if a program is needed are frequency and intensity. If many people have a need for a program (frequency), then public support can be elicited, as in the case of the child abuse education program. In addition, if the need is seen as intense or grave, the program will receive support as well. There are some questions that researchers should consider when they are about to undertake a needs assessment (Anderson & Ball, 1978, p. 20):

1. What made us think that there were needs requiring investigation?
2. Whose needs are we talking about?
3. How can we find out whether the needs are frequent or intense enough to justify intervention?
4. How much frequency or intensity is sufficient, and how much discrepancy between acceptable state and observed state is undesirable?

Once researchers have determined to undertake a needs assessment, it becomes a fairly straightforward matter. The need has been determined; there is a discrepancy between an acceptable condition and one that now exists. Let us assume that our case study began at the needs assessment stage. Sarah was asked to evaluate a cardiac rehabilitation program. The major design would be to survey the important figures (as previously mentioned) and perhaps interview a smaller, select group. The survey would be designed so that as many issues relevant to the program would be discerned to elicit an analysis, which would compare the status of the current program with the desired program.

The final report that Sarah submits to Rosewood Hospital's board of directors and chief of staff should enable the decision-makers to be better informed about the cardiac rehabilitation program. Many specific objectives and goals of the program can be determined by the outcome of the analysis of the results.

Formative Evaluation

Scriven (1967) distinguished between two forms of evaluation: formative and summative. Formative evaluation occurs when data are being collected. This process provides information so that revisions and improvements can be made for the program. Formative evaluation can occur when instructional programs or curricula are to be evaluated. The cardiac rehabilitation program would have been a good target for formative evaluation. Industry also utilizes this type of evaluation when evaluating products during particular stages of development.

Baker (1974) describes four stages of concern when an evaluation of a new program (formative evaluation) is undertaken:

1. Determine the results of the program.
2. Diagnose the weak areas.

3. Limit the number of subjects exposed to the new, unproven program.
4. Limit the costs of the program.

Keeping these guiding principles in mind, the evaluator should then decide on what kinds of data are to be collected. Outcome data is the first category of data collection. Here, the researcher is concerned with how the program affects those people directly involved in the program. A second type of data that is to be collected is that of program implementation. How does the program operate? Is the sequence adequate? What about the presentation of the format? At this stage, weaknesses of the program may be enlightened, and thus serve as targets for revision. So the revisions will have a high probability of success, it is suggested that the data collected on program effects should be correlated with those concerning its implementation. The data collected are usually in the form of observations, questionnaires, and interviews.

Formative evaluations are usually conducted by an in-house or internal evaluator. Formative evaluators are concerned with several important questions when conducting the review (Baker, 1974). The first to consider is: *Are the instructional materials accurate?* This leads evaluators to examine the curriculum materials, instructional guides, plans, and activities to ensure that the concepts are properly presented and are accurate. For example, in the cardiac rehabilitation program, all the materials and subsequent examples would be scrutinized.

A second major concern is: *Does the content reflect an appropriate range?* The researchers would look for a broad range of materials, rather than a set of materials that represents only one point of view. For example, in our case study, it would be inappropriate for the materials to contain an overabundance of information about hydrotherapy, if that took away from a well-rounded program.

A third consideration is: *Is the product well designed instructionally?* The evaluation team has to determine if the prescribed goals and objectives of the program are being met. In addition, if the program planners had designed the program to utilize a certain learning theory, were the principles of that theory ascribed to in the delivery process of the program?

A fourth question to be asked is: *Does instruction account for all planned outcomes?* In this situation, the evaluator is faced with determining whether the outcomes, or goals, as stated by the program developers have been accomplished. In health science, we must ensure that all domains—cognitive, affective, behavioral, skills, and decision-making—are taken into account when developing and evaluating a program.

A fifth consideration is: *What is the instruction's level of quality?* Here, the program activities are judged to see if they are effective. An evaluator can determine, by assessing the participants' levels of activity and consequent outcomes, if learning opportunities meet their objectives.

A final question in the internal review of a program is: *Do things fit together?* The evaluator must ask when reading through a program: *Do references match, are page numbers accurate, are the objectives clearly met, are there typographical errors, and can the program be easily utilized by the intended user?* Once the internal review has been completed and is communicated to the program planners, it is up to them to institute the changes or make revisions.

Preliminary Field Test.   After the internal review process has been completed, the program is tried out on a small sample of potential program participants. Two areas of concern are of importance here: the *effects* of the program on the participants and the *implementation process* of the program. At this phase of the evaluation, questionnaires, observations, and tests are used to collect the data.

Participant tests are utilized to determine the outcomes of the program. These can be used in a pretest-posttest manner, or any other experimental design that is appropriate. The use of standardized tests is not recommended here, because those tests would not necessarily reflect the anticipated outcomes of a particular program. Tests also can be in the form of observing behavior and attitudes, or observing skills in decision-making.

To obtain data concerning the implementation process of the program, the evaluator can collect items completed by the participants during the program. These materials can be in the form of assignments, memos, letters, fieldwork situations, and so on. The data can be related to the participant's postprogram scores to determine any weaknesses in the program or any areas that need revision. Observational data become very useful at this stage because the evaluator can pinpoint when certain activities work, are helpful, provide enrichment, and the like. The data collected during the preliminary field test enable the evaluator to gather information regarding the program participants' reactions and to detect unplanned outcomes of the program (Baker, 1974). The evaluators then prepare a report for the program planners so that they can debug the program and get it ready for an operational field test. In this context, the program is then placed in the situation for which it was intended. At this stage, the evaluation is not as concerned with meeting program goals and objectives, but rather attention is directed toward issues of program utility, integration, and access. In our case study, Sarah must ask if the cardiac rehabilitation administrators and health care workers would become actively involved in the evaluation process.

Summative Evaluation

Once the program has been evaluated in the formative manner, summative evaluation can take place. The purpose of this type of evaluation is to access the overall effectiveness of a program and the extent to which the program is worthwhile in comparison to other, similar programs. The results of the evaluation assist decision-makers in terms of whether to adopt a particular program, utilize a product, or implement a procedure. An external evaluator usually is employed to conduct the summative evaluation. This person should be as impartial as possible and have no connection to the program whatsoever. In our case study, Sarah is conducting a summative evaluation in that she is concerned with evaluation of the cardiac rehabilitation program after it has been in effect for two years. Once Sarah completes the evaluation process, administrators and the Rosewood Hospital board will be able to determine if the program is worthwhile and if it is cost-effective for the hospital. Thus, summative evaluation can provide the consumer with an independent assessment of a program.

Summative evaluation is concerned with the impact of a program, and because of this, the researcher has to ask: impact with respect to what? Many evaluators set about conducting a summative evaluation with a behavioral objectives approach, and yet others advocate employing a goal-free approach. Once the criteria against which the program's effectiveness will be measured are chosen, the evaluator then chooses measures that reflect the chosen criteria. The researcher also is concerned with the target population, sampling, and the study design. An evaluation report usually is rendered to those who called for the evaluation. This report should indicate the successes and weaknesses of the program and should be able to point to those program features that influence successes or failures (Anderson, Ball, Murphy, & Associates, 1975).

Planning Summative Evaluations.   There have been many summative evaluations in the health sciences, especially in the area of program evaluation. There also have been summative evaluations in the medical field in which a product or procedure has been evaluated for its effectiveness. No matter the context of the evaluation, planning is a very important and vital aspect in summative evaluation. Because external evaluators are utilized, the process can be costly and very time-consuming.

Purposes of Summative Evaluation.   Anderson and Ball (1978) have delineated the various purposes of summative evaluation, which include the *monitoring of the continuing needs for the program.* At times, it can be shown that the program has met its original intent and should be disbanded. This is true in some health maintenance programs, for example, in which hypertension is under control, smoking has ceased, or weight loss has been achieved. This purpose can be achieved through collecting survey data, conducting personal assessments of the participants, and gathering expert judgments about the program.

A second purpose for summative evaluation is the *assessment of the cost-effectiveness of the program.* Sometimes it appears that it may be impossible to evaluate human effectiveness in terms of costs; for example, if a medical procedure saves one life at a high cost, is this cost-effective? An example is the use of heart transplants in very ill people. If the evaluator were to ask the recipients' family about the cost-effectiveness and then survey the general public, disagreement about the outcome would certainly become apparent. In terms of our case study, the evaluators of the cardiac rehabilitation program would address one of the following decisions:

1. Determine the least-expensive means of achieving a specified level of performance.
2. Determine the greatest level of performance that can be obtained for a specified cost.

In cost-effectiveness analysis, it is easier to determine the cost-effectiveness of a program when it is evaluated against another, similar program than it is to evaluate a program as an absolute. Sarah will have to determine which approach to take when determining the cost-effectiveness of the cardiac rehabilitation program. Methods to utilize in determining these factors include surveys and correlational status studies.

A third purpose of summative evaluation is to determine the *global effectiveness of the program in meeting the goals and objectives of that program*. Most programs have predetermined goals and objectives, and, as discussed previously, criteria and measures by which to determine the success of the programs. Factors such as long- and short-term effects also should be considered. If a program was instituted as a precursor to a more advanced program (e.g., Phase I before Phase II), the effects of the first program should be evaluated at the end of the program. On the other hand, if one of the aims of the Phase I program was to teach patients to utilize cardiac rehabilitation programs, this cannot be evaluated until the patients have a chance to choose their type of health care delivery. Long-term effects are much more difficult to evaluate because of the impracticality of following subjects over a long period of time. Methodologies that are utilized for this purpose include experimental and quasi-experimental studies.

The fourth purpose of summative evaluation involves *determining the possible side effects of a program*. Although program objectives may have been clearly delineated at the outset, other positive and negative effects may occur because of that program. For example, the cardiac rehabilitation program may have had a positive effect in keeping patients from high rates of absenteeism from the program because of their interest in the program. On the other hand, a negative, and unintended, side effect may be that some patients enrolled in the program resented it because of the time commitment they were supposed to give. Side effects can be determined by using the case study, experimental, or quasi-experimental approaches.

Responsive Evaluation

Responsive evaluation research focuses on the issues and concerns of the persons who have a stake in the evaluation, or the *stakeholders*. The evaluator *responds* to what different audiences wish to know. Stake (1998) was the first to use the term *responsive evaluation* and says the following about the method:

> An educational evaluation is responsive evaluation if it orients more directly to program activities than to program intents; responds to audience requirements for information; and if the different value perspectives present are referred to in reporting the success and failure of the program. To do a responsive evaluation, the evaluator conceives of a plan of observations and negotiations. He arranges for various persons to observe the program, and with their help prepares brief narratives, portrayals, product displays, graphs, etc. He finds out what is of value to his audiences and gathers expressions of worth from various individuals whose points of view differ. Of course, he checks the quality of his

records, he gets program personnel to react to the accuracy of his portrayals; and audience members to the relevance of his findings. He does most of this informally—iterating and keeping a record of action and reaction. He chooses media accessible to his audiences to increase the likelihood and fidelity of communication. He might prepare a final written report, he might not—depending on what he and his clients have agreed on. (p. 16)

What organizes an evaluation utilizing the responsive approach? As Stake has alluded, it is the issues and concerns of those persons the evaluator has had conversations with that will receive the attention. He has referred to other evaluation approaches as *preordinate*. The following are suggested steps that Stake (1991) enumerated. They are to be used in progression, but also may interchange as the evaluation progresses:

1. The evaluator talks with program staff, clients, and anyone else involved in the program to gain a sense of their posture with respect to the purposes of the evaluation.
2. The evaluator then places limits on the scope of the program. In addition, documents and official records will have been reviewed to help set these limits.
3. The evaluator personally observes the program in action.
4. As a result of Steps 1 through 3, the evaluator begins to discover, on the one hand, the stated and real purposes of the program, and on the other hand, the concerns that various audiences may have with it and/or the evaluation.
5. The evaluator begins to conceptualize the issues and problems that the evaluation should address.
6. Once issues and problems have been identified, the design takes some form. (This occurs very late, as is not true of other evaluation approaches, and is called an *emergent design*.)
7. The evaluator selects methods for gathering data. Stake considers the instrument as humans, in that they will be observers.
8. The data collection procedures are accomplished.
9. Once the data have been collected and processed, the evaluator goes to an information-reporting mode. The information is organized into themes, and the evaluator prepares portrayals designed to communicate naturally and provide as much direct personal experience as possible. Portrayals, in this sense, include case studies, plays, artifacts, and videotapes.
10. The evaluator matches issues and concerns to audiences in deciding what form the report will take.
11. The format of the report must be decided when reporting to each audience. The reports may be in the form of written statements, discussions, newspaper articles, and films.
12. The final step is completed when the evaluator assembles any formal reports.

It is obvious that this type of evaluation is continuous and interactive, in that at any point the evaluator could begin again because of the results found so far in the

TABLE 9.2 Comparison of Preordinate and Responsive Evaluation Models

Comparison Item	Type of Evaluation	
	Preordinate	**Responsive**
Orientation	Formal	Informal
Value perspective	Singular; consensual	Pluralistic; possibility of conflict
Basis for evaluation design (organizer)	Program intents, objectives, goals, hypotheses; evaluator preconceptions such as performance, mastery, ability, aptitude, measurable outcomes; the instrumental values of education	Audience concerns and issues; program activities; reactions, motivations, or problems of persons in and around the evaluation
Design completed when?	At beginning of evaluation	Never—continuously evolving
Evaluator role	Stimulator of subjects with a view to testing critical performance	Stimulated by subjects and activities
Methods	Objective; "taking readings" (for example, testing)	Subjective; negotiations and interactions (for example, observations and interviews)
Communication	Formal; reports; typically one-stage	Informal; portrayals; often two-stage
Feedback	At discrete intervals; often only once at end	Informal; continuously evolving as needed by audiences
Form of feedback	Written report, identifying variables and depicting the relationships among them; symbolic interpretation	Narrative-type depiction, often oral (if that is what the audience prefers), modeling what the program is like, providing vicarious experience, "holistic communication"
Paradigm	Experimental psychology	Anthropology, journalism, poetry

Note. From *Fourth-Generation Evaluation* by E. Guba & Y. Lincoln, 1999, Newbury Park, CA: Sage. Copyright 1989 by Sage. Adapted by permission.

process. There may be new issues and concerns that have been discovered through the evaluation process. Table 9.2 summarizes the preordinate evaluation approaches in comparison to those of responsive evaluation.

Methodological Approaches in Evaluation Research

Although we have discussed the various methodologies used in other types of research, it is important that methodological approaches be explained with specific respect to those used in evaluation research. The methods that will be discussed include: experimental and quasi-experimental designs, correlation, surveys, personnel assessment, expert judgment, and case study.

Experimental and Quasi-Experimental Designs

True experimental designs will enable evaluators to assess absolute answers to questions they have conceived. If, for example, a curriculum was being evaluated for teaching students the cognitive skills in anatomy, then a true experimental design should be utilized. Randomization, an issue discussed at great length elsewhere in this text, also should be employed. The evaluator should decide to use the classroom, client, program, or school as the unit of randomization, because this provides a much stronger design than a nonrandomized study.

Quasi-experiments are usually used when randomization is not feasible. As an alternative to randomizing subjects, matching them or using a statistical technique (analysis of covariance) may suffice. Evaluators may want to generalize their results to other, similar groups, such as the success (or failure) of a preschool program. Therefore, in this instance, generalizability is very important and should be carefully considered when setting up the study design. Quasi-experimental designs include time series and the pretest-posttest nonequivalent control group design. The regression-discontinuity design (Anderson et al., 1975) is frequently utilized in evaluation research. Here, comparison groups that differ from the treatment group in one significant and continuous dimension are chosen. An example of this would be a control group that differed significantly in family income.

Correlation

Correlational methods are utilized frequently by evaluators, and sometimes without justification for the reported results. Correlations do not imply cause and effect, and researchers must take precautions not to make such inferences. Regression analyses, however, have proved to be helpful in determining the formative evaluation aspects of a study in which the positive and negative aspects of the program can be compared. Correlations can be utilized in the typical experimental control group design, in which measures are compared to the pretest scores. In addition, correlations between costs and program-effectiveness indices across several programs, or even parts of a program, could be utilized to determine the continuation or modification of a program (Anderson & Ball, 1978).

Surveys

Surveys, which are a major type of evaluation research, are the primary instruments utilized to collect the necessary data in a needs assessment. Surveys can include interviewing (telephone, individual, group), observations, questionnaires, and analysis of program records. There are some general facets to interviewing, questionnaire design, and observations that should be regarded by evaluation re-searchers:

1. Provide the appropriate reading level in the questionnaire.
2. Avoid sensitive or ambiguous questions.
3. Match the interviewer with the interviewee.
4. Ensure that the questions are relevant and remain on task as to the purpose of the survey.

These are discussed in greater detail in Chapter 6, on survey research.

Personnel Assessment

Personnel assessment is especially useful for determining the context of the program being evaluated. The administrative structure and procedures of the program can be ascertained by surveying (as above) the personnel involved in the practice of administration. Data about staff roles, relationships, responsibilities, in-service training, hiring and firing procedures, policies for internal evaluation for remuneration, and the like can be gathered using personnel assessment.

The actual collection of this type of data varies from program to program and within the context of that program. There are many cognitive, affective, behavioral, psychological, and physiological instruments available for use. However, even though these tests may be standardized, we recommend them with caution, and ascribe to the tenet that most instruments for program evaluation should be tailored for each program.

Expert Judgment

Expert judgment can come in three or more forms, including: (1) the evaluators as experts; (2) the program staff as experts; and (3) outside panels of experts. The evaluation researcher and the evaluation team can and should be considered experts. They will have to make important decisions concerning design, data collection, interpretation, and the like. With their experience and education, they should be, and usually are, accountable and responsible for the decisions they render.

The program staff that is being evaluated can serve as experts as well. They can give first-hand observations, thoughts, and beliefs about the program. Although they at times may appear to be too close to the program to be objective, recurrent themes can be deduced from the many data sources. These themes will provide invaluable information to the evaluation team.

External experts can be very helpful to the evaluation process. They can be especially useful when the goal is to estimate cost-effectiveness of programs. In these instances, economists or other social scientists familiar with cost-effectiveness determinations can be called upon for their expert advice and judgment. In addition, if documented support for the program is necessary, outside experts, political and professional, may be called upon to provide documentation of the merits and the worth of the program.

Case Study

The case study approach has been discussed in detail elsewhere. In evaluation research, as in other types of research, the case study is very valuable in determining the effectiveness, merit, and worth of programs or organizations. Usually, the evaluator or the team will determine how the case study should be conducted, when it should occur, and which elements are necessary for inclusion in this methodological approach.

A case study can help determine if a program should be initiated, continued, or expanded. It can also help diagnose weaknesses and strengths of a program so that modifications can be instituted. And finally, this methodology can enable the evaluator to establish the process of how and why the program operates.

The methodological approaches discussed in the preceding chapter were illuminated in light of evaluation research. While these approaches are useful and important in other types of research, their uniqueness is apparent to evaluation research. It should be noted here that several methods may be used in any one evaluation project, as they each contribute to the total process.

New Methodological Approaches

Evaluation researchers have recently begun to use several methodologies in their studies. These include simulation modeling, cost analysis, and contextual evaluation. While these methodologies may have been utilized in other types of research, evaluation researchers have seen the advantages of these methods.

Simulation Modeling. A simulation model enables one to understand how and why an intervention works or should work. Several characteristics make simulation modeling a valuable tool for evaluation research (Cooper & Huss, 1981). The first is that simulation modeling requires the investigator to make explicit assumptions regarding the system to be studied. Simulation modeling assists this effort by simulating alternatives or variations to raise assumptions. The second characteristic is that the model can create conditions that would otherwise be difficult, hazardous, or unlikely to occur. These types of models are frequently used in nuclear reactor coding systems. A third use of simulation modeling is that events not under the control of social scientists can be studied. The barriers may be costs or ethics that are beyond the control of the investigator. And finally, the simulation model can be utilized to forecast future conditions, guide future allocations of funding, select optional populations for the program, or evaluate additional program alternatives before implementation. Simulation modeling usually begins from theory, builds up the causal links, and then produces results that can be compared with other data to test the reasonableness of the modeled theory. An example of simulation models that have been utilized in the health sciences is the health risk appraisal. The health risk appraisal is a tool that can describe an individual's chance of becoming ill or dying from some cause over a period of time. Most health risk appraisals are statements of probability of a disease, rather than detection or diagnosis. These kinds of appraisals have been in existence since the eighteenth century, when health professionals began associating specific illnesses with certain occupations. These appraisals did not have a scientific base, as they were made by observing patients. Since that time, the creators of the health risk appraisals have improved the scientific base of the tools in demonstrating the relationship between certain risk factors and specific causes of death or disability. A health risk appraisal is:

1. A method or tool that describes an individual's chance of becoming ill or dying from a select cause over a specific period of time, as compared to either (a) the population as a whole; or (b) some similar subset of the population, such as those people of the same age, race, and sex
2. A technique that is in a relatively early stage of development and most useful for middle-class white people
3. Is most often intended to:
   a. Raise an individual's and/or group's level of awareness and knowledge of personal risk factors and potential health outcomes.
   b. Serve as a vehicle for health education and counseling in order to promote voluntary health-related behavior change.
   c. Serve as a group needs assessment instrument for planning health education/health promotion programs.

There are two major types of health risk appraisals: self-scored and computer-analyzed. The computerized health risk appraisal gives an estimate of risk based upon physiological (e.g., blood pressure), biochemical (e.g., cholesterol), and health habit (e.g., smoking) data. It can provide an estimate of the risk of dying and/or having a serious adverse health effect from a certain cause within a specified time period. The appraisal also compares risk with the "average" risk for the same age and sex and provides an appraised age as well as an achievable age. In addition, it also can provide group analysis based on participants in the appraisal process.

Cooper and Huss (1981) recommend that an evaluator develop a simulation model with the help of a systems analyst if the evaluator is not familiar with computer capabilities. The steps in the construction and utilization of a simulation model for evaluation purposes include:

1. Determine that a simulation model is an appropriate device. Where the system is simple and all interactions are clear, other techniques may be more cost-benefit effective. With a large number of observations and few variables, standard causal analyses are a possible preliminary or alternative approach.

2. Define the boundaries of the simulation. The scope must draw the line between events to be simulated in the model and those assumed to be externalities or inputs to the model.
3. Specify the key interactive components. These may be the individual program participants, the service units, or any decision-maker. If the reaction of a group as a group is a key event, then that group is a necessary component.
4. Define the actions (outputs) of each component as a list of possible "events." These become the effect of previous system events and the cause of other system events.
5. Specify which components will be affected immediately and directly by an event. An example from our model is that the event of gasoline purchase fills the automobile tank, lowers the tank level for the station, and occupies the station's availability to pump gasoline.
6. Define the effect, on a component, of the events that component "receives." This frequently requires an assumption or working hypothesis. If a number of outcomes is possible, then assign a probability to each and have the program select at random to match the probabilities.
7. Begin simulating to see how the model operates. This involves making systematic changes in variables and any constants to see how the model responds. This process is sometimes referred to as a sensitivity analysis. (Cooper & Huss, 1981, pp. 28–29)

Cost Analysis. Statistical significance of program benefits have long sufficed for determining the effectiveness of a program. Evaluation researchers began to realize that the public and the funding sources were not satisfied with numbers of statistical importance. Instead, what was wanted was a demonstration of the practical benefits of the program. To accomplish this, researchers showed that the benefits exceeded all adverse program effects, including budgetary costs; hence the term *benefit-cost analysis*. Thompson, Rothrock, Strain, and Palmer (1981) found that there was a problem using benefit-cost analysis in the realm of evaluation research. This problem concerned the evaluation of main program effects. For example, evaluators in hypertension control programs cannot value, monetarily, statistical decreases to control rates. In a situation such as this, researchers rely on the principle of cost-effectiveness; even if we do not know the value of achieving an objective, we do know that we wish to achieve the objective in a way that minimizes costs.

Cost-effectiveness analysts determine the ratio of monetary to nonmonetary program effects (e.g., the amount in dollars required per hypertensive patient who achieves control). These ratios do not determine if the programs should be implemented, but are used comparatively by decision-makers who would choose the least expensive program that produces the same result.

The cost-effectiveness ratio for social programs is expressed as follows (Thompson et al., 1981):

$$\frac{ML - MG}{B - R}$$

ML = monetary losses (program costs plus some induced costs)
MG = monetary gains (monetary costs that are averted)
B = benefits
R = risks (adverse side effects of the program)

For example, in a mammography screening program, the costs (ML) could be $200,000; the monetary gains (MG) could be $20,000 in savings of hospitalizations for patients; 15 could be the number of breast cancer deaths prevented (B); and 2 could be the mortality number for those dying from the chemotherapy and radiation treatments (R). The ratio then is

$$\frac{\$200,000 - \$20,000}{15 - 2} = \$13,846 \text{ per life saved due to the mammography screening program}$$

In cost analysis, the numerator of the ratio is the focus of attention. Determining the *costs* of a program is extremely important and can have important implications for program evaluation. In determining the costs of a program, the following must be considered: *direct costs*, which include budgetary and nonbudgetary direct costs; *indirect costs*; and *opportunity costs*. (For a complete discussion of these main categories of costs, see Thompson et al., 1981.)

Contextual Evaluation. We have chosen to discuss ethnography here within the context of program evaluation. To reiterate the difference between experimental and contextual evaluations, *experimental evaluations* validate simplified causes and effects through controlled comparisons, and *contextual evaluations* attempt to understand the complexity of a program.

Contextual evaluations assume that social interventions have several facets and relationships that relate to multiple outcomes (Britan, 1981). These evaluations seek to determine how programs work, how they fit into settings, how they achieve results, and how they can be improved. Contextual evaluations are inductive and describe program implementation—how treatments occur, and how program activities relate to formal rules, informal goals, participant understandings, and environmental pressures. The major methodology for a contextual evaluation is ethnography.

Ethnography encompasses the use of observations and interviews and relies very heavily on participant observation. The hallmark of ethnography is the observation, recording, and analysis of behavior in context. It includes systematic descriptions of social systems that look for interrelationships among particular behaviors, customs, rituals, beliefs, and values in terms of broader patterns of cultural understanding, social structure, and environment (Britan, 1981). The usual format for an ethnographer is a case study in which an analysis of program implementation and impact is conducted.

There are certain advantages to using experimental evaluations: in cases in which program goals are clearly stated, treatments are straightforward, and theoretical constructs are unambiguous. On the other hand, contextual evaluations are more useful when the goals are broadly stated, treatments are complex, and theoretical constructs are vague. Therefore, the choice of an evaluation methodology may depend upon the type and setting of the program.

Case Discussion

The cardiac rehabilitation program was judged by Sarah's evaluation team from the University of Dover to be a cost-effective venture for the hospital. Their recommendation to the chief of staff of Rosewood Hospital was to retain the program. This decision was based upon a variety of material gathered by the study team. The major approach used by the Dover team was conducting a case study enhanced by survey data, meeting with hospital personnel, conducting patient interviews, and conducting a cost-analysis of the cardiac rehabilitation program.

Summary

This chapter has attempted to provide a condensed version of the field of evaluation research. This area of research generates much discussion and experimentation in the social sciences, with specific emphasis in educational evaluation. The case study depicted such a project in which a program for cardiac rehabilitation patients was to be evaluated. A broad, general definition of evaluation research was established as the process of determining the effectiveness of a program.

The purposes of evaluation vary, depending upon the vantage point: administrator, consumer, evaluator, or organization. Almost anything can be evaluated, especially if there is support from one of the aforementioned groups.

There are many evaluation models, including behavioral objectives, systems analysis, decision-making, goal-free, connoisseurship, case study, and accreditation. A discussion of the advantages and disadvantages of each model led us to the conclusion that perhaps a combination of models might be necessary for many program evaluations. The following steps were enumerated to aid the evaluator in conducting an evaluation: determine the client, the purposes of the evaluation, the methodology to be utilized, the nature of the contact, how the evaluation should be conducted, and who will use the results of the evaluation.

The major types of evaluation research used in the health sciences include needs assessment, formative, summative, and responsive. Each type has its inherent strengths, weaknesses, and best area of suitability. It is generally up to the contractor to determine the type of evaluation, and this is accomplished by the nature of the evaluation research contract and the question that needs to be answered by the investigator. Methodological approaches utilized in evaluation research are experimental, quasi-experimental, correlation, surveys, personnel assessment, expert judgment, and case study. Though these approaches are used in other research paradigms, they are discussed with specific reference to evaluation research. New and innovative research methodologies were discussed, including simulation, cost analysis, and contextual evaluation.

Evaluation research is a valuable tool for the health sciences. Programs have been asked to be accountable, and through a well-designed evaluation, that accountability can be assessed.

Suggested Activities

1. Refer to the list in the section *What Can Be Evaluated?* and add to the evaluation possibilities.

2. From the list in Activity 1, choose one topic and briefly describe the steps you would take in the evaluation process.

3. Interview a program administrator to assess that program's evaluation status (i.e., when was it last evaluated, by whom, why, and so on).

4. You have been asked by your employer to locate the most recent references with regard to health program evaluation. Utilizing your university's online computer system, determine at least ten references that would be beneficial to you in this assignment. Annotate each reference, then rank-order them with a view to their importance and helpfulness.

5. Utilizing the Web, evaluate any health-related program that is complete. The program should be of some interest to you and somewhat interactive. In doing your evaluation, state what type of evaluation methodology you will use, describe the evaluation plan, and predetermine the possible outcome of your evaluation.

References

Anderson, S., & Ball, S. (1978). *The profession and practice of program evaluation.* San Francisco: Jossey-Bass.

Anderson, S., Ball, S., Murphy, R., & Associates. (1975). *Encyclopedia of education evaluation.* San Francisco: Jossey-Bass.

Baker, E. (1974). Formative evaluation of instruction. In W. Popham (Ed.), *Evaluation in education.* Berkeley: McCutchan.

Bloom, B. (1984). *Taxonomy of educational objectives.* New York: Longman.

Britan, G. (1981). Contextual evaluation: An ethnographic approach to program assessment. In R. Conner (Ed.), *Methodological advances in evaluation research.* Beverly Hills: Sage.

Chelimsky, E. (1978). Differing perspectives of evaluation. In C. Rentz & R. Rentz (Eds.), *Evaluating federally sponsored programs: New di-*

rections for program evaluation (Vol. 2, Summer). San Francisco: Jossey-Bass.

Cook, T., & Campbell, D. (1994). The design and conduct of quasi-experiments in field settings. In M. Dunnette (Ed.), *Organizational psychology* (2d ed.). Chicago: Rand McNally.

Cooper, R., & Huss, W. (1981). Simulation as an evaluation tool. In R. Conner (Ed.), *Methodological advances in evaluation research*. Beverly Hills: Sage.

Eisner, E. (1994). *The educational imagination* (3rd ed.). New York: MacMillan.

Guba, E., & Lincoln, Y. (1994). *Fourth-generation evaluation* (2d ed.). Newbury Park, CA: Sage.

Harless, J. (1973). An analysis of trend analysis. *Improving Human Performance: A Research Quarterly, 3*, 229–244.

House, E. (1999). *Evaluating with validity.* Beverly Hills: Sage.

Mager, R. (1962). *Preparing objectives for programmed instruction.* San Francisco: Fearon.

Patton, M. (1990). *Qualitative evaluation and research methods.* Newbury Park, CA: Sage.

Popham, W. (1993). *Educational evaluation.* Boston: Allyn & Bacon.

Rossi, P. H., Freeman, H. E., & Lipsey, M. W. (1999). *Evaluation* (2d ed.). Thousand Oaks, CA: Sage.

Rutman, L. (Ed.). (1984). *Evaluation research methods.* Beverly Hills: Sage.

Scriven, M. (1967). *The methodology of evaluation* (AERA Monograph Series on Curriculum Evaluation No. 1). Chicago: Rand McNally.

Scriven, M. (1973). Goal free evaluation. In E. House (Ed.), *School evaluation: The politics and process.* Berkeley: McCutchan.

Shortell, S., & Richardson, W. (1978). *Health program evaluation.* St. Louis: C. V. Mosby.

Stake, R. (1991). Responsive evaluation and qualitative methods. In W. Shadish, T. Cook, & L. Levison (Eds.), *Foundations of program evaluation: Theories of practice.* Newbury Park, CA: Sage.

Stake, R. (1998). *Evaluating art programs in community centers.* Stamford, CT: JAI Press.

Streuning, E., & Brewer, M. (Eds.). (1983). *Handbook of evaluation research.* Beverly Hills: Sage.

Stufflebeam, D. (1971). *Educational evaluation and decision making.* Itasca, IL: Peacock.

Suchman, E. (1976). *Evaluative research.* New York: Russell Sage Foundation.

Thompson, E., Rothrock, J., Strain, R., & Palmer, R. (1981). Cost analysis for program evaluation. In R. Conner (Ed.), *Methodological advances in evaluation research.* Beverly Hills: Sage.

Tyler, R. (1949). *Basic principles of curriculum instruction.* Chicago: University of Chicago Press.

Windsor, R., Baranowski, T., Clark, N., & Cutter, G. (1994). *Evaluation of health promotion, health education, and disease prevention programs.* Mountain View, CA: Mayfield.

Chapter *10*

Analytical Epidemiologic Studies

Case Study A: Cohort Study

Fraser enjoyed working with adolescents and young adults. He found them to be challenging, humorous, and full of energy. From a health perspective, however, he had difficulty in dealing with teenage suicide. His local data were no different than national data; suicide had become second only to accidents and homicide as a leading cause of death. It was particularly disconcerting in knowing that some teens in his community health and activity program had taken their own lives. Hindsight revealed that there were perhaps some dissimilarities between those who committed suicide and those who didn't, but there was nothing he could really put his finger on. He decided to investigate it further through reading and tracking those who came through his community program. Fraser knew from years of experience that most of "his kids" entered his program at age 13 and stayed there until they finished high school. He could follow them for at least five years in most instances. He had to think of some way to organize his ideas. He really wanted to find out what the cause was so that he could prevent any more teen suicides in his community.

Case Study B: Case Control

In looking over the clinic data, Meg was concerned about the rising rate of cervical cancer in young women. The rate had risen about one year ago, and clinic records proved that the increased rate was not only being maintained but was on a slight rise again. In her work, Meg knew that several factors could influence the rate for cervical dysplasia and cervical cancer. The principal factors, she believed, were cigarette smoking; early sexual intercourse; multiple partners; prior sexually transmitted disease (STD), especially human papillomavirus (HPV) type 16; and possibly oral contraceptive use. She wondered how her patients diagnosed with high-grade cervical intraepithelial neoplasia (CIN III) and cervical cancer differed from those patients who displayed no such symptoms. Perhaps she could pull medical records for patients over the past two years to find the answer. This would be a lot of work, and she speculated as to whether she could prove anything.

The Nature of Epidemiology

As a discipline, epidemiology knows few, if any, boundaries. This is to be expected, since health is multidimensional. Therefore, epidemiologic investigations are connected to the biomedical sciences, behavioral sciences, computer sciences, engineering, and other disciplines. Rockett (1994) has embraced this concept by stating that epidemiology is "the study of our collective health" (p. 2). As such, it comprises two facets, one of which is descriptive, involving the identifying of patterns, trends, and disease and injury differentials. The second facet moves beyond the descriptive approach to embrace causation or etiology. This latter approach is called *analytic epidemiology*.

Analytic Methodologies in Epidemiology

There are two major analytic methods used in epidemiologic investigations: cohort and case control. The purpose of each is to test the hypothesized cause-effect relationship between a suspected risk factor and a disease, injury, or even a social condition such as welfare status.

Cohort studies, sometimes called prospective studies, work from a postulated cause to an effect. Therefore, the general design is to begin with a group of people (a cohort) and observe them over a period of time. Selection for the group can be based upon the presence or absence of a characteristic (e.g., diabetes, spinal cord injury, welfare) or at random. The individuals within the group, as to be expected, will vary in exposure to one or more of the factors being observed. The epidemiologist watches to determine the differences in the rate at which the characteristic occurs (disease, injury, behavioral problem) in relation to exposure to the factor(s).

Case-control investigations, or retrospective studies, start with a group of people who already have the characteristic (health problem) and compare them with people who do not have that health problem (characteristic). The people who have the health problem are referred to as "cases," while those in the other group are termed "controls." In searching for the "cause," the case-control method determines if the two groups differ in the degree of exposure to different factors. Figure 10.1 illustrates the timing differences between cohort and case-control studies.

Another way to compare the similarities and differences between these two analytic methods is shown in Figure 10.2. Herein, a 2 × 2 table shows how groups

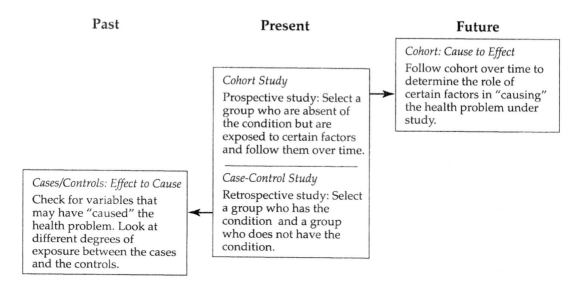

FIGURE 10.1 Timing Schematic for Cohort and Case-Control Prospective and Retrospective Investigations

can be categorized as well as the timing direction of the particular method. Once again, note how the cohort study moves forward (cause-to-effect), similar to an experimental design. The case-control approach, sometimes referred to as *ex post facto*, moves backward in time (effect-to-cause).

Figure 10.2 shows that when a positive relationship exists between the health problem (behavioral, medical, public) and the exposure factor(s), those who

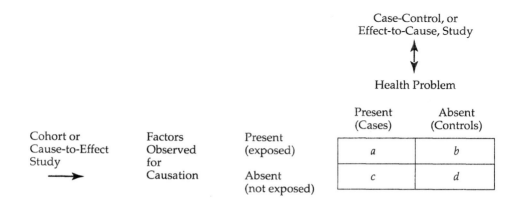

FIGURE 10.2   A 2 × 2 Table Illustration of Cohort and Case-Control Methodologies

are exposed (Group *a*) will be greater in number than those who are not exposed (Group *d*). Logically there should be a larger concentration of subjects in Cells *a* and *d* than in Cells *b* and *c*. This holds true with both the cohort and case-control methods.

Both Figures 10.1 and 10.2 are basic models. Complexity can arise when the health problem is subdivided into categories or when the risk factors are analyzed in degrees of exposure rather than all or none. Examples of subdividing health problems include drug abuse, which can be subdivided into alcohol, cocaine, tobacco, and so forth. Similarly, coronary heart disease (CHD) can be broken into angina pectoris, myocardial infarction, and sudden death subcategories.

Cohort or Prospective Investigations

A cohort is simply a group of people with a common experience over a defined period of time. For example, a marital cohort consists of all people married within a certain time period. A disease (e.g., juvenile diabetes) cohort may be all those patients with juvenile diabetes who presented at Hospital A during a particular time frame. All members of the cohort are assumed to be free of the health problem at the commencement of the investigation. They are divided into two or more groups, according to exposure to the risk factors under investigation. Using hemodialysis as a risk factor, Kutner, Brogan, Hall, Haber, and Daniels (2000) conducted a three-year study with one group comprising older hemodialysis patients and the other group age-matched controls. Simon, Peters, Christiansen, and Fletcher (2000) investigated the effect on patient satisfaction of medical student participation in care and the presence of medical student teaching. One group of patients were involved with medical students, while another group was not. In another educational study, Chok and Gomez (2000) examined the effect of a neck care talk to patients receiving physiotherapy at a neck pain clinic. Two groups were used, with one receiving the educational intervention.

In our case example with Fraser, we find that his cohort group is all the adolescents who go to his community health and activity program. He knows that he can follow them for a five-year period, beginning at age 13. In epidemiological terms, he would conduct a *current cohort study,* which means that selected subjects are followed from the beginning of the study for a period of time. This is in contrast to a *historical cohort study,* in which the events have already taken place and data are collected retrospectively (Schlesselman, 1982). Both are prospective in nature; the principal difference is the starting point. Current cohort studies have the advantage of greater researcher control over data collection.

There are several ways to select a cohort. One way is simply by accessibility, as in Fraser's case, while other ways include history of exposure or availability of medical records. A researcher can take a random sample of exposed and unexposed individuals. The cohort is then divided according to their exposure to the risk factor(s). This sample is random in that, among exposed and unexposed partici-pants, there is an equal chance of studying subjects who will develop the health

TABLE 10.1 Advantages and Disadvantages of the Cohort Strategy

Advantages
1. The cohort is categorized by exposure to the risk factor(s) before the health problem occurs.
2. Provides for the study of multiple potential effects of exposure, both positive and negative.
3. Permits calculation of incidence rates among those exposed and those not exposed. Specifically, exposure-specific incidence rate, attributable risk rate, relative risk, and odds ratio can be determined.
4. Provides flexibility in variable selection.
5. Allows for a large degree of quality control in the research effort.

Disadvantages
1. Large numbers are generally required, which can increase expense and time requirements.
2. Study duration is usually long.
3. Lengthy duration can present problems with attrition and change in subject status as it relates to the risk variables (e.g., smoking, residence).
4. Follow-up can be difficult as the length of the study increases.
5. Difficult to control extraneous variables.
6. Almost impossible to study detailed mechanisms.

problem and subjects who will not develop the health problem. In our case study with Fraser, he could use his accessible population and group them according to exposure to such risk factors as psychosocial distress (e.g., disrupted family relations, loneliness, hopelessness), drug involvement, or exposure to suicide by a family member or very close friend.

At the conclusion of the study, the researcher compares the two groups for the incidence rate of the health problem. In a cohort study, estimations can be made for exposure-specific incidence rates, attributable risk, relative risk, and the odds ratio. These will be discussed in a later section. The advantages and disadvantages of the cohort method are outlined in Table 10.1.

Case-Control or Retrospective Investigations

One of the most important aspects of case-control studies is the delineation of study groups—cases and controls. The researcher must establish criteria so that no ambiguity exists. For example, in our case study, Meg would need to be definitive in her criteria about the stages of cervical intraepithelial neoplasia. Meg's choice for case and control groups should be dictated by validity rather than generalizability. While it is good to be able to generalize to the entire population, it is more important to establish an etiologic relationship between the cervical cancer and the risk factor(s).

As a general rule, it is best to select the case group from newly diagnosed cases that meet the criteria within a designated time frame. Incident cases are preferred to prevalent cases (Mausner & Kramer, 1985). Sources for case groups can be records of physicians and employers, HMO groups, hospital records, death certificates, and so forth. Of course, information can be gathered from subjects themselves or even from proxies for the subjects or patients. Oftentimes a combination of records and actual subjects are used (Landmark & Abdelnoor, 2000).

In regard to control groups, a study may have more than one control group. Sources are hospital records of patients with different diagnoses, relatives or friends of the cases, the general population, and so forth. The bottom line is that controls should be representative of the general population in terms of probability of exposure to the risk factor(s). Preferably, they should have had the same opportunity to be exposed. As you would logically expect, it is important that sources and methods of data collection are similar for both cases and controls.

Meg could select other clinic patients for her control group. In selecting patients from the same clinic, she should nullify certain effects. For example, it is likely that these patients come from similar geographic locations, have similar socioeconomic characteristics, are alike in ethnicity, and so forth. On the other hand, she would need to be certain that this group of controls is similar to the general population and that they do not have any diseases that share risk factors with cervical cancer. In her study, a plausible control group would be women who attended the clinic for their annual Pap exam who had negative findings for cervical cancer. Table 10.2 summarizes the advantages and disadvantages of the case-control method.

TABLE 10.2 Advantages and Disadvantages of the Case-Control Method

Advantages
1. The number of subjects can be small. This is because the study starts with identification of cases and a like number of controls.
2. A study can be planned quickly, carried out in an expedient manner, and analyzed in a short period of time.
3. More than one risk factor can be identified in the same data set.
4. Requires few subjects, making it excellent for studying rare diseases.
5. There is no risk to subjects.
6. Subjects do not need to volunteer.
7. Minimal ethical problems.
8. Relatively inexpensive.

Disadvantages
1. The information necessary to the investigation may be unavailable or inaccurate.
2. May be difficult or impossible to validate some records.
3. Recall by a subject or informant for the person with the health problem may be quite different than that of controls.
4. Selection of an appropriate control group can be difficult. For example, selection from hospital or clinic records can introduce bias depending upon the risk factors and the nature of the controls.
5. Rates of disease in exposed and nonexposed subjects cannot be determined.
6. The odds ratio is the only calculation available to case-control studies. In cases of rare diseases (health problems), the relative risk can be calculated because in these instances the odds ratio approximates relative risk.
7. Difficult to control extraneous variables.
8. Difficult, if not impossible, to study detailed mechanisms.

Establishing Causation

As noted at the outset of this chapter, analytic epidemiology attempts to establish causation between the health problem and selected risk factors. In the absence of experimentation, the following can be of value in determining causation (Rockett, 1994; Schlesselman, 1982):

Temporal sequence: Causative factors occur before effects (events). This seems obvious but is not always readily identifiable. For example, is endometriosis the cause or consequence of the disease process that leads to infertility?

Consistency: If the association of the health problem and risk factor(s) is evidenced in several different conditions of the study, it gives credence to causation.

Strength of association: Generally, the larger the association between risk exposure and the health problem, the less likely the relationship is spurious. In other words, the larger the value of relative risk, the more likely is causation.

Specificity of effect: This is rather simplistic in that the effect should be specific to the risk factor(s). If the risk factor is removed, the effect should be also. Of course, most events do not stem from a singular cause, which makes this approach weak, but it may be of some value when combined with other approaches to causation.

Biological gradient: A dose-response relationship makes an excellent argument for causation.

Existing data and theory: When the relationship between risk factor(s) and the health problem is consistent with previous research efforts or perhaps theoretical constructs, then causation is more likely to be established.

Although causation may never be fully proven in the experimental sense (e.g., smoking and lung cancer), analytic epidemiology can assess the likelihood of causation. In a real world with many research constraints, we often cannot ask for any more.

Problems of Error

Like other research approaches, analytic investigations can succumb to error. Rockett (1994) describes three principal types of error: bias, random variation, and random misclassification. This section addresses these errors along with suggested ways to prevent them.

Bias

Bias refers to any error in design, conduct, or analysis of a study that makes the estimate of an exposure's effect on the risk of disease inaccurate. One way this can happen is through *selection bias.* In this instance, poor research design brings about a difference in comparison groups (e.g., diseased and nondiseased, exposed and not exposed) that misrepresents true results. As you would expect, bias is a threat to internal validity. To prevent this source of error, cohort groups should be homogeneous in as many factors as possible, except for the risk factors under investigation. In Fraser's study, his two groups should differ only in his chosen risk factors—psychosocial distress, drug involvement, or exposure to the suicide of a friend or relation. In case-control studies, the only difference between the two groups should be their disease status or health problem. For Meg, this would mean that her control group consisting of patients from the clinic would be similar in almost all respects to her case group—with similar geography, socioeconomic status, health care plans, and so forth. The only difference should be their diagnosis of cervical cancer. Matching is one technique to assure similarity of several factors and will be discussed in a later section.

A second form of bias is *information bias,* which occurs in cohort studies when information about disease outcome is not collected uniformly across groups. In case-control studies, information bias occurs when exposure information is not collected uniformly for cases and controls. The prevention step is obvious—collect information uniformly. This means that you must monitor those people who are helping you collect data. Another way to reduce information bias is to "blind" the study to both the subjects and the data collectors. In other words, do not reveal any more about the study than you have to for both ethical and data collection reasons.

A third form of bias is termed *confounding.* Confounding variables are extraneous variables that are (1) risk factors for the health problem under investigation; and (2) factors that are associated with the exposure of interest but that are not a consequence of exposure. For example, in Meg's case-control study, if she were to study just the relationship between cervical cancer and HPV 16, at least one confounding variable exists. In comparing cases and controls, she could find that the case group had a greater number of subjects who had multiple partners than the control group, since multiple partners are a risk factor for cervical cancer. At the same time, multiple sexual partners is known to be associated with HPV. Therefore, if she conducts her study this way, Meg could find that an apparent increase in cervical cancer found to be associated with HPV 16 might in fact be a result of multiple partners (Robinson, 2000; Murthy & Mathew, 2000). A study by Kjellberg et al. (2000) shows how cigarette smoking can play a role as a confounding factor in the etiology of cervical cancer. The two principal ways to control for confounding variables are by matching and by using statistical techniques. These are discussed in the section entitled *Control in Epidemiologic Research.*

Random Variation

As the name implies, random variation means chance differences between groups. This source of error affects the ability to generalize to a larger population—external validity. It generally occurs because of unrepresentativeness in the comparison groups. Fraser and Meg can minimize random variation in their studies by increasing the size of their study and comparison groups.

Random Misclassification

Errors can be made when determining a subject's exposure status or disease (health problem) status. In other words, a subject could be misclassified. In Fraser's cohort investigation, he could misallocate an adolescent who has been exposed to the nonexposed group or vice versa. In Meg's situation, misclassification refers to whether subjects have cervical cancer (lab results could be in error). If this happened in either investigation, the results are likely to underestimate the real association between exposure and effect. The possibility of finding a strong causal-like relationship between risk factor and health problem is greatly reduced, if not eliminated, in the presence of random misclassification.

Control in Epidemiologic Research

While the preceding section addressed some ways to control for error in analytic epidemiologic research, this section expands on some of the more complex methods.

Matching

One of the most common methods to reduce error is to match on a subject-to-subject basis. For example, in a case-control study like Meg's, each case individual can be matched with each control individual on confounding factors. So, a 32-year-old black female whose lab results are positive for cervical cancer (a case individual) would need to be matched with a 32-year-old (give or take a year or two) black female who has negative lab results. They should match on all confounding variables. Age, gender, and race are the most commonly matched variables. According to Schlesselman (1982, p. 107): "Variables to be considered for matching are those that independently of exposure are risk factors for the study disease. A matching variable need not be a 'cause' of the disease, but may derive its risk-factor status as a result of associations with other causal variables, excluding the study exposure."

If subject-to-subject matching is not feasible, group matching may be the next best choice. For example, Meg could go with a mean age or perhaps with age categories (e.g., ten-year age groups). Group matching at least keeps cases and controls in similar proportions. Sometimes more than one control individual needs to be matched to a case individual. When matching multiple controls to each case, a constant ratio should be used, such as 1:2 or 1:3 (Schlesselman, 1982). Like many aspects of research, however, this looks great on paper but may not be functional in the real world, as seen by studies that attempt this and end up with incomplete matching.

While the intent of matching is to eliminate biased comparisons, researchers must be careful not to overmatch. Overmatching reduces validity or statistical efficiency. Remember that a matched factor cannot be evaluated for its etiological role. Another problem with overmatching is cost—depending on the factor, matches can be difficult to locate.

Logically, if matching is part of the overall design, then the analysis should reflect that design. In other words, matching has two steps: (1) matching the design; and (2) matching the analysis. If Step 2 is not carried out, the estimated relative risk is likely to be biased.

Homogenous Grouping

Another procedure is to use groups that are as homogeneous as possible. In this approach, you would select a sample in which all the subjects would be homogeneous on the variable(s) in question. For example, if level of education were a confounding variable, its effect could be controlled by the use of subjects who all have the same education (e.g., high school). In this manner, the effects that are found can be justified as stemming from the independent variable more readily (Ary, Jacobs, & Razavieh, 1972).

The use of homogeneous groups is not always possible, however, because some of the extraneous variables either may not be identified or may not be present in large enough numbers to carry out the research. Further, if control is accomplished on only one variable, such as level of education, you cannot generalize findings to other levels of education.

Stratified Sampling

This strategy is similar to homogeneous grouping in that subgroups are formed by separating the ranges of selected variables and sampling a predetermined number of cases and controls within cells made from the multiple cross-classification. Using the education example from above, you could look at education as a whole and subdivide it into three groups: elementary school, high school, and college. It would then be a matter of determining how many should be in each educational cell, or subgroup. Controls should be in a constant ratio to the case subgroup—1:1, 1:2, and so forth. The actual numbers may vary across the strata, but the case-control ratio would be the same.

Poststratification

Matching, homogeneous grouping, and stratified sampling demand that you identify variables to control before commencing the study. Poststratification, as well as regression analysis, avoids this requirement. Simply, poststratification means that you classify unmatched cases and controls by their values on one or more variables determined during the study. This strategy is similar to stratified sampling except that (1) the variables used for grouping do not have to be selected ahead of time; (2) the case-control ratio does not have to be identical across strata; and (3) not all subgroups will contain both cases and controls, making comparison impossible in some instances. Needless to say, this would be a definite drawback for some research efforts.

Multivariate Analysis

Like poststratification, multivariate analysis is conducted after the data have been collected. Research has shown that we can rarely rely on a two-variable study to explain, predict, or control relationships or variables. Instead, we must deal with several variables simultaneously. To do so, we must use multivariate procedures. While several of these are discussed in detail in Chapter 12, on inferential analysis, the outline below describes their usage.

Analysis of Covariance. The dependent variable is continuous in nature, whereas the independent variables are a mixture of nominal and continuous variables. The continuous variables are used as control variables.

Multiple Regression Analysis. The dependent variable is generally continuous, as are the independent variables, although in the research world this technique is used with any type of independent variable. For example, in Meg's investigation, her dependent variable is continuous, for Pap smear (histological) results. Her independent variables are continuous: number of sexual partners, age at first intercourse, number of previous STDs, and so forth. The principal objection to linear regression is that the parameters have a limited range of validity and interpretation (Schlesselman, 1982).

Logistic Regression. Also called logit analysis, logistic regression analyzes relationships between several independent variables and a dependent variable that is nominal. Remember, a nominal variable is categorical (e.g., gender). It is an either/or classification system with no ranking. Logistic regression uses maximum likelihood estimation for analysis, thereby transforming the likelihood (probability) of an event occurring into its odds (e.g., coming up with the odds that a woman who has multiple sexual partners will develop cervical cancer).

Schlesselman (1982) describes logistic regression as:

$$y = b_0 + b_1 E = b_2 X$$

where E is the study exposure
X is the confounding variable to control
$y = \ln p/q$ is the logarithm of the odds of "disease" or "case"

Therefore, for exposed subjects $E = 1$ and the logarithm, the odds of disease becomes:

$$y = b_0 + b_1 + b_2 X$$

In comparison, the unexposed subjects are $E = 0$, and the log odds of disease becomes:

$$y_o = b_0 + b_2X$$

In this manner, there is the assumption that the log odds of disease (health problem) has the same dependence on X for both exposed and unexposed individuals (b_2 is constant). The adjustment for multiple confounding factors is handled as in multiple regression.

Some investigators use logistic regression with an ordinal dependent variable. Hillis, Marchbanks, and Peterson (1995) researched the effectiveness of hysterectomy for chronic pelvic pain, with the latter being subdivided into a trichotomous variable—no pain, continued but decreased pain, and unchanged or increased pain.

Logistic regression is preferable to discriminant function analysis (Cleary & Angel, 1984). One reason is that logistic regression is more theoretically appropriate, and a second is that it addresses probability of an outcome rather than just prediction. The odds ratios developed through logistic regression are meaningful and can be illustrated graphically, making them easier to interpret. Nonetheless, logistic regression is often not used in medical research because the outcome variable cannot be assumed to have a normal distribution (Matthews & Farewell, 1996).

Linear Structural Relation Analysis (LISREL).   This is a complex statistical procedure that like logistic regression analysis, is based on maximum likelihood estimation. It is a versatile approach and is often used much like path analysis. It is often a better approach than path analysis, however. Since the data collected by health researchers usually contain some type of error, LISREL is preferred over least-squares regression in doing path analysis. Further, least-squares regression operates on the assumption that residuals in the various regression equations are not correlated, an assumption that is difficult to accept. Finally, path analysis usually assumes a unidirectional flow in causation, and we know that in the area of health, cause and effect are often iterative or reciprocal. Joreskog and Sorbom (1989) and Hayduk (1987) offer more information on this technique.

Proportional Hazards Regression.   In many health investigations, the end point of interest is survival. This is particularly so when studying chronic disease. Educators and researchers alike use estimated survival curves for teaching or explaining survival data. The Kaplan-Meier estimate of a survival curve, referred to as an *actuarial estimate,* has long been used. However, specific regression models have been developed to consider the simultaneous influence of several explanatory variables on survival time. Matthews and Farewell (1996) provide a detailed usage of proportional hazards regression with an example of two lymphoma groups. One group presented with clinical symptoms, while the other was asymptomatic. The regression is used to determine why the asymptomatic group has a longer survival rate. Specifically, what factors played a role to create this difference? These authors also discuss this regression technique in terms of time-dependent covariates.

Analysis of Results in Analytic Epidemiology

As discussed at the outset of this chapter, the purpose of both cohort and case-control studies is to test the hypothesized cause-effect relationship between a suspected risk factor(s) and a disease, injury, or social/health condition. This section presents information about measures of association for each type of investigation.
     It is important to understand some basic terms prior to discussing the analyses.

Prevalence

Prevalence is a measure of the proportion of individuals within a population who have a specific health problem, disease, injury, or other health event at a particular point in time. It can be expressed as:

$$\text{prevalence} = \frac{\text{number of people who have the health problem at a point in time}}{\text{number of people in the study program}}$$

Incidence

A subcategory of prevalence is incidence, in that it is the number of new cases in a population at risk during a specified time period (e.g., a calendar year or duration of a study). Rosner (1990) interprets the incidence rate as "the probability an individual with no prior disease will develop a new case of the disease over some specified time period" (p. 58). The incidence rate is expressed as:

$$\text{incidence} = \frac{\text{number of new cases over a period of time}}{\text{population at risk}}$$

The incidence rate formula is sometimes modified to fit the nature of the study. For example, the numerator could be the number of conditions rather than the number of people. This would reflect the fact that a person may get the condition more than once during the specified time period. For example:

$$\text{incidence} = \frac{\text{number of colds in a 6-month period}}{\text{number of people at risk}}$$

Similarly, for some cohort (prospective) investigations, the denominator can be changed to reflect the problem of attrition. For example, in Fraser's study some individuals will move away, drop out of the program, or somehow get lost for follow-up. Also, other individuals will enter the study after it is initiated. Both these

TABLE 10.3 Person-Years Calculation for Incidence

Adolescent	Number of Years Observed
1	4
2	5
3	1
4	4
5	2
6	5
7	5
8	2
9	3
10	5
11	4
12	3
13	5
14	4
15	1
Total Person-Years	53

situations mean that there will be an unequal period of observation time for subjects. As a result, subjects will contribute unequally to the calculation of population at risk. To overcome this dilemma, epidemiologists use the idea of "person-time." This is often, but not always, shown as person-years and is used in the denominator of the incidence formula. Table 10.3 is a hypothetical example of person-years calculation for incidence in Fraser's study.

From Table 10.3 we find that 15 people were followed for a period of 53 person-years. If 2 of the 15 adolescents committed suicide, the incidence rate would be 2 in 53 person-years, or 0.0377 per person-year. This can be expressed as 3.77 per 100 person-years of observation. The calculation is as follows:

$$\text{incidence} = \frac{\text{number of adolescents who committed suicide over 5 years}}{\text{person-time at risk}} \times 100$$

$$= \frac{2}{53} \times 100 = 3.77$$

Of course, the multiplier could be 1,000 or 100,000 rather than 100 person-years.

The use of person-years rather than population units should bring greater accuracy to the measurement. However, in using person-years the following three conditions must be met (Mausner & Kramer, 1985). First, the risk of the condition must be constant throughout the period of study. Second, the rate of the condition for those who are lost to follow-up should be about the same as for those who remain in the study. Third, if the condition under study is a rapidly fatal disease, the rate could be artificially high if certain subjects are studied for less than the full period of time.

Analyses for Cohort Investigations

In cohort studies, investigators measure the strength of the association between exposure and the disease or health outcome by means of the rate ratio or relative risk. Relative risk (RR) is defined as the ratio of the incidence rate for persons exposed to a risk factor to the incidence rate for those not exposed to that same risk factor. It can be expressed as:

$$\text{relative risk} = \frac{\text{incidence rate for those exposed to risk factor}}{\text{incidence rate for those unexposed to risk factor}}$$

Table 10.4 illustrates a typical 2 × 2 table for a cohort study using population units rather than person-time units.

Using the cells in Table 10.4, relative risk would be:

$$RR = \frac{a/(a+b)}{c/(c+d)}$$

Relative risk, or risk ratio, shows the extent to which it is more (or less) likely that a health problem or condition will occur in the exposed group as compared to the unexposed group. If *RR* equals 1, there is no relationship between exposure and the condition or health problem. If *RR* is greater than 1, a positive association exists, meaning that those exposed are so many times more likely to contract the health problem. In contrast, if *RR* is less than unity, there is a negative association, implying that the exposed group is less likely to contract the health problem.

If person-time units rather than population units are employed in the study, the 2 × 2 table would need to reflect this change, and the relative risk formula would be modified (Rockett, 1994). Table 10.5 shows the change.

TABLE 10.4   A 2 × 2 Cohort Table for Determining Relative Risk Based on Population Units

Risk Factor	Disease Present	Disease Absent	Total	Incidence Rate
Exposed	*a*	*b*	*a + b*	*a/a + b*
Not exposed	*c*	*d*	*c + d*	*c/c + d*

TABLE 10.5   A 2 × 2 Cohort Table for Determining Relative Risk Based on Person-Time Units

Risk Factor	Disease Present	Disease Absent	Person-Time Unit	Incidence Rate
Exposed	a	b	e	a/e
Not exposed	c	d	f	a/f

Note. Person-time unit replaces population unit in the denominator for incidence rates.

Using the cells in Table 10.5, a relative risk would be:

$$RR = \frac{a/e}{c/f}$$

To illustrate this further, Table 10.6 presents hypothetical data for Fraser's cohort study on teen suicide. In other words, imagine that after five years of investigation, his results would be those in Table 10.6.

Note that person-time units in years are used to develop the incidence rates, which in turn are multiplied by 100,000 to develop the incidence rates per 100,000 person-years. The relative risk or rate ratio, using our formula for person-years, is:

$$RR = \frac{466}{77} = 6.05 \text{ per } 100,000 \text{ person-years}$$

This is interpreted as a positive association between the risk factor and suicide. While it cannot be said that this risk factor "causes" teen suicide, Fraser can say that those exposed to the risk factor in question are six times more likely to commit suicide than those who were not exposed to that risk.

Another rate that can be used in cohort studies is the attributable risk rate, which is simply the difference between incidence rates. Specifically, it is the incidence rate for the exposed group minus the incidence rate for the unexposed group. This rate, also called the risk difference, indicates the magnitude of the absolute change

TABLE 10.6   Hypothetical Results from a Cohort Study of Teen Suicide

Risk Factor	Suicide Status Yes	No	Person-Time Units	Incidence Rate	Incidence Rate per 100,000
Exposed	10	560	2,148	0.00465	466
Not exposed	2	610	2,590	0.00077	77

Note. Relative risk = 6.05 per 100,000 person-years.

brought about by exposure. Suppose we have two people who are at equal risk for the health problem except for the presence or absence of exposure to the risk factor. The risk of disease for the exposed person is the incidence rate for exposure, while the incidence rate for nonexposure is the rate for our other individual. If the exposure did not exist, then the risk for our first person would be the same as for the second. Subsequently, the difference between the two incidence rates represents the increase (or decrease) in risk owing to the exposure. In our example with Fraser's data in Table 10.6, we would have the following:

$$\text{attributable risk} = \text{incident rate for exposed group}$$
$$- \text{incident rate for unexposed group}$$
$$= a/e - c/f$$
$$= 466 - 77$$
$$= 389 \text{ per } 100,000 \text{ person-years}$$

These two methods of calculating rate ratio or relative risk need to be modified if matching was used in the epidemiologic study design (Fleiss, 1981; Mausner & Kramer, 1985). As noted in the section on matching, in such studies the unit of analysis is the matched pair. Table 10.7 illustrates the possible outcomes for a matched cohort investigation.

In Table 10.7, those in Cells a and d are concordant pairs, whereas those in Cells b and c are discordant. Only the latter are used for the relative risk ratio, which becomes Cell b divided by Cell c, or, in other words, b/c. McNemar's test is generally used to test significance.

Analyses for Case-Control Investigations

The odds ratio is the most common measure of association between exposure and the health outcome in case-control or retrospective investigations. The odds ratio

TABLE 10.7 A 2 × 2 Table for Relative Risk in a Matched Cohort Investigation

Exposed Subjects	Not Exposed Subjects	
	Diseased	Disease Free
Diseased	a	b
Disease Free	c	d

where

Cell a = exposed who get the disease + nonexposed who get the disease
Cell b = exposed who get the disease + nonexposed who are disease free
Cell c = exposed who are disease free + nonexposed who get the disease
Cell d = exposed who are disease free + nonexposed who are disease free

TABLE 10.8 A 2 × 2 Table for a Case-Control Study

Exposure to Risk Factor	Disease Status	
	Diseased (Cases)	Disease Free (Controls)
Exposed	a	b
Not exposed	c	d
Proportion exposed	a/a + c	b/b + d

can be seen as an estimate of the relative risk. Specifically, the odds ratio is the ratio of the odds of disease in exposed individuals relative to the odds of disease in unexposed individuals. Table 10.8 illustrates a typical 2 × 2 table for a case-control study.

The odds ratio, signified by the sign ψ, is calculated as:

$$\text{odds ratio } (\psi) = \frac{ad}{bc}$$

Interpretation is similar to relative risk in a cohort study. That is, an odds ratio of 1 implies no association between outcome and exposure. However, when the odds ratio is greater than unity, the exposure is positively related to the outcome (thereby contributing to it). On the other hand, a negative relationship between the exposure and the outcome exists when the odds ratio is less than 1. Let's use some hypothetical data from Meg's investigation of cervical cancer. Table 10.9 illustrates her hypothetical data.

The risk factor selected is prior infection with human papillomavirus (HPV). Using the formula, the odds ratio is:

$$\text{odds ratio } (\psi) = \frac{40 \times 33}{15 \times 20} = 4.4$$

TABLE 10.9 Hypothetical Data from a Case-Control Study of Cervical Cancer

Exposure to Risk Factor (Papillomavirus Infection)	Disease Status	
	Diseased (Cases)	Disease Free (Controls)
Exposed	40	20
Not exposed	15	33
Total	55	53

Note. Odds ratio = 4.4

**TABLE 10.10 A 2 × 2 Table for Odds Ratio in a
Matched Case-Control Study**

	Controls	
Cases	Exposed	Not Exposed
Exposed	*a*	*b*
Not exposed	*c*	*d*

where

Cell *a* = cases exposed + controls exposed
Cell *b* = cases exposed + controls not exposed
Cell *c* = cases not exposed + controls exposed
Cell *d* = cases not exposed + controls not exposed

This is greater than unity, so Meg can say that those women exposed to HPV (prior infection) have four times the odds of getting cervical cancer as compared to women who have not been exposed to HPV.

As with cohort investigations, this formula must be modified if matching has occurred. Once again, the analysis unit is the matched pair, and the odds ratio becomes Cell *b* divided by Cell *c*, which represent discordant pairs. Table 10.10 illustrates a 2 × 2 table for the odds ratio in a matched case-control (retrospective) study.

In Table 10.10, those in Cells *a* and *d* are concordant pairs and do not contribute to the results. McNemar's test is generally used to test significance (Fleiss, 1981).

Confidence Intervals

Statistical inference can be in the form of hypothesis testing or estimation of parameters. While hypothesis testing is more pronounced in the literature, parameter estimation can play a major role. The two forms of estimation are point estimation and interval estimation. The former is single statistic (or point) to estimate the population parameter. For example, if you calculated the mean score of the national examination of the Council on Resident Education in Obstetrics and Gynecology (CREOG) for a sample of 64 ob/gyn residents and found it to be 510, that mean would be the point estimate of the population mean (μ). Similarly, relative risk and odds ratios are point estimates. The problem with all point estimates is that they fail to convey the accuracy of the estimation. Just how accurate is the relative risk of 6.05 per 100,000 person-years in Fraser's study or the odds ratio of 4.4 in Meg's investigation?

A confidence interval (*CI*), or interval estimation, provides a range of values within which the population parameter has a specified probability of falling. That is, a *CI* sets a range or interval of numbers in which we have a designated degree (usually 95% or 99%) of assurance that the population parameter lies within the upper and lower limits of the *CI*. The degree of probability is established by the researcher.

Using our CREOG example, we can calculate the *CI* for our sample mean of 510. The calculations involve both the standard error of the mean (*SEM*) and the principles of the normal curve or distribution. Suppose that our sample of 64 ob/gyn residents had a standard deviation of 80. This being the case, the SEM of our sample would be:

$$SEM = \text{standard deviation} = \frac{80}{\sqrt{64}} = 10$$

Given this information you can determine the 95% *CI* as follows:

$$95\% \; CI = (510 \pm (1.96 \times 10))$$
$$= (510 \pm (19.6))$$
$$= (490.4 \leq \mu \leq 529.6)$$

Given this result, you can say that you are 95% confident that the population mean is greater than or equal to 490.4, but equal to or less than 529.6. In other words, if the study were repeated 100 times, with a *CI* for each, you can be assured that 95% of the *CI*s calculated would contain the population mean (or whatever population parameter was being presented).

There are several methods for determining the *CI* for an odds ratio, and they are beyond the scope of this text. (Schlesselman, 1982, explains six techniques.) However, the same principles apply as in our illustration with the sample mean, and it is important to understand them in order to interpret epidemiological results. If we have a 95% *CI* for an odds ratio, we can be assured that there is a 95% chance that the true exposure-disease parameter (true measure of association) is contained within the confidence limits (upper and lower ends of the confidence interval). A general rule of thumb when reading the literature is that "the wider the confidence interval, the larger is the variability of the point estimate and the less likely that the point estimate is accurate" (Peterson & Kleinbaum, 1991, p. 715).

In reading epidemiologic studies, you will find that the *CI* is used to ascertain statistical significance. This is a two-tailed significance test allowing the epidemiologist to recognize that the exposure either increases or decreases the risk of disease. The investigator establishes the significance level; for example, $\alpha = .05$. The null hypothesis is rejected when the $100(1 - \alpha)\%$ *CI* does not overlap the null value being tested. Remember that for relative risk and odds ratio, the null value equals 1. Consequently, if a 95% *CI* for the relative risk or odds ratio fails to overlap 1.0, we reject the null hypothesis that there is no association between the risk factor and the health outcome. It is rejected at the .05 significance level.

In this manner the confidence level is used in place of the p value to test the hypothesis.

Suppose that in Meg's study, with an odds ratio of 4.4, the 95% CI is 1.8–6.2. This does not overlap with 1.0; therefore, she would reject at the .05 significance level the null hypothesis that there is no relationship between prior HPV infection and cervical cancer. She would arrive at the same result if $p \leq .05$. In contrast, if her 95% CI were 0.75–6.2 she could not reject the null hypothesis, because it overlaps 1.0. She would have the same conclusion if $p > .05$.

Computer programs are available to establish relative risk, odds ratio, and CIs. While it would be good to have that knowledge, as a minimum you should be able to interpret the results of analytic epidemiology investigations, including CIs and levels of significance.

Case Discussion

Case Study A: Fraser's Cohort Study of Teenage Suicide

In this investigation Fraser decided to follow those adolescents who entered his program for a period of five years—a current cohort investigation. Cohort selection was through accessibility. He determined the risk factors to be psychosocial distress, drug involvement, and exposure to suicide by a family member or close friend. Fraser's null hypothesis would be that there is no association between psychosocial distress, drug involvement, or exposure to suicide and committing suicide. Since the adolescents who frequent his program come from the same geographic area, it is likely that they will be homogeneous in several respects. This will help control for confounding variables. He can use logistic regression for analysis since it deals with a nominal dependent variable and several independent variables while controlling confounding variables. The results, as discussed in the chapter, should be based on person-years, since he will have subjects exiting and entering at different points over the five-year investigation. To solidify his relative rate finding of 6.05 per 100,000 person-years, Fraser should establish a confidence interval and use it to test for significance. In addition, he can further support causation through temporal sequencing and use of existing data and theory.

Case Study B: Meg's Case-Control Study of Cervical Cancer

In her retrospective study, Meg wanted to review records of clinic patients to determine the strength of the relationship between selected risk factors and cervical cancer. Her null hypothesis could be written as: There is no relationship between cigarette smoking, early sexual intercourse, number of sexual partners, prior HPV infection, and cervical intraepithelial neoplasia (CIN) diagnosis. As described in the text, her choice of controls—patients with negative findings—supports homogeneity between cases and controls as well as the use of a similar source and data collection technique. Because Meg has several variables and because there is the likelihood of confounding factors, logistic regression is probably her best choice. As in the cohort study, she should determine the *CI*s surrounding her odds ratio of 4.4 and check for significance at the .05 level.

Summary

The two principal directions for epidemiologic studies are descriptive and analytic. The focus of this chapter was analytic epidemiologic investigations. One of type of analytic methodology is the prospective or cohort study, while the other is the retrospective or case-control investigation. The task for both is to test the hypothesized cause-and-effect relationship between a suspected risk factor and a health condition. The principal difference between the two approaches is the commencement or timing of the study (going forward or backward in time). The advantages and disadvantages of each are outlined in detail.

The cohort in a prospective study is simply a group of people with a common experience over a defined period of time. Some of the ways to select a cohort include accessibility, history of exposure, and availability of needed records. The cohort is divided according to their exposure to the risk factor (exposed versus not exposed, or gradients of exposure). At the end of the study, the two groups are compared to measure the strength of association between the risk factor(s) and the health outcome. In comparing the two groups, it may be more accurate to use person-years rather than population units in the data. Several methods of analysis are available, each dependent upon the study design and nature of the data.

In regard to the case-control technique, the researcher must establish criteria so that no ambiguity exists between cases and controls. The cases must clearly have the condition or disease, while the controls must be disease- or condition-free. Generally, it is best to select the case group from newly diagnosed cases that meet the criteria and took place within the specified time frame. Sources can include physician and employer records, hospital records, death certificates, birth certificates, and the like. As in the cohort study, once the data are collected, the cases and controls are compared to determine the strength of the association between exposure and health condition. The odds ratio gives us that answer.

While analytic epidemiologic studies do not show causation, they do approximate it. In addition to the rates (relative risk, odds ratio, attributable risk) that can be developed, the researcher can look at temporal sequence, consistency, specificity of effect, biological gradients, and existing data or theory.

Like any research effort, analytic epidemiology can have problems of error. The major ones are bias, random variation, and random misclassification. Bias refers to any error in design, conduct, or analysis of a study. Subsequently, bias includes selection bias, information bias, and confounding. All sources of error need to be controlled as much as possible. Some ways to do this include matching, homogeneous grouping, stratified sampling, poststratification, and multivariate analysis. Logistic regression is quite common because it avoids the problems of matching.

Confidence intervals (CI) can be established for relative risk and odds ratios. A confidence interval sets a range or interval of numbers in which we have a designated degree (usually 95% or 99%) of assurance that the population parameter lies within the upper and lower limits of the CI. The CI is important not only to ensure confidence that the rate represents the true association but to test the hypothesis at a preset level of significance.

Suggested Activities

1. You are interested in studying the attitudes of pediatricians about using e-mail to communicate with their patients (or their guardians) for non-life-threatening conditions. You decide to survey the pediatricians who began to practice in the city in the year 2000. You plan to repeat the survey annually with a random sample of this group of pediatricians through 2004. Would you describe your study as longitudinal, cohort, or case-control? Explain your answer.

2. One of your responsibilities at the hospital is to educate women about the need for a colposcopy if they have an abnormal cytologic smear. You wonder if women who are HIV-infected might be less likely to adhere to their physician's recommendation for a colposcopy. The data show the findings below:

	Colposcopy	
	No	**Yes**
HIV-infected	120	50
Not infected	30	170

   a. Calculate the odds ratio.
   b. Are the odds greater or less that HIV-infected women adhere to the recommendation to obtain a colposcopy?
   c. To what might you attribute these results?
   d. What do these results imply regarding an educational program?

3. If you elected to change your teaching style based on a review of the literature, which of the following would provide the best evidence to change: cohort study, case-control investigation, meta-analysis study, or random-controlled study? Why?

References

Ary, D., Jacobs, L. C., & Razavieh, A. (1972). *Introduction to research in education.* New York: Holt, Rinehart and Winston.

Chok, B., & Gomez, E. (2000). The reliability and application of the neck disability index in physiotherapy. *Physiotherapy-Singapore, 3*(1), 16–19.

Cleary, P. D., & Angel, R. (1984). The analysis of relationships involving dichotomous dependent variables. *Journal of Health and Social Behavior, 25,* 334–348.

Fleiss, J. L. (1981). *Statistical methods for rates and proportions* (2d ed.). New York: John Wiley & Sons.

Hayduk, L. A. (1987) *Structural equation modeling with LISREL: Essentials and advances.* Baltimore: John Hopkins University Press.

Hillis, S. D., Marchbanks, P. A., & Peterson, H. B. (1995). The effectiveness of hysterectomy for chronic pelvic pain. *Obstetrics & Gynecology, 86,* 941–945.

Joreskog, K. G., & Sorbom, D. (1989). *LISREL ® 7: User's reference guide.* Mooresville, IN: Scientific Software.

Kjellberg, L., Hallmans, G., Ahren, A., Johansson, R., Bergman, F., Wadell, G., Angstrom, T., & Dillner, J. (2000). Smoking, diet, pregnancy, and oral contraceptive use as risk factors for cervical intra-epithelial neoplasia in relation to papillomavirus infection. *British Journal Cancer, 82*(7), 1332–1338.

Kutner, N. G., Brogan, D., Hall, W. D., Haber, M., & Daniels, D. S. (2000). Functional impairment, depression, and life satisfaction among older hemodialysis patients and age-matched controls: A prospective study. *Archives of Physical Medicine and Rehabilitation, 81*(4), 453–459.

Landmark, K., & Abdelnoor, M. (2000). Current smokers develop more posterior myocardial infarctions probably due to increased tendency to thrombosis. *Scandinavian Cardiovascular Journal, 34*(1), 73–78.

Matthews, D. W., & Farewell, V. T. (1996). *Using and understanding medical statistics* (3rd ed.). Basel, Switzerland: S. Karger.

Mausner, J. S., & Kramer, S. (1985). *Epidemiology— An introductory text.* Philadelphia: W. B. Saunders.

Murthy, N. S., & Mathew, A. (2000). Risk factors for pre-cancerous lesions of the cervix. *European Journal of Cancer Prevention, 9*(1), 5–14.

Peterson, H. B., & Kleinbaum, D. G. (1991). Interpreting the literature in obstetrics and gynecology: I. Key concepts in epidemiology and biostatistics. *Obstetrics & Gynecology, 78,* 710–717.

Robinson, W. (2000). Invasive and preinvasive cervical neoplasia in human immunodeficiency virus-infected women. *Seminar Oncology, 27*(4), 463–470.

Rockett, I. R. H. (1994). Population and health: An introduction to epidemiology. *Population Bulletin, 49*(3).

Rosner, B. (1990). *Fundamentals of biostatistics* (3rd ed.). Boston: PWS-Kent.

Schlesselman, J. J. (1982). *Case-control studies: Design, conduct, analysis.* New York: Oxford University Press.

Simon, S. R., Peters, A. S., Christiansen, C. L., & Fletcher, R. H. (2000). The effect of medical student teaching on patient satisfaction in a managed care setting. *Journal of General Internal Medicine, 15*(7), 457–461.

Chapter *11*

Analyzing and Interpreting Data: Descriptive Analysis

Case Study

Manuel, chief health educator for the county, left the meeting knowing that he had a large task ahead of him. The county health board wanted some facts and figures about the apparent rise in teenage pregnancy. The local media were purporting that teen pregnancy was having a large negative impact on schools, the economy, and families. However, they were using national data rather than data from this small, rural county. County board members requested that Manuel calculate the number of pregnancies, the number of deliveries, the frequency of abortions and adoptions, the average age of the pregnant teens and the number that were in stable relationships, contraceptive usage, and the frequency of perinatal complications. He was to have this information prepared for the next county board meeting, one month from now. He knew that he had access to most of the information; it was a matter of procuring it and then making some statistical sense out of it so his description of the pregnant teenage population would meet the needs of the county board.

The Meaning of Statistics

Statistics is a language that can be employed to express concepts and relationships that cannot be communicated in any other way. To the neophyte health researcher, it is a language to be in awe of, or to fear; in contrast, the seasoned health scientist who understands the logic of statistics and appreciates its expressive power views it as a language to organize, analyze, and interpret numerical data.

Another approach to looking at statistics is in terms of its functional aspects. On the one hand, it can function to describe data: to explain how the data look, what the center point of the data is, how spread out the data may be, and how one aspect of the data may be related to one or more other aspects. For example, Manuel wants to describe the total number of pregnancies in the teenage population, the average age at the time of pregnancy, the age range of the group, the relationship between age at first coital experience and age at the time of pregnancy, and the number of perinatal complications. His primary concern, then, is to describe this group of teenagers. Subsequently, this branch of statistical analysis is called *descriptive statistical analysis*. No conclusions can be extended beyond this immediate group, and any similarity to those outside the group cannot be assumed.

A different function of statistics is to infer. *Inferential statistical analysis* involves observation of a sample taken from a given population. Conclusions about the population are inferred from the information obtained about the sample. Suppose you were to observe the health habits of a random sample of poor inhabitants from the Appalachian region. You could then make inferences about the health habits of the total population of poor persons in the Appalachia. Unlike descriptive data analysis, generalizations can be made from the sample to the respective population. Note that Manuel will not do this in his study because he is using descriptive data analysis.

Inferential data analysis can be used for estimation and prediction. For example, scores obtained on the Graduate Record Examination may predict how well an incoming candidate may perform in a graduate health science program. Extrapolation is a component of inferential statistics but not of descriptive statistics.

Statistical Analysis and Data

Levels of Measurement

While there are several ways to classify variables, one of the principal techniques is the preciseness of measurement of the variable. We will discuss four levels of measurement.

The first and weakest measure is called *nominal*. At this level, variables are simply placed into different categories. For example, "gender" is nominal data since 1 or 0 can be assigned to male and female, respectively.

The next higher level measures both groups and ranks the data through ordering of categories. This is called *ordinal* data or measurement. Examples of ordinal measurements in the health sciences are abundant—dosage levels, degree of education, severity of illness, and even social class. The limitation to some categories may be the amount of information available to do the ordering. For example, how much difference is there between lower middle class and upper middle class? In short, the rankings may be relative rather than absolute.

The next level of measurement categorizes, orders, and provides a meaningful measure of the differences in the ordering. That is, *interval* variables can be separated by how much they differ from one another. These variables are not nebulous, unlike socioeconomic status. Examples of interval variables include height, weight, blood pressure, and the like; their intervals are equal. Celsius temperatures are another example, with the temperature difference between 5 and 15 degrees Centigrade (10 degrees Celsius) being the same as that between 20 and 30 degrees Centigrade.

When interval variables have a true zero point, they may be called *ratio* variables. Height is an example of a ratio variable, as is measure of temperature in Kelvin. As a point of note, Celsius temperature is an interval measurement because the zero is an arbitrary point.

Parametric and Nonparametric Data

Two types of data are recognized in the application of statistics: parametric and nonparametric. *Parametric* data are either interval or ratio data. Parametrical statistical tests assume that the data are normally or near normally distributed. In comparison, data that are either counted (nominal scale) or ranked (ordinal scale) are called *nonparametric* data. Nonparametric statistical tests, often referred to as distribution-free tests, do not require the more restrictive assumption of a normally distributed population.

Frequently parametric tests are considered the more powerful of the two. However, this is only the case when all the assumptions and restrictions of parametric data have been met. If there is lack of homogeneity of variances, unequal n's, and oppositely skewed distributions, using the t-test is not as powerful as converting the data to ordinal scale and applying nonparametric tests. Generally, nonparametric tests have wider applications and are less difficult to compute.

Population and Sample

A *population* can be defined as the set of elements we are planning to study. In the health sciences it usually refers to a group of people—all the patients in the hospital, all those living in the county, all graduate students in the health sciences, and so on. However, the population can be something other than a group of people, such as all daily maximum temperatures or all automobiles produced in a given time frame. A *sample* is a subset of the population.

Parameters and Statistics

A *parameter* is a characteristic of a population, whereas a *statistic* is a characteristic of a sample. Although different texts often employ different symbols, some of the more common ones are:

	Sample Statistic	Population Parameter
Mean	$M, \overline{X}$	μ
Standard deviation	s, sd	σ
Variance	s^2	σ^2

Descriptive Data Analysis Techniques

There are several statistical techniques available to the health science researcher who wishes to describe the observed research group:

- Measures of central tendency
  Mean
  Median
  Mode
  Geometric mean
- Measures of spread or variation
  Range
  Standard deviation
  Variance
  Coefficient of variation
- Standard measures
- Measures of relationship
  Spearman rank order correlation
  Pearson product-moment correlation

It is the responsibility of the health science reseacher to select the technique that best fits the data and that will explain the data in a manner comprehensible to the intended audience.

Measures of Central Tendency

Manuel, in our teenage pregnancy example, was asked to describe the group using averages—average age, average grade level, average number of sexual partners, and so on. This is a typical request, because most people wish to find a value about which the observations tend to cluster. The three most common measures used to describe the centering point of a set of data are the mean, median, and mode. Collectively, they are called measures of central tendency.

Mean.   The mean (M or $\overline{X}$) of a set of data is commonly referred to as the arithmetic mean or average. It is computed by summing all the observations in the group and dividing by the number of observations. The formula is:

$$M = \frac{\Sigma X}{N}$$

where M = mean
$\quad\quad X$ = scores in a distribution
$\quad\quad \Sigma$ = sum of
$\quad\quad N$ = number of scores

TABLE 11.1 Current Age and Arithmetic Mean of Pregnant Teenagers

Teenager	X
1	11
2	15
3	18
4	12
5	11
6	16
7	14
8	13
9	19
10	14
11	16
12	17
13	15
14	16
15	15
16	15

$$M = \frac{237}{16} = 14.81$$

$\Sigma X = 237 \qquad N = 16$

For example, Manuel recorded the ages of 16 pregnant teens and computed the average age. His data are displayed in Table 11.1.

The arithmetic mean, which may be considered the fulcrum or balance point of a distribution, is one of the most useful statistical measures because it provides much information; is affected by all the scores; and serves as a basis for the computation of other important measures, such as variability.

Median. The median is a measure of position in that it is the point above and below which one-half of the scores fall. In other words, it is the middle-most position. If Manuel examined the number of sexual partners for an odd number of the pregnant teens to determine the median point, he would find that it is the midscore. For example:

7
6   2 scores above
4 = median
3   2 scores below
1

If Manuel had an even number of subjects, the median would be the middle point between the two middle scores:

```
10
 3                    2 scores above
 2.5 = median
 2                    2 scores below
 1
```

Unlike the mean, the median is not influenced by extreme scores. Therefore, in some instances it may be a more realistic measure of central tendency than the mean. Our second example with four scores and a median of 2.5 illustrates this concept. However, the median is usually reserved for when a quick measure of central tendency is needed or when distributions are markedly skewed.

Mode. The mode is simply the most frequently occurring score. By examining the ages of the 16 pregnant teenagers in Table 11.1, it can be seen that the most frequently occurring age is 15. Subsequently, the modal age for this group is 15. The mode is the quickest estimate of central value and shows the most typical case.

Geometric Mean. The geometric mean is often used in laboratory data. This is especially true with data in the form of concentrations of substances. An example might be the concentration of penicillin in urine for *N. gonorrhea*. The geometric mean is calculated using the antilogarithim of log *x*. Rosner (1990) provides an excellent illustration for infectious disease.

Measures of Spread or Variation

The measures of central tendency are useful, but oftentimes more information is needed for an accurate description of the sample or population. This is particularly true in a comparison of two groups whose means are identical. In such situations, it is important to know whether the scores or observations for each group tend to be quite similar (homogeneous) or spread apart (heterogeneous). Measures of variation, to include range, variance, and standard deviation, may be employed to show the degree of spread or variation among scores. As an example, Manuel reviewed the data for two groups of pregnant teenagers in regard to the total number of sexual partners. The first group comprised those currently in a committed relationship, whereas the members of the second group were not presently in a committed relationship. Table 11.2 illustrates his findings. A comparison of the two groups shows that the average total number of sexual partners for each group is identical: 4. This information has little value if he presents it as is to the county board. However, if he examines the measures of spread or variation within each group, differences are apparent. This illustrates the need for measures of variation or spread.

Range. The range is the simplest measure of variation. It is the difference between the highest and lowest scores. For example, from Table 11.2, Group 1 has a range of 14 (15 – 1), while Group 2 has a range of 5 (6 – 1). The range may be used justifiably

TABLE 11.2 Current Relationship Commitment and Total Number of Sexual Partners

Group 1: Committed Relationship	Group 1: Number of Sexual Partners	Group 2: Uncommitted Relationship	Group 2: Number of Sexual Partners
Marge	15	Kim	1
Sarah	1	Terri	5
Karen	1	Louise	5
Teresa	4	Tamara	6
Wendy	4	Venessa	4
Liz	3	Caitlin	1
Emily	1	Freda	5
Mary	3	Anna	5
	$\Sigma X = 32$		$\Sigma X = 32$
	Mean = 4		Mean = 4

as a hasty measure of variability, but since it takes into account only the extremes and not the bulk of observations, it is not generally employed.

Standard Deviation and Variance. The most useful measures of variation are standard deviation and variance. Deviation is defined as the distance of the measurements away from the mean. In a study dealing with a sample, the variance is the sum of the squared deviations from the mean, divided by $N - 1$. Although it will be discussed later, it is important to understand that the variance is obtained from squared deviations from the mean, thereby making the variance a different unit of measurement than the mean. The formula is

$$s^2 = \frac{\Sigma(X - M)^2}{N - 1}$$

or

$$s^2 = \frac{\Sigma x^2}{N - 1}$$

where $x = (X - M)$

Using the information in Table 11.2, the variance for Group 1 is calculated as:

$$s^2 = \frac{150}{7} = 21.43$$

The complete calculations are shown in Table 11.3. Using the same formula, the variance for Group 2, as shown in Table 11.4, is 3.71. In comparing the variances,

TABLE 11.3 Variance of Group 1: Committed Relationship

X	x or (X – M)	x^2
15	+11	121
1	–3	9
1	–3	9
4	0	0
4	0	0
3	–1	1
1	–3	9
3	–1	1
$\Sigma X = 32$	$\Sigma x = 0$	$\Sigma x^2 = 150$

TABLE 11.4 Variance of Group 2: Uncommitted Relationship

X	x or (X – M)	x^2
1	–3	9
5	+1	1
5	+1	1
6	+2	4
4	0	0
1	–3	9
5	+1	1
5	+1	1
$\Sigma X = 32$	$\Sigma x = 0$	$\Sigma x^2 = 26$

Manuel would find that the number of partners for the pregnant teens in Group 1 varied much more than those in Group 2. That is, the data for Group 1 are heterogeneous, while the data for Group 2 are homogeneous.

The standard deviation is computed by obtaining the square root of the variance. Notice that this takes away the squaring of deviations, thereby making the standard deviation the same unit of measurement as the mean. By formula, standard deviation is:

$$s = \sqrt{\frac{\Sigma x^2}{N-1}}$$

Therefore, the standard deviations for Groups 1 and 2, respectively, are:

$$\text{Group 1} \quad s = \sqrt{\frac{\Sigma x^2}{N-1}} = \sqrt{\frac{150}{7}} = \sqrt{21.43} = 4.63$$

$$\text{Group 2} \quad s = \sqrt{\frac{\Sigma x^2}{N-1}} = \sqrt{\frac{26}{7}} = \sqrt{3.71} = 1.93$$

As with the variance data, comparison of the standard deviations reveals that the spread of scores (total number of sexual partners) is much greater in Group 1 than in Group 2. As stated previously, the variance is the sum of squared deviations, whereas the standard deviation is not squared, thereby leaving it in the same measurement units as the arithmetic mean. This holds true whether the measurement is in centimeters, units of blood, people, or whatever. This is one of the principal reasons why the standard deviation is reported more often than the variance as a measure of spread.

When the health science researcher is working with data from an entire population, there is a slight change in the formula along with different symbols. The population mean, μ (*mu*), is the sum of all values divided by N (the total number in the entire population). By comparison, the sample mean, M or $\bar{x}$, is an estimation of the population mean. Similarly, the sample variance (s^2) is an estimate of the population variance (σ^2), which is determined by the formula:

$$\sigma^2 = \frac{\Sigma x^2}{N}$$

The standard deviation of the population is ascertained by:

$$\sigma = \sqrt{\frac{\Sigma x^2}{N}}$$

The difference between formulas and samples is the use of $N-1$ rather than N for division in the sample formula. The reason for employing $N-1$ in the sample formula is to provide an equation that gives an unbiased sample variance. In other words, $N-1$ allows for a more accurate estimate of the population variance and standard deviation.

Coefficient of Variation. As noted previously, the arithmetic mean and standard deviation are usually reported together to describe data. This is important because, for example, a standard deviation of 10 would mean something different if the arithmetic mean were 20 rather than 500. Also, the standard deviation and the mean are in the same units. However, there are occasions when the health science researcher wishes to compare the variability of different samples, each having different arithmetic means and perhaps differing units of measurement.

In our example with Manuel, suppose he wanted to compare birth weights of the infants of the pregnant teens based upon their site for prenatal care and delivery.

However, he finds that one site recorded the birth weights in grams and the other in ounces. Because the standard deviation for each group is based on the unit of measurement, this would be an inaccurate comparison. To overcome this problem, Manuel would use the coefficient of variation (*CV*). It is calculated as:

$$CV = 100\% \times \frac{s}{M}$$

If the birthweights at the site using grams as the measurement unit had a mean and standard deviation of 3121.8 grams and 432.6 grams, respectively, the *CV* would be:

$$CV = 100\% \times \frac{432.6}{3121.8} = 13.9\%$$

The site using ounces as the unit of measurement had a mean of 89.9 ounces and a standard deviation of 12.2 ounces. The calculation is:

$$CV = 100\% \times \frac{12.2}{89.9} = 13.6\%$$

The comparison shows little difference in the variability of birth weights between the two sites.

Standard Measures

Standard scores are equal units of measurement and are very useful in reporting test scores or doing research involving test results. For example, if a subject scored a 75 on a health science test and 85 on a statistics test, which one is really better? Obviously the raw data are of little use, since the tests may differ in the number of items and scaling. For comparison, the scores must be transformed to a common equal-interval scale in which they are called *standard scores*. The standard score, also called the *z*-score, is calculated by subtracting the mean from the observed score and dividing the result by the standard deviation:

$$z = \frac{X - M}{s}$$

where M = mean
X = observed score of the observed distribution
s = standard deviation of the observed distribution

Suppose the health science test had a mean (*M*) of 70 with a standard deviation (*s*) of 3, whereas the statistics test had a mean (*M*) of 88 with a standard deviation (*s*) of 6. Using the formula, the *z*-score for the health science test would be +1.67 and for the statistics test –0.5. The comparison shows the health science test score is much better than the statistics test score. Note that z-scores can be negative as well as positive.

Since z-scores can be expressed in negatives and decimals, oftentimes they are converted so as not to be cumbersome. For example, the subtests of the SAT scores are simply converted z-scores. The mean is set at 500, and the standard deviation is 100. To transform the score, simply multiply the z-score by the standard deviation and then add the mean. Conversion of the health science score to this system is as follows:

$$\text{Transformed score} = z(100) + 500 = 1.67(100) + 500 = 667$$

Intelligence test scores (IQ) have means of 100 with a standard deviation of 15.

Standard scores rather than raw scores can be used by teachers in summing test results for the semester. These give each measure or test the same weight. If the distribution is normal in shape, the standard score can be converted to a percentile rank from a table in most statistics books.

Measures of Relationship

Some of the most interesting questions posed in health science research revolve around the relationship of one variable to another, such as smoking and lung cancer. The method used most frequently to describe the relationship between two or more variables or between two or more sets of data is linear correlation. The degree of relationship is expressed by the coefficient of correlation, symbolized by *r*.

Some of the unique characteristics of the correlation coefficient are that it is a pure number, it is nondimensional, and it may take on values between –1.00 and +1.00. A correlation coefficient of zero indicates no relationship between the variables in question. The closer the *r* is to 1.00 (negative or positive), the stronger the relationship. A perfect positive correlation of =1.00 specifies that for every unit increase in one variable, there is a proportional unit increase in the other variable. Concomitantly, a perfect negative correlation of –1.00 means that for every unit increase in one variable, there is a unit decrease in the other variable. Perfect correlations are highly unlikely in dealing with human health concerns.

The scattergram is a means of displaying the relationship between variables and is developed by graphically plotting each pair of variables that correspond to the X and Y axis, respectively. The line drawn through or near the coordinate points is referred to as the line of best fit or regression line. Figure 11.1 demonstrates several correlations and their regression line.

The beginning health science reseacher must be careful not to fall into the trap of attributing a cause-and-effect relationship to variables that might be related. For instance, Kuzma (1984) reports a strong relationship between a child's foot size and handwriting ability. As explained, however, this is likely because both increase with age rather than being a direct cause-and-effect relationship. Spurious relationships must be viewed with caution and interpreted judiciously.

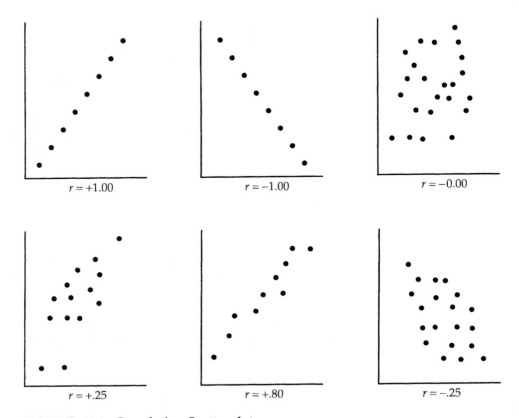

FIGURE 11.1   Correlation Scatterplots

Spearman Rank Order Correlation. The Spearman rank order correlation is used to determine the relationship between two ranked variables (rather than interval or ratio variables). That is, the Spearman rank order correlation, signified by r_s, is designed for nonparametric data. Frequently, a health science investigator may employ it to compare judgments by a group of judges on two objects or the scores of a group of subjects on two measures (for further information on this usage, consult Siegel, 1956). A less frequent but valuable usage is to compare judgments by two judges on a group of objects or items. Hays (1973) discusses the Spearman rank order correlation for assessing interjudge equivalence. In cases of multiple judges and multiple objects, the Friedman two-way analysis of variance or Kendall coefficient of concordance would be used.

The equation for Spearman rank order correlation coefficient is:

$$r_s = 1 - \frac{6 \, \Sigma d^2}{n(n^2 - 1)}$$

where n = number of pairs
      d = difference between paired ranks
   Σd^2 = sum of the squared differences between ranks

If Manuel, in our case example, were to have two independent physicians rank 10 teenage mothers according to the severity of perinatal complications (teen pregnancies are typically associated with a 25% increase in the risk of perinatal mortality), he would use the Spearman technique. Table 11.5 displays the data. Note that ties in ranks are handled by averaging the ranks. Using the formula, Manuel would obtain:

$$r_s = 1 - \frac{6(63.75)}{10(99)} = .62$$

The Spearman rank order correlation procedure is an acceptable method for parametric data when there are fewer than 30 but greater than 9 paired variables. The ease of computation allows it to be used by health teachers for a single classroom of students.

Pearson Product-Moment Correlation. The Pearson product-moment correlation, the most often used and most precise coefficient of correlation, is used with parametric data. The basic formula, symbolized by r, is:

$$r = \frac{N\Sigma XY - (\Sigma X)(\Sigma Y)}{\sqrt{N\Sigma X^2 - (\Sigma X)^2}\ \sqrt{N\Sigma Y^2 - (\Sigma Y)^2}}$$

TABLE 11.5 Ranking of Severity of Perinatal Complications by Two Independent Physicians

Patient Number	Physician 1's Rank Order (X)	Physician 2's Rank Order (Y)	d ($x - y$)	d^2 ($x - y)^2$
1	1	2	1	1.00
2	4	1	3	9.00
3	7.5	9.5	-2.5	6.25
4	2	3	-1	1.00
5	7.5	8	-0.5	0.25
6	3	4	-1	1.00
7	5	9.5	-4.5	20.25
8	6	6	0	0.00
9	9	5	4	16.00
10	10	7	3	9.00
				$\Sigma d^2 = 63.75$

This is the raw score equation that is convenient for both calculator and computer use. Statistics books can be explored to obtain equations written in a different format (Kuzma, 1984).

Manuel wished to investigate the relationship between the pregnant teenagers' ages at the time of becoming pregnant and their first coital experience. Table 11.6 illustrates the data and necessary calculations for 16 pregnant teenagers. The process involves five columns.

TABLE 11.6 Age at Pregnancy and Age at First Intercourse

Age at Pregnancy X	Age at First Intercourse Y	X^2	Y^2	XY
11	11	121	121	121
15	12	225	144	180
18	12	324	144	216
12	11	144	121	132
11	11	121	121	121
16	13	256	169	208
14	13	196	169	182
13	12	169	144	156
19	11	361	121	209
14	10	196	100	140
16	15	256	225	240
17	14	289	196	238
15	13	225	169	195
16	16	256	256	256
15	13	225	169	195
15	14	225	196	210
$\Sigma X = 237$	$\Sigma Y = 201$	$\Sigma X^2 = 3589$	$\Sigma Y^2 = 2565$	$\Sigma XY = 2999$

$$r = \frac{16(2999) - (237)(201)}{\sqrt{[16(3589) - (237)^2][16(2565) - (201)^2]}}$$

$$r = \frac{47{,}984 - 47{,}367}{\sqrt{[57{,}424 - 56{,}169][41{,}040 - 40{,}401]}}$$

$$r = \frac{617}{\sqrt{[1255][639]}}$$

$$r = \frac{617}{\sqrt{801{,}945}}$$

$$r = \frac{617}{895.51} = 0.69$$

Personal Computers and Information Delivery Systems

As computer technology has increased, the cost of hardware and, in many instances, of software has decreased. Consequently, most entry-level health science researchers are able to analyze their data on desktop or laptop PCs. The power of these computers has grown significantly, allowing very sophisticated computations through a myriad of software programs. In addition to the obvious data analysis, several software packages have an integrated suite to address issues of data access, management, and presentation. Examples of computer programs that can be employed by the health science researcher include: Statistical Analysis System (SAS), Statistical Package for the Social Sciences (SPSS for Windows), Minitab, Statistica, and S-Plus.

Selection of a statistical analysis package can be an arduous process. Some considerations for selection and possible purchasing are:

1. Know what statistical analyses you need to do now or in the near future. The package you purchase is likely to be updated in the future (for ease of use and so forth), so you can probably plan on getting another package as your needs change. Table 11.7 illustrates some of the procedures that can be found in various programs.
2. Know whether you need a full database system.
3. Think about your knowledge of variables, variable labeling, and variable manipulation, and select a program that meets or slightly exceeds your knowledge level.
4. Display of data is important, and you should consider the nature of the graphic displays you would like to have as well as the look of tables. For example, do you need plotting capabilities? Do the tables generated by the program indicate all the necessary variables and labels?
5. Does the package have a tutorial segment? If so, does it allow you to exit and then reenter where you left off, rather than having to start at the beginning again?
6. Is online help readily available in the package, and is it understandable?
7. Is technical support service available locally, through a help line, on the Internet or World Wide Web, or by fax or e-mail?
8. If you plan to buy, know how much money you have to spend and be careful not to be sold something you neither need nor can afford.

Computer software can take the drudgery out of many research tasks. However, as the world becomes more mobile, access to information in a portable and simple manner is becoming more important. Wireless technologies extend information delivery as well as advanced data analysis. Instead of computers, health science researchers can use lightweight devices such as cell phones, pagers, handheld PCs, and Palm Pilots for computing. Accessing data from CDC while on the golf course

TABLE 11.7 Typical Statistical Procedures Available in Software for the PC

Statistical Component	Typical Usage
Frequencies	Counts, percentages, central tendencies, dispersion, distributions
Descriptives	Central tendencies, geometric mean, variance, standard deviation, standard error of the mean, coefficient of variation, N and $N-1$ denominators
Confidence intervals	User-specified, such as one group mean, paired mean difference, unpaired mean difference, variance, t-test
t-tests	One group, two group paired, two group unpaired, one sample to compare sample mean to reference mean of choice
Cross-tabulation	Two-way contingency tables, summary statistics, Fisher's exact test, continuity correction, *phi* coefficient for 2×2 tables, Cramer's *V*, Mantel-Haenszel's *chi*-square, Goodman and Kruskl's *lambda, tau, gamma*
ANOVA and ANCOVA	Balanced and unbalanced designs, several covariates, several independent variables, post-hoc tests such as Duncan's multiple range, Scheffe's test, Student-Newman-Keuls, Tukey's procedure
Correlation	Bivariate to include Pearson's *r*, Kendall's tau-b, Spearman, cross product deviations and covariances; partial correlation
Regression	Several methods: forced entry; forced removal; backward elimination; forward entry; stepwise procedures; polynomial; plots such as scatterplots, outlier, normal probability, partial, histogram
Nonparametric tests	*Chi*-square; one sample tests such as Kolmogorov-Smirnov, Poisson; two independent samples Mann-Whitney, Kolmogorov-Smirnov Z; *k*-independent samples Kruskal-Wallis; two related samples Wilcoxon, sign, McNemar; *k*-related samples Kendall's *W*, Friedman
Survival analysis	Actuarial estimates, linear rank tests, Kaplan-Meier; plots like cumulative survival, hazard
Graphing capabilities	Importing and exporting files; chart production directly from statistical results; graphs; automatic templates; page layout; interface with several printers

or at the gym will be simple. Crucial to mobile computing as well as more standard computers are packages available on the Internet. Appendix B provides further information about these resources.

Case Discussion

To describe the pregnant teenagers in the county, Manuel needed to analyze the data so that they could be presented in an understandable fashion. This required using descriptive data analysis with several of his variables, which were nominal or ordinal. Other data, such as age, however, were interval data. Central tendencies provided averages for the data, but he found it necessary to employ measures of variation (range and standard deviation) to better describe this group of pregnant teens. Relational measures were used with both ordinal and interval variables. Using any or all of these statistical analysis procedures, Manuel can work through each variable to arrive at a very descriptive report for the county board.

Summary

This chapter discussed descriptive analysis. Statistics, it was seen, is simply a language to express concepts and relationships that cannot be communicated in any other way. As we saw, statistics can be divided into descriptive and inferential. Descriptive statistics describe the population or sample. Inferential statistical analysis involves observation of a sample taken from a population, and conclusions about that population are then inferred from the sample.

Statistical analysis takes several things into consideration. One is the level of measurement, which can be nominal, ordinal, interval, or ratio. Another issue is the type of data—parametric and nonparametric. The researcher must know the differences between parameter and statistic as they apply to a population and sample.

The measures of central tendency examined included the mean, median, mode, and geometric mean for laboratory data. Measures of spread or variation discussed were the range, standard deviation, variance, and coefficient of variation. Relationship measures presented were Spearman rank order correlation and Pearson product-moment correlation.

Computer software is readily available in either abbreviated student packages or packages for professionals. Many of the major companies have packages for basic statistics and other packages for advanced statistics. The WWW has several computer resources and support services, some of which are connected directly with universities, while others connect directly to the software company.

Suggested Activities

1. What measure of central tendency would you use to describe a group of people with normal blood pressure as compared to a group experiencing severe hypertension? Why?

2. Go to the website www.math.yorku.ca and review the statistical resources available. As you move further into the site, seek www resources and, in particular, software available to students and professionals, such as SPSS, SAS, Minitab, and others. Appendix B contains website addresses for several statistical packages.

3. Use a calculator, a software package, or Microsoft Excel to calculate the mean, median, mode, variance, and standard deviation for each of the following two groups of scores, which represent student performance on a health science test, with the highest possible score being 50. (Microsoft Excel has several statistical tests that can be used for descriptive analysis and often comes bundled with other packages.)

Group A		Group B	
35	21	20	25
49	28	50	44
33	41	16	29
44	37	21	40
45	39	23	26

   a. Which group has the greatest variability in scores?
   b. Which group has the highest mean score?
   c. How would you describe each group when comparing it to the other?

4. Visit the website http://ebook.stat.ucla.edu/textbook/calculators/ and go to two-test sample calculator (http://ebook.stat.ucla.edu/textbook/calculators/twosamp/), enter the data from Activity 3 above. This is from Statistics UCLA (the general website is www.stat.ucla.edu/) and allows you to input two sets of numbers; it gives a one-sided or two-sided t-test for paired or independent samples. It can either look up the P value for t or compute the P value using the randomization distribution.

References

Hays, W. L. (1973). *Statistics for the social sciences* (2d ed.). New York: Holt, Rinehart, & Winston.

Kuzma, J. (1984). *Basic statistics for the health sciences.* Palo Alto, CA: Mayfield.

Rosner, B. (1990). *Fundamentals of biostatistics* (3rd ed.). Boston: PWS-Kent.

Siegel, W. (1956). *Nonparametric statistics.* New York: McGraw-Hill.

Analyzing and Interpreting Data: Inferential Analysis

Case Study

Schyler, a resident in internal medicine at Harbor Hospital, has been assigned a research project to complete her MSN. Her advisor has asked her to conduct a study to determine if the effects of a new patient education program for AIDS patients can be generalized to all AIDS patients in the state.

Inferential Analysis

After reading Schyler's assignment you will probably ask: How can we make such inferences about the patient education program from just one sample of patients? Inferential statistics use procedures that allow researchers to make those inferences about the population based on the descriptive statistics obtained from analyzing the data collected on the sample. The descriptive measures from the sample are the statistics, while the descriptive measures from the population are the parameters. Inferences are thus made about the parameters from the statistics.

Testing Statistical Significance

To analyze data utilizing inferential statistics, two procedures may be employed: testing hypotheses or estimating parameters. Hypothesis testing is more generally used and is a statement about one or more parameters. The estimating of a parameter is done by point or interval estimation, also known as a confidence interval (CI). A point estimate is a single-value estimate of the parameter and is the value of the corresponding statistic from the sample. An interval estimate (or CI) is an interval on the scale of measurement that contains estimates of the parameter (Wiersma, 2000). It seems that intervals are used more often than point estimation in the type of research that Schyler is conducting.

Estimation of Parameters

We use estimation procedures when we have no pre-established hypothesis about the value of a population characteristic. In our case study, Schyler might make an estimate of our AIDS patients' beginning T-cell count, using an average count for similar patients. As mentioned before, CIs are the ranges of values within a parameter. The upper and lower limits of the range values are *confidence limits.*

Constructing a confidence interval around a sample mean establishes a range of values for a population parameter in addition to a certain probability of being correct. This degree of confidence we have is arbitrary; however, researchers usually use either a 95% or 99% CI.

Hypotheses Testing

Hypotheses or significance testing is used to determine whether all observed difference (the sample) provides enough evidence to believe that there is a corresponding difference in the population. A *significance test* is a procedure to determine whether:

1. The difference between a sample value and another value should be attributed simply to random error or chance, in which case the sample difference is said to be *not statistically different*, or;
2. The difference is large enough for us to conclude that the corresponding population values are different, in which case the sample difference is said to be *statistically significant* (Boniface, 1999).

There are two competing hypotheses in hypothesis testing: the *null hypothesis* and the *alternative hypothesis*. The null hypothesis (H_0) is that a certain population's values are not different from each other. In our case study, the null hypothesis would be stated:

H_0 = There is no difference in T-cell counts between the AIDS patients exposed to the new patient education program and the patients not using the new patient education program.

If we find that the data are unlikely to have occurred in the null hypothesis, we reject the null hypothesis, and conclude that the values, in this case T-cell counts, are different from each other. Here we have a difference that is statistically significant. On the other hand, if it is found that the data are reasonably likely to occur in the patient education program, as proposed by the null hypothesis, we do not reject it, and we attribute the difference to chance (not statistically significant).

Once the null hypothesis is rejected, an *alternative hypothesis* (H_1) is used:

H_1 = The T-cell counts of both groups of AIDS patients are not equal.

This alternative hypothesis is nondirectional because it does not state which group's T-cell count will be lower. A *directional hypothesis* specifies the direction of the expected findings:

H_1 (directional) = The T-cell counts of the patients in the experimental program
will be lower than the T-cell counts of patients in the
control group.

Once the null hypothesis is stated, you should select an appropriate test statistic to be used. A listing of these can be found in Appendix A. You need to determine if a parametric test should be utilized and what the level of measurement was used for the measures. Most researchers apply *two-tailed* tests of significance. This means that each "tail," or end, of the sample distribution is used to determine the range of improbable values (Polit & Hungler, 1999). A *one-tailed* test should be used when there is a directional hypothesis. However, use of one-tailed tests has met with much criticism; therefore you might assume that two-tailed tests have been utilized unless specified by the researcher.

Level of Significance

The acceptance or rejection of a hypothesis is based upon a level of significance (*alpha* level, or α), which corresponds to the area in the critical region. Many research efforts in health science establish the level of significance at the 5% (.05) *alpha* level, although it may be set at the .025, .01, or .001 levels. Rejecting the null hypothesis at the .05 *alpha* level suggests a 95% probability that the differences between the two variables is real, that is, not the result of chance. In other words, there is a less than 5% probability that the differences are caused by error or chance.

In a two-tailed test of significance, the 5% area of rejection is split between the upper and lower tails of the curve since the null hypothesis is nondirectional. By comparison, in the directional one-tailed test, the 5% area of rejection is at either the upper end or the lower end of the curve. As a general rule of thumb, the following probabilities and interpretations are widely accepted by health science researchers (Kuzma & Bohneneblust, 2001):

Probability Value	Interpretation
>.05	Result is not significant.
<.05	Result is significant.
<.01	Result is highly significant.

Critical Region

The critical region is the far end of the distribution as seen in the normal curve. In a one-tailed test, only one end of the distribution is used, whereas in a two-tailed test, both ends of the distribution are used (Figure 12.1). For example, if Schyler were to hypothesize that knowledge about AIDS is the same for AIDS patients as for the general public (null, no difference), a two-tailed test would be employed. On the other hand, Schyler could hypothesize either of the following:

1. AIDS patients have greater AIDS knowledge than the general public, or;
2. AIDS patients have less AIDS knowledge than the general public.

FIGURE 12.1 Two-Tailed and One-Tailed Regions

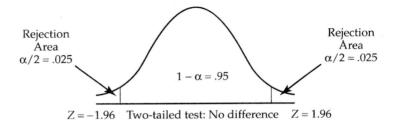

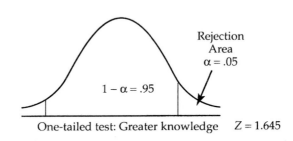

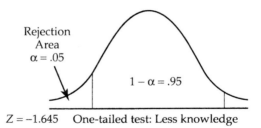

Both hypotheses indicate direction of difference and would therefore require a one-tailed test.

Type I and Type II Errors

Type I error is the rejection of a null hypothesis when it in fact is true. The *alpha* level of significance determines the probability of a Type I error. If the health science researcher rejects a null hypothesis at the .01 level, there is a 1% risk of rejecting it when it is actually true. Similarly, using the .05 *alpha* level of significance, the researcher is taking a 5% risk of rejecting the null hypothesis even when it is true.

However, if the null hypothesis is accepted when in fact it is false, a Type II error occurs. Therefore, if the health science researcher establishes the *alpha* level of significance as high as .01, the possibility of a Type I error is reduced, but the chance of a Type II error increases.

As an example, suppose that Schyler compared two educational techniques to be used with the AIDS patients—Technique A and Technique B. If she rejected the null hypothesis and claimed that Technique B was the preferred method for teaching, new equipment may be purchased and additional personnel budgeted. Later, in subsequent experimentation or in actual programs, it may be found that Technique B failed to bring about the expected results. Although the ultimate truth about the falsity of the null hypothesis would still be unknown, evidence supporting the null hypothesis would be abundant, leaving Schyler humiliated and with a depleted budget. She probably committed a Type I error.

On the other hand, if she accepts the null hypothesis and it is later found that there is a difference between Techniques A and B in that one brings about better results, she again may be embarrassed. Typically, Type I errors lead to unwarranted changes, whereas Type II errors maintain the status quo when a change should occur.

Inferential Data Analysis Techniques

The t-Test for Two Independent Sample Means

Health science research workers frequently draw two samples from a population and assign them to a control group or to an experimental group. After the experimental group has been exposed to the treatment, the researchers may wish to compare the experimental to the control group. Because the mean is likely the most satisfactory measure for characterizing a group, health scientists find it important to determine if there is a difference between the mean of the experimental group and the mean of the control group. To accomplish this, a *t*-test is used to determine the probability that the difference between the means is a real difference rather than a chance difference.

In such a situation, the null hypothesis is expressed as:

$$H_0: M_1 = M_2 \quad \text{or} \quad H_0: M_1 - M_2 = 0$$

The alternative hypothesis is:

$$H_1: M_1 > M_2$$

The formula for the *t*-test is as follows:

$$t = \frac{M_1 - M_2}{\sqrt{\dfrac{s_1^2}{N_1} + \dfrac{s_2^2}{N_2}}}$$

where M_1 = mean of experimental group
M_2 = mean of control group
N_1 = number in experimental group
N_2 = number in control group
s_1^2 = variance of experimental group
s_2^2 = variance of control group

When the samples are greater than 30 subjects, the *t* critical values are expressed as *z* scores. Therefore, the obtained *t*-value from the formula is compared with the *z* distribution for acceptance or rejection of the null hypothesis. If the obtained *t*-value exceeds the *z* score of 1.96 (two-tailed test), the researcher may conclude that a significant difference exists between the two means at the .05 level. Concomitantly, an obtained *t*-value greater than a 2.58 *z* score (two-tailed test) allows the researcher to reject the null hypothesis at the 0.1 level of significance.

One of the concerns that Schyler may have about an educational program for AIDS patients is a reduction in the fear and panic displayed by many such patients. If she had two randomly selected groups, with one being experimental and the other being control, she could compare the mean of the two groups on a measure designed to reflect fear. To obtain the necessary data to test the null hypothesis that there is no difference between the experimental and the control, she could compare the mean of the two groups on a measure designed to reflect fear. The necessary data to test the null hypothesis that there is no difference between the experimental and control groups at the .01 level would be

Experimental Group	Control Group
$N_1 = 34$	$N_1 = 32$
$M_1 = 75.25$	$M_2 = 70.25$
$s_1^2 = 21$	$s_1^2 = 22$

$$t = \frac{M_1 - M_2}{\sqrt{\dfrac{s_1^2}{N_1} + \dfrac{s_2^2}{N_2}}} = \frac{75.25 - 70.25}{\sqrt{\dfrac{21}{34} + \dfrac{22}{32}}}$$

$$t = \frac{5}{\sqrt{.62 = .69}} = \frac{5}{\sqrt{1.31}} = \frac{5}{1.14}$$

$$t = 4.39$$

Because the obtained *t*-value from the formula exceeds the z score of 2.58, Schyler may reject the null hypothesis at the .01 level of significance. Table 12.1 shows the *t*-critical values for the rejection of the null hypothesis in samples with an *N* greater than 30.

When the samples are fewer than 30 in number (small samples), a *t*-table is used rather than the normal probability table. The reason for this is that the distribution curves of small samples are different from the normal curve.

The formula for testing the significance of the difference between two small sample means is:

$$t = \frac{M_1 - M_2}{\sqrt{\dfrac{(N-1)\,s_1^2 + (N-1)\,s_2^2}{N_1 + N_2 - 2}\left(\dfrac{1}{N_1} + \dfrac{1}{N_2}\right)}}$$

The *t*-value, which is obtained from the formula, is then compared with the *t*-value from a *t*-table with $N_1 + N_2 - 2$ degrees of freedom. If the *t*-value obtained through the formula exceeds the table *t*-value at a specific probability level, then the null hypothesis is rejected at that level.

The t-Test for Two Nonindependent Sample Means

Often the health science researcher is involved with samples in which the composition of one group has bearing on the composition of the other group. For example, the subjects may be matched on one or more characteristics, or the same subjects may be in a pretest-posttest experiment. In such cases, the two groups are no longer independent, so a special *t*-test for nonindependent or correlated means is required. The measure to be analyzed is the difference between the paired scores.

The formula used is:

$$t = \frac{M_D}{\sqrt{\dfrac{\Sigma D^2 - \dfrac{(\Sigma D^2)}{N}}{N(N-1)}}}$$

where D = the difference between the paired scores
M_D = the mean of the differences
ΣD^2 = the sum of the squared difference scores
N = the number of pairs

The *t*-value obtained is compared to those in the *t*-table with $N - 1$ degrees of freedom at the appropriate level of significance.

Analysis of Variance (ANOVA)

When comparing the mean of two groups, the health science researcher employs the *t*-test. However, if two or more groups are involved, one of the most powerful methods for comparing means is analysis of variance (ANOVA). For example, a health science investigator may want to determine whether there is a significant difference in blood pressure among three groups of students—those under conditions of high stress, moderate stress, and no stress (assuming there are students with no stress). It is possible to compute a *t*-test between the means of each pair, but the problems with this approach are (1) the need to ascertain a level of significance to compensate for "over-testing," (2) the necessity of computing several tests, and (3) the possibility of errors in calculating so many tests. This is particularly so if several groups are involved—five different groups would require 10 separate *t*-tests. ANOVA is able to avoid these problems.

In analysis of variance, as in the *t*-test, a ratio of observed differences/error is used to test hypotheses. The ratio, call the *F*-ratio, uses the variance of group means as a measure of observed differences among groups. The within-groups variance (V_w), simply the sum of the variances of each of the groups, is the denominator in the *F*-ratio. The between-groups variance (V_b), which measures the variation among the means of the groups, is the numerator in the *F*-ratio:

$$F = \frac{V_b}{V_w} = \frac{\text{between-groups variance}}{\text{within-groups variance}}$$

The total groups variance (V_{vt}) equals the scores for all groups combined into one composite group.

The rationale of the *F*-ratio is a follows. The between-groups variance shows the influence of the experimental variable or treatment, while the within-groups variance represents the sampling error in the distributions. If the between-groups variance fails to be much greater than the within-groups variance, the health scientist would conclude that the difference between the means is likely caused by

TABLE 12.1   Critical Values for Large Samples

	0.5 Level	.01 Level
Two-tailed test	1.96	2.58
One-tailed test	1.64	2.33

sampling error. On the other hand, if the *F*-ratio is substantially greater than 1, it would appear that the difference is likely the result of the treatment.

To determine whether the *F*-ratio is great enough to reject the null hypothesis at the predetermined level of significance, the researcher must consult an *F*-table. Like the *t*-table, it contains the critical values necessary for testing. In entering an *F*-table, the appropriate degrees of freedom must be used. The between-groups variance (V_b) has $k - 1$ degrees of freedom (where k is the number of groups), and the within-groups variance (V_w) has $k(N - 1)$ degrees of freedom (where N is the number of observations in each group).

The analysis of variance is the first step in the analysis of such designs. If a significant *F*-ratio is obtained, it is only known that somewhere in the data something other than chance is operating. The researcher must employ a special form of the *t*-test to isolate the presence, nature, and extent of the influencing variable. Examples of such special *t*-tests are Duncan's multiple range test and tests by Newman-Keuls, Tukey, and Scheffe.

Because ANOVA is a complex tool with several applications, variations, and limitations, it is suggested that the health science investigator consult statistical texts that outline it in detail. The only additional comment to make here is a delineation of the assumptions made when using ANOVA:

1. Observations must be independent.
2. The observations in each group must be normally distributed.
3. The variances of the groups are homogenous; that is, the variance of each group must be equal to that of any other group.

These can usually be accomplished with well-planned random sampling.

Multivariate Analysis of Variance (MANOVA)

The statistical test usually referred to as multivariate analysis of variance (MANOVA) determines whether several groups differ on more than one dependent variable. It is similar to ANOVA and the *t*-test. Each subject in a MANOVA will have a score on two or more dependent variables. These scores are represented by an expression called a *vector*. Each subject has a vector score. A mean vector score can be calculated for a group of subjects. This mean vector score is called a *centroid*. The MANOVA determines whether there are statistically significant differences between the centroids of different groups (Borg & Gall, 1999). In our case study we'll consider two groups: the experimental and control groups, who have been measured on T-cell count and knowledge about AIDS. The purpose of the MANOVA that Schyler will use is to determine if the differences are significant between the scores for these patients.

The first step when conducting a MANOVA is to test the assumption of the equality of group dispersions (Borg & Gall, 1999). The assumption is satisfied if a nonsignificant F is obtained. The next step involves a statistical significance test of the difference between the group centroids. Wielks *lambda* (Λ) is generally utilized for this procedure. The Wielks *lambda* yields an *F*-value, and the level of statistical significance is determined. (In your printout significant *F*-ratios will be noted.) If a significant MANOVA *F* is obtained, an ANOVA can then be computed on each dependent variable to determine which variables are statistically significant and therefore contributing to the overall MANOVA *F*. You can refer to Appendix A for brief descriptions of some common statistical procedures.

Nonparametric Tests of Significance

We have discussed tests of statistical significance known as *parametric statistics*. A parameter is a population score, whereas a static is a score for a sample that is randomly drawn from the population. There are assumptions made when using parametric statistics:

- Scores in the population are normally distributed about the mean.
- Population variances of the groups are approximately equal.

When deviations from these assumptions are in the data, parametric statistics should not be used, but rather one of the nonparametric statistical tools should be selected. These techniques do not make any assumptions about the population variance or shape of the data (Borg & Gall, 1999).

The advantages of nonparametric tests are (1) they do not have the many restrictions required for parametric tests; (2) they are very suitable for health surveys and experiments in which outcomes are difficult to quantify; and (3) they offer ease of computation. On the other hand, they (1) are less efficient, (2) are less specific, and (3) fail to deal with all the special characteristics of a distribution. Some of the most frequently used nonparametric tests are presented in this section.

The Chi-Square Test. The chi-square test (χ^2) is generally employed in causal comparative studies and in comparison of observed and theoretical frequencies. As a test of independence, it is used not to measure the degree of relationship but rather to estimate the likelihood that some factor other than chance accounts for the apparent relationship. It is used when the research data are in the form of frequency counts.

The Mann-Whitney Test (*U*-Test). The Mann-Whitney test is the nonparametric counterpart of the parametric *t*-test. Simply, it is designed to test the significance of the difference between two randomly drawn samples from the same population. Usually each sample has less than 20 subjects, because more than that allows the sampling distribution of *U* to approach a normal distribution wherein the *t*-test may be used.

The Sign Test. The sign test is a procedure for determining the significance of the differences between two correlated or nonindependent samples. For example, experimental and control groups may be matched on several variables, or the subjects may be matched with themselves in a pretest-posttest situation wherein they act as a control group in one instance and an experimental group in another. The sign test is particularly useful when the treatment effect cannot be measured but only judged to result in inferior or superior performance.

The Median Test. The median test, a nonparametric test, determines the significance of the difference between the medians of two independent groups, whereas the sign test operates with two correlated groups. It is an application of the χ^2 test with a 2×2 table and one degree of freedom.

The Wilcoxon Matched-Pairs Signed Rank Test. The Wilcoxon matched-pairs signed rank test is employed by the health researcher to ascertain whether two samples differ from each other to a significant degree when there is a relationship between the samples. Although similar to the sign test, it is more powerful because it tests not only direction but also magnitude of difference between matched groups.

The Kruskal-Wallis Test. Developed along the same lines as the Mann-Whitney U-test, the Kruskal-Wallis test is the nonparametric correspondent to the parametric one-way analysis of variance procedure. This would be used when the researcher wished to determine the significance of difference among three or more groups.

The Kendall Coefficient of Concordance. This coefficient of concordance, frequently referred to as Kendall's concordance coefficient W or the concordance coefficient W, is used in research efforts involving rankings made by independent judges. The Kendall coefficient shows the degree to which such judges agree in their assignment of ranks.

Advanced Data Analysis Techniques

We will briefly describe four data analysis techniques that are more advanced than those previously studied. While we believe these to be important, we must caution that the statistical test must fit the data, and the best fit is usually the least complicated.

Multiple Regression. This is a multivariate technique that determines the correlation between a criterion variable and a combination of two or more predictor variables. This technique can be very versatile and also enables the researcher to gain information about relationships among variables. The tool can handle interval, ordinal, or categorical data. It can also produce estimates of both the magnitude and the statistical significance of relationship among variables. Computer programs for both Macintosh and IBM compatibles are available to help with the data analysis. The first step is usually to compute the correlation between the best predictor and the criterion variable. This yields a multiple correlation coefficient (R). Borg and Gall (1999) have explained the next steps:

- The computer program will start the multiple regression analysis with the most powerful predictor of the criterion variable (see Table 12.2).
- The computer program will continue to search for the next best predictor variable, unless you have specified otherwise. The second predictor is chosen on the basis of how well it improves upon the prediction achieved by the first variable.
- The overlap between two predictor variables, or the extent to which they intercorrelate with each other, is called *colinearity*.
- The third predictor entered in the analysis is determined by whether it improves upon the prediction made by the first two predictors.
- The larger the R, the better the prediction. If R is squared, it will yield a statistic known as the coefficient of determination (R^2).
- The R^2 increment is a statistic that expresses the additional variance in the criterion variable that can be explained by adding a new predictor variable to the multiple regression analysis.

Analysis of Covariance.   On occasion, intact rather than random groups must be used by the researcher. For example, in an educational setting the health science investigator must employ intact classes for research rather than selecting students randomly and assigning them to control and experimental groups. In such situations, without several pretests, it is difficult to know the initial difference between the groups. To work around this, the analysis of covariance (ANCOVA) can be used to equate the preexperimental status of the groups. That is, ANCOVA statistically removes the differences in initial status of the groups so that they are equal with respect to one or more control variables. Therefore, if a difference is found between the groups after experimentation, the control variable(s) cannot be used to explain the effect.

ANCOVA is useful to the health science researcher when comparison groups can only be matched on the principal variable and not on others. It is a post hoc technique of matching on such variables as prior education, age, and socioeconomic status. Any computer program for the PC will be able to get you through this technique.

Discriminant Analysis.   This statistical procedure is very similar to regression. It uses predictor variables to classify subjects into two or more distinct groups, such

TABLE 12.2 Typical Multiple Regression Table Printout

Variables	Beta	Correlation Coefficient (r)	Multiple Correlation (R)	R^2	R^2 Increment

as drug abusers versus nondrug abusers. The criterion is a person's group membership, and the computer program will result in an equation known as the *discriminant function*, where the scores on the predictor are multiplied by weights to permit classification of subjects into groups (Ary, Jacobs, & Razavieh, 1996). The intent is to develop an equation that can be used to predict membership for new subjects for whom only measures of the independent variables are available. Thus, the discriminant function will indicate to which group every subject might belong (Polit & Hungler, 1999).

Factor Analysis. This is another statistical procedure that is based upon correlation. It analyzes the intercorrelations among a large set of measure so that a smaller number of common factors can be identified. These factors can be said to go together. As an example, Peshkin (1989) did a factor analysis that is depicted in Table 12.3.

Percent variance explained was as follows: Factor 1, 24.12%; Factor 2, 10.02%; Factor 3, 8.91%; Factor 4, 6.74%; Factor 5, 6.05%; total variance explained was 55.84%.

TABLE 12.3 Factor Analysis for Female Self-Efficacy Items

Factor 1: The ability to communicate about sexual matters and using contraception

Item	Question	Factor Loading
2	Even if my sex partner can talk about sex, I can't tell a man how I really feel about sexual things.	0.46
9	Sometimes I just go along with what my partner wants to do sexually because I don't think I can take the hassle of trying to say what I want.	0.74
5	If my partner didn't talk about the sex that was happening between us, I couldn't either.	0.59
14	I could excuse myself to put in a diaphragm or foam (if I used it for birth control).	0.54
16	I could stop before intercourse if I could not bring up the subject of protection.	0.52
17	There are times when I should talk to my sex partner about using contraceptives, but I can't seem to do it in the situation.	0.70
18	Sometimes I end up having intercourse with a sex partner because I can't find a way to stop it.	0.52

Factor 2: Strong feelings of sexual arousal and obtaining contraception

Item	Question	Factor Loading
8	There are times when I'd be so emotionally or sexually involved that I could have sexual intercourse even if we weren't protected.	0.66
12	It would be difficult for me to go to the drugstore and ask for foam, a diaphragm, a pill prescription, etc., without feeling embarrassed.	0.72

Continued

TABLE 12.3 *Continued*

Factor 3: Assumption of responsibility for the direction of sexual activity

Item	Question	Factor Loading
13	I could easily ask him if he had protection.	0.73
15	I could tell him I was on the pill or had an IUD (if I used it for birth control).	0.67

Factor 4: Assertiveness in preventing sexual intercourse in a highly involved situation

Item	Question	Factor Loading
4	If my partner and I are getting turned on sexually and I don't really want to have sexual intercourse, I can easily tell him "no" and mean it.	0.80
7	If my partner and I are getting turned on sexually and I don't really want to have sexual intercourse, I can easily stop things so that we don't have intercourse.	0.80

Factor 5: Conscious acceptance of sexuality and sexual activity

Item	Question	Factor Loading
1	When I am with a sex partner, I feel that I can always be responsible for what happens sexually with him.	0.68
3	When I have intercourse, I can enjoy it as something that I really wanted to do.	0.57
6	When I think about what having sex means, I can't have sex as easily.	0.51
10	If there were a man to whom I was very attracted physically and emotionally, I could feel comfortable telling him that I wanted to have sex with him.	0.42
11	I couldn't continue to use a birth control method if I thought that my parents might find out.	0.50

A factor, mathematically, is a linear combination of the variables in a data matrix. A data matrix contains the scores of N people on k different measures. As Polit and Hungler (1999) express it:

$$F = b_1 X_1 + b_2 X_2 + b_3 X_3 + \ldots + b_k X_k$$

where F is a factor score, X_1 to X_k are original variables from the matrix, and b_1 to b_k are weights. The development of such an equation for a factor permits reduction of the X_k scores to one or several factor scores.

Table 12.4 depicts a summary of some of the statistics tests we have discussed.

TABLE 12.4 Statistical Procedures

Name of Procedure	Test Statistic	Parametric or Nonparametric	Purpose
t-test for independent samples	t	P	To test the difference between the means of two independent samples
t-test for dependent (paired) samples	t	P	To test the difference between the means of two related groups or sets of scores
Median test	X^2	NP	To test the difference between the medians of two independent groups
Mann-Whitney *U*-test	U (Z)	NP	To test the difference in the ranks of scores of two independent groups
Wilcoxon matched-pairs signed rank test	Z	NP	To test the difference in the ranks of scores of two related groups or tests of scores
ANOVA	F	P	To test the difference among the means of a number of groups
Kruskal-Wallis test	H (X^2)	NP	To test the difference in the ranks of scores of three or more independent groups
Chi-square test	X^2	NP	To test the difference in proportions in two or more groups
Kendall's coefficient of concordance	T	NP	To test that a correlation is different from zero

Note. From *Nursing Research* by D. Polit & B. Hungler, 1995, New York: Lippincott. Copyright 1995 by Lippincott. Adapted by permission.

The PC for Data Analysis

The previous discussion may have left you a little daunted as to how you might analyze the data you collect. Computers, once again, have enabled that task to be simplified. There are several PC programs available for data analysis, including:

- Statistical Package for the Social Sciences (SPSS-X)
- Statistical Analysis System (SAS)
- BMDP Statistical Software

All of these programs provide excellent manuals and are usually available at computer centers. These programs provide easy and thorough mechanisms for data entry and analysis. We strongly recommend that you utilize these or similar programs, and that you avoid the do-it-yourself approach.

Meta-Analysis

Meta-analysis is a method developed by Glass (1977) to synthesize quantitative data from many primary sources. The data focus on the same question and use similar variables. The purpose of using meta-analysis is to statistically integrate the findings from a broad population of individually conducted projects. The statistic used to integrate the findings of these studies is the magnitude of the effect of the treatment. The *effect size* (Δ) is computed by subtracting the mean score of the control group on the dependent variable from the experimental group mean and dividing by the control group standard deviation:

$$\Delta = \frac{X_e - X_c}{SD_c}$$

where Δ = effect size
        e = experimental group
        c = control group
       SD = standard deviation

The mean of the effect sizes for all studies included in the research review is then calculated to estimate the typical effect of the problem being studied. For example, a meta-analysis of pretext sensitization effects in experimental design was conducted by Wilson and Putnam (1982). The authors wished to investigate if subjects' posttest scores were affected by a pretest. They gathered results from 32 studies and computed those outcomes as standardized differences between pretested and nonpretested groups. The average effect size was +.22, indicating a general positive (elevated) effect of pretest on posttest. Cognitive results were elevated .43, attitude results .29, and personality .48. Of all effects, 64% were positive, and 81% of the cognitive effects were positive. The investigators concluded that researchers should use the pretest as a design variable (if present) and should estimate its effect.

There are several limitations of meta-analysis, including (1) inclusion of poorly conducted studies in the equation, (2) cost of conducting the study, (3) criteria being used for including primary sources are difficult to agree upon, and (4) incomplete data are sometimes used because they are the only data available. However, meta-analysis has been and will continue to be a valuable aid in helping scholars keep up with the relevant research. Although it will not replace the literature review, it does provide a method for reviewing the studies mentioned in the literature review.

According to Daly, Kellehear, and Gliksman (1997), the advantages of meta-analysis include (1) being able to identify a finding in a diverse array of similarly designed studies, (2) providing a systematic overview of findings in a particular area of study, (3) determining larger research questions, (4) enabling an alternative method when other methods are inappropriate, and (5) being able to conduct methodological assessments of research designs.

Case Discussion

Schyler was able to report to her advisor that, based on the project she conducted to determine the generalizability of the AIDS patient education program, the program should become available to other hospitals in the state similar to Harbor Hospital. Schyler made this determination because there was a statistically significant difference between the patients' T-cell counts in the experimental group and those in the group that did not get the patient education program. Recall that Schyler is recommending that only hospitals similar to Harbor should invest in this program.

Summary

Chapter 12 began with a general discussion about inferential analysis and testing statistical significance. The differences between estimation of parameters and hypothesis testing were elucidated. The null and alternative hypothesis were reviewed. In regard to tests of significance, the critical region, level of significance, and Type I and Type II errors were discussed. Inferential data analysis techniques were explained and included the *t*-tests for independent and nonindependent sample means, analysis of variance, and multivariate analysis of variance. The nonparametric tests of significance that were discussed included *chi*-square, Mann-Whitney, sign, median, Wilcoxon matched-pairs, Kruskal-Wallis, and the Kendall coefficient. Advanced data analysis techniques of multiple regression, analysis of covariance, discriminant analysis, and factor analysis were briefly reviewed. The chapter concluded with a discussion of the PC for data analysis and meta-analysis.

Suggested Activities

1. Read three articles on a topic that is of interest to you and critique the data analysis utilized in each article.

2. Attempt to enter data and complete a data analytic technique on your PC. This can be for a hypothetical data set.

3. Describe some topic areas where you might use meta-analysis.

4. You have been assigned a research project to determine the smoking habits of preteen males in North America. Using the Web, obtain 15 pertinent articles and determine if they could be included in a meta-analysis.

5. Using government websites, attempt to conduct your own meta-analysis of any public health issue that interests you.

References

Ary, D., Jacobs, L, & Razavieh, A. (1996). *Introduction to research* (2d ed.). Fort Worth: Harcourt.

Boniface, R. (1999). *Statistics*. Boston: Allyn & Bacon.

Borg, W., & Gall, M. (1999). *Educational research: Applying a practical guide*. New York: Longman.

Daly, J., Kellehear, A., & Gliksman, M. (1997). *The public health researcher*. New York: Oxford.

Glass, G. (1977). Integrating findings: The meta-analysis of research. In L. Schulman (Ed.), *Review of research in education* (Vol. 5). Itasca, IL: Peacock.

Kuzma, J., & Bohneneblust, S. (2001). *Basis statistics for the health sciences*. Mountain View, CA: Mayfield Publishing Company.

Peshkin, F. (1989). Contraceptive self-efficacy in adolescents: A comparative study of male and female contraceptive behavior. Unpublished master's thesis, University of Illinois, Urbana-Champaign.

Peshkin, F., & Rubinson, L. (1997). Contraceptive self-efficacy in adolescents: A comparative study of male and female contraceptive practices. *Journal of Sex Education and Therapy, 22*(2), 23–29.

Polit, D., & Hungler, B. (1999). *Nursing research* (2d ed.). Philadelphia: Lippincott.

Wiersma, W. (2000). *Research methods in education*. Boston: Allyn & Bacon.

Wilson, V., & Putnam, R. (1982). A meta-analysis of pretest sensitization effects in experimental design. *American Journal of Research, 19*(2), 249–258.

Chapter 13

Techniques for Data Presentation

Case Study

Caleb, a senior at Newtown University, is enrolled in a health sciences research course. The major semester assignment is to conduct a research study using the components learned in the course. In other words, Caleb is to state the problem, derive hypotheses, conduct a literature search, conceive the methodology, actually carry out the experiment, present and analyze the data, and summarize the project, including conclusions and recommendations. If he has read the text to this point, Caleb will be equipped with the necessary knowledge to complete the assignment. This chapter will enable Caleb to present the data he collects for his study. Usually, the form of data presentation includes tables, figures, and graphics. ·

Table Presentations

The first part of this chapter will discuss the presentation of tables in manuscripts for publications, reports, books, term papers, master's theses, and doctoral dissertations. The purpose for including tables and several types of tables will be described. In addition, we will discuss the relationship between the table and the text, which is a very important consideration. Finally, the format of tables will be detailed so that you can construct a proper table. The section concludes with guidelines for including tables.

Purpose of Tables

Tables usually represent quantitative material, and sometimes words that present qualitative comparisons or descriptive information. As an example of a word table,

Caleb could use a table to depict some of the questions and their responses in the questionnaire he used. Word tables should not repeat what has been discussed in the text, but rather illuminate that discussion. Using tables to depict collected data enables the reader to have a clear understanding and comprehension of the masses of numbers that have been collected during the project. The analysis of original data should be presented in these tables so that readers are not burdened with long lines of numbers that disrupt the smooth flow of the text. Data should be presented so that their significance is easily recognized by the reader.

Tables are used to present information in the form of totals and subtotals, rank-order relationships, and results of statistical analyses (Slade, Campbell, & Ballou, 2000). Once you have decided what data belongs in the table, there are a few additional considerations:

1. Rounded-off values may display patterns more clearly than precise numbers.
2. It is easier to compare numbers down a column than across a row.
3. Row and column averages can provide a visual focus that allows the reader to inspect the data easily.
4. Ample spacing between rows and columns can improve a table because the white space creates a perceptual order to the data. (American Psychological Association [APA], 1994, p. 121).

It should be noted here that some institutions of higher education suggest or mandate use of a particular style or publication manual. You should consult with the appropriate personnel to determine which, if any, style manual is utilized. Many university health science departments use the *Publication Manual of the American Psychological Association* (APA, 1994), because it is preferred for most journals to which potential social sciences authors might submit their projects for publication.

Relating the Tables to the Text

A good table should supplement the text of the paper. However, you should refer to all tables and their data in the text. A discussion of the highlights of the table is all that is necessary in the paper, and each table should have a brief introduction that explains the manner in which the data are presented and suggests their general meaning. Two rules apply to the inclusion of tables:

1. Each table should be understandable without reference to the text.
2. The text should be complete so that the reader may follow it without referring to the tables.

In the text, tables are referred to by their numbers. They are numbered consecutively, using arabic numerals; for example:

Table 4 shows . . .
. . . behavioral scores with no pretest (see Table 4)

The actual placement of the table is sometimes a difficult decision. Should it go after the analysis? Before? Here are some rules that may be helpful:

1. Each table should be placed entirely on one page when possible.
2. Text material may be placed on the same page with a table of about one-half page or less.
3. A table should be separated from the text by four spaces above and below (Table 13.1).
4. A page containing both a table and text should begin with the text material.
5. If all the preceding conditions cannot be met, a table should be placed between paragraphs (Slade et al., 2000).

Single-Variable Tables

Single variables are usually used in a descriptive or explanatory study. Measurements such as the range, mean, mode, or median may be depicted in such a table. In addition, frequency distributions and grouped data may be presented. Table 13.1 is an example of a single variable table in that one score was reported. Table 13.2 depicts the frequency distribution for the scores on the health science knowledge test.

Percentage Tables

Percentages can provide an efficient way to summarize information. These data can be reported in single or multiple variable form. The listing of percentages as presented in Table 13.3 should be summed. An indication of sample size is also

TABLE 13.1 Mean Knowledge Scores of Pretested and Unpretested Students

This summarizes the mean knowledge scores of the students who took the health science test. The students were asked about their health knowledge in regard to smoking, nutrition, and exercise. In both the pretested and unpretested groups, girls achieved slightly higher scores on the test. However, scores of both groups were very similar and showed no difference between the pretested and unpretested groups.

	Group	*N*	Health Science Test
Girls	Pretested	120	18
	Unpretested	110	20
Boys	Pretested	118	17
	Unpretested	108	19

Note. Maximum score was 30.

TABLE 13.2   Frequency Distribution of Scores on Health Science Knowledge Test

Score	Frequency	Score	Frequency	Score	Frequency
1	0	11	18	21	38
2	0	12	20	22	20
3	0	13	22	23	17
4	0	14	20	24	14
5	0	15	25	25	13
6	0	16	35	26	7
7	6	17	36	27	4
8	7	18	40	28	0
9	15	29	41	29	0
10	14	20	44	30	0

important so that the percentages will not be misleading. There is an important question you might be asking here: What happens to the nonrespondents? Should they be included in the computation for the percentages? There are two methods that you could choose to answer this dilemma. The first is to subtract the number of nonresponses from the total sample size and use this new figure as the base for the percentages. In our example, Caleb may have a sample size of 456, but only 411 students reported their gender. In this case, the 45 nonrespondents would be omitted, and 411 rather than 456 would be the base for computing the respective percentages. A second method of dealing with nonrespondents is to use the total sample size (456) as the base and include the nonrespondents as a percentage. In our case study of 456, assume that 205 were males, 206 were females, and 45 were nonrespondents. If we used the first method (using 411 as a base), we would be able to write that 50% were males and 50% females. By the second method (456 as base), we would have 45% males, 45% females, and 10% nonrespondents. If we continue to use nonrespondents as part of the analysis, the base number remains constant and adds stability to all the analyses.

TABLE 13.3   Sex Distribution for Students Taking Health Science Knowledge Test

Sex	Percentage
Males	45
Females	55
Total	100
	(N = 456)

Contingency (Bivariate) Tables

Health science studies, as well as other social science investigations, sometimes focus upon the relationship between two variables. Tables are used to display the way the values of the variables are associated. Interrelationships are examined and are thus called *cross-tabulations* or *contingency tables*. In these kinds of tables, all combinations of categories of all the variables are presented. However, the most usual form is the two-variable table, with each variable being dichotomous. Therefore, two dichotomous variables present a table with four cells, sometimes labeled a *four-fold table*. Through evolution, one variable has been termed the *column variable* and is labeled across the top so its categories form vertical columns down the page and usually represent the independent variable. The other variable, the *row variable*, is labeled on the left margin, forming categories of rows across the page and thus is the dependent variable. The intersections of the categories of these two variables form the interior of the table.

An easy way to construct this contingency table is to list the total frequencies in each category for each variable. The simplest dichotomous variables and those most frequently used are gender and race. If we had 100 respondents to a survey concerning health risk factors, we would have 100 as a total for gender and race (each person has a gender and race). Table 13.4 shows that we have 50 males: 30 blacks and 20 whites. The numbers outside the square are referred to as *marginals*. The row marginals are 60 and 40, and the column marginals are 50 and 50. The row and column marginals provide no information about each other, but are found in the interior of the cells. You should, once again, be sure to note the N (100) in the lower right-hand corner, which is attained by adding either the row or column marginals.

Absolute numbers should be used in the cells when a statistical analysis will be conducted. This analysis is always placed at the bottom of the table. If, however, no statistical analysis will be used, then percentages should be used in the cells. Usually, the independent variable is presented in percentages; thus the columns become percentaged.

TABLE 13.4 Race by Gender

Race	Male	Female	
Black	30 (Cell a)	30 (Cell b)	60 $a + b$
White	20 (Cell c)	20 (Cell d)	40 $c + d$
	50	50	
	$a + c$	$b + d$	
		$100 = a + b + c + d$	

TABLE 13.5 Correlation Matrix-Multivariable Table

Variable	B	C	D	E
A	.10	.30	.40	.35
B		.72	.50	.62
C			.21	.41
D			.48	.48

Multivariable Tables

Multivariable tables contain three or more variables and are similar to those presented in the previous sections. Caleb would use such a table in his paper if he wanted to report on a number of variables and their association or correlation. The format is typically a correlation matrix, which presents the correlations between all the pairs of variables in the analysis. If we had five variables, we would want to show the relationship between each pair of variables. The matrix, as in Table 13.5, would list all the variables along the left-hand margin of the table, except for the last one. At the top of the table, the variables are listed beginning with the second variable. The obtained correlations are presented once for each pair of variables. The dependent variable should be placed in the last column, column E in Table 13.5. Now you can easily determine the relationship between the dependent variable and each of the independent variables.

Another type of multivariable table that is frequently used is the analysis of variance table (ANOVA). Table 13.6 is an example of how to set up the ANOVA table.

Word Tables

Some tables may consist mainly of words. These tables present qualitative comparisons or perhaps descriptive information. An example can be found in Chapter 9 (see Table 9.1), where various evaluation models were described. Word tables should explain the discussion in the text, but not repeat that discussion. When preparing a word table, you should maintain the same format as you would use in other tables, and be sure to double-space all parts of the word table.

TABLE 13.6 Analysis of Variance Table

Source of Variance	SS	df	MS	F	Level of Significance
Between groups	261.1	2	100.1	21.0	.01*
Within groups	687.8	144	477.7		
Total	888.9	146	577.8		

*$p < .01$

Table Format

As we have mentioned previously, each institution will have a set of guidelines for personnel to use when submitting reports, articles, and the like. Caleb would need to find out what is needed for his class and institution. The following discussion should enable you to ascertain the many different terms associated with constructing a table. Table 13.7 has been devised to depict these many terms.

Table Numbers

All tables should be numbered consecutively with arabic numerals. In a book chapter, use sequential numbers preceded by the chapter number and a decimal point. We have used this method throughout this book. In the text of your report, paper, or thesis, refer to the tables by number, not by the title. If your manuscript includes an appendix with tables, identify the tables of the appendix with capital letters and arabic numerals: Table B.1, for example, would be the first table of Appendix B.

Table Titles

The title of a table should be clear and brief and should explain the table. *Avoid* using information contained in the headings of the table; such as the following for Table 13.7:

TABLE 13.7 Mean Scores of Students with Pretesting and | *table number* and *table title*
Without Pretesting

stub head	Group	N^a	7	8	9	column heads
					Grade *column spanner*	
	Knowledge Tests *table spanner*					
stub column	Boys *row stubs*					
	Pretested	118	17	18	20	
	Unpretested	108	19	22	21	
	Girls					*columns*
	Pretested	120	18	19	20	
	Unpretested	110	20	21	20	
	Attitude Tests *table spanner*					
	Boys					
	Pretested	118	18	20^b	22	
	Unpretested	108	20	22	23	
	Girls					
	Pretested	120	19	20	21	
	Unpretested	110	22	24	23	

Note. Maximum score on each test was 30.
[a]Numbers of students out of 125 in each group who completed both tests.
[b]Two boys had identical answers.

Relation Between Attitude and Knowledge Tests

This would be unclear and not tell what data are contained in the table. Another bad title would be:

Mean Health Science Knowledge and Attitude Scores of Girls and Boys in Grades 7, 8, and 9 Who Were Pretested and Not Pretested

This is too detailed and duplicates the information in the table headings. A better example is:

Mean Scores of Students with Pretesting and Without Pretesting

This is a *good* table title in that it explains clearly what the data will tell the reader.

Table Body

The body of a table contains the data. Mullins (1983) suggests the following guidelines when constructing the body of a table:

1. Use as few entries as possible without eliminating vital information.
2. Within each table, use the same rules for retaining decimals and for rounding.
3. Arrange entries so that the most important comparisons are between adjacent numbers.
4. To prevent confusion of percentages and numbers, place a percent sign (%) after the first number in a column of percentages that add up to 100%. Also, use "percentage" in the column heading.
5. If a column head does not apply to an item in a row stub (this is called a *cell*), leave the cell blank.
6. If rounding prevents the sum of percentages in an additive column from being 100%, use a footnote to explain why this is so.
7. Do not use intersecting lines to connect items in different columns.

Stub

Stub is the name for the rows in the far left-hand column of the table. The names of these columns should be short, clear, and grammatically consistent. The stubs usually present the independent variables. If you use abbreviations, use them consistently in all tables and use a note to explain the abbreviations in your first table.

Stub Column

The stub column is the column of row stubs and their subcategories. In Table 13.7 these rows are labeled *Boys, Girls, Pretested,* and *Unpretested.* The subcategories should be indented at least one space from the margin to distinguish them from the row stubs.

Stub Head

The stub head is the title of the stub column. In Table 13.7, *Group* is the stub head.

Column Head

The column head names the column and should be grammatically consistent with others in the table. These heads usually name the dependent variables, dependent upon the discipline and guidelines followed. In Table 13.7, for example, *7*, *8*, and *9* are the column heads.

Column Spanner

The column spanner identifies two or more columns, each of which has its own column head. In Table 13.7, *Grade* is the column spanner.

Table Spanner

Table spanners cover the entire width of the body of the table, allowing for further divisions within the table. *Knowledge Tests* and *Attitude Tests* in Table 13.7 denote table spanners. Table spanners can also be utilized to combine two tables into one, as they are in Table 13.7.

Notes

Tables have three types of notes: general notes, specific notes, and probability level notes. These are always placed below the table.

General Note

General notes explain, qualify, or provide information relating to the entire table. This may include an explanation of abbreviations, symbols, and so on. These notes are designated by the word *Note* (italicized, followed by a period). In Table 13.7, it reads:

Note. Maximum score on each test was 30.

In addition, general notes indicate that if a table has been reprinted from another source. To do this, you must obtain permission to reproduce or adapt all or part of a table from a copyrighted source. Give credit to the original author and to the copyright holder.

Example of Note from Book

Note. From *Contemporary Human Sexuality* (p. 42) by J. Turner & L. Rubinson, 1993, Upper Saddle River, N.J: Prentice-Hall. Copyright 1993 by Prentice-Hall. Reprinted by permission.

Example of Note from Article

Note. From "Acquaintance rape: The influence of alcohol, fraternity membership, and sport team membership" by M. Frintier and L. Rubinson, *Journal of Sex Education and Therapy, 19*(4), 272–284.

Specific Note. A specific note refers to a particular column or to an individual entry. Specific notes are indicated by superscript lowercase letters (superscript *a* in Table 13.7, for example). Within the headings and body of the table, the superscripts are ordered horizontally from left to right across the table by rows, beginning at the top left. Each table is independent of any others; therefore, notes always begin on each table, with superscript *a*.

Probability Level Note. A probability level note indicates the results of significance tests. Asterisks indicate the probability levels of tests of significance. When more than one level appears in a table, use one asterisk for the lowest level, two for the next, and so on. These levels and the number of asterisks do not have to be consistent from table to table. Table 13.8 is an example of a probability level note.

Note Format. The ordering of the notes in a table is (1) general; (2) specific; and (3) probability level.

Example of Order of Notes

Note. Maximum score on each test was 30.
[a]Numbers of students out of 125 in each group who completed both tests.
*$p<.05$
**$p<.01$

TABLE 13.8 Example of a Probability Level Note

E
1.70*
3.86**

*$p < .05$
**$p < .01$

Each type of note begins at the margin on a new line below the table, beginning with the general note. The first specific note begins flush left on a new line, and all subsequent specific notes follow one after the other. The first probability level notes follow one another. These parts of a table have been presented so that you can easily construct a good, coherent, and useful table. The following are some guidelines you might use when constructing your tables:

- Is the table necessary?
- Is the entire table—including the title, headings, and notes—double-spaced?
- Are all comparable tables in the manuscript consistent in presentation?
- Is the title brief but explanatory?
- Does every column have a column heading?
- Are all abbreviations, underlines, parentheses, dashes, and special symbols explained?
- Are all probability level values correctly identified, and are asterisks attached to the appropriate table entries? Is a probability level assigned the same number of asterisks if it appears in more than one table?
- Are the notes in the following order: general note, specific note, probability note?
- Are all vertical rules eliminated?
- Will the table fit across the width of a journal column or page?
- If all or part of a copyrighted table is reproduced, do the table notes give full credit to the copyright owner? Have you received written permission from the copyright holder and sent a copy to the APA production office?
- Is the table referred to in text? (APA, 1994, pp. 140–141)

Figure Presentations

This section describes how figures should be utilized in a manuscript. The various types of figures will be discussed, as well as how to cite figures in the text. A general discussion of instructions for preparing figures with an accompanying list of guidelines completes the section. We have determined, for use in this text, that figures encompass any type of illustration other than a table. These may be in the form of charts, graphs, photographs, maps, drawings, and some kinds of computer printouts. The author provides these materials for the publisher to photograph.

Purpose of Figures

Figures, as mentioned, refer to charts, graphs, drawings, maps, and photographs. They are used to present data very clearly and concisely. The inclusion of a figure should be carefully considered, because figures are expensive to produce, both for the author and publisher. Therefore, figures should be used only when they actually contribute something to a paper. Some points to consider when including a figure are:

- What idea do you need to convey?
- Is the figure necessary? If it duplicates text, it is not necessary. If it complements text or eliminates lengthy discussion, it may be the most efficient way to present the information.
- What type of figure (e.g., graph, chart, diagram, drawing, map, or photograph) is most suited to your purpose? Will a simple, relatively inexpensive figure convey the point as well as an elaborate, expensive figure? (APA, 1994, p. 140)

Sometimes it becomes confusing to decide if you should use a table or a figure. A good rule of thumb might be, if the data shows trends, it could be better augmented by a figure rather than a table. Remember that a good figure should not duplicate what is contained in the text, should be easy to read and understand, and should be carefully prepared. You can employ a professional artist to do the work, or you can attempt the project yourself. Check the guidelines from your college or university, or from the publisher (if you are submitting a manuscript for publication).

Types of Figures

There are many types of figures. Those we will discuss here include graphs, charts, dot maps, drawings, and photographs.

Graphs. Graphs usually show how things are compared or distributed. These come in the form of percentages or absolute values. There are several types of graphs: line graphs, bar graphs, circle graphs, and scatter graphs.

Line Graphs. Line graphs are used to show trends or results of a line series experiment. The independent variable is plotted on the x axis (horizontal), and the dependent variable is plotted on the y axis (vertical). See Figure 13.1 for an example. The length of the y axis should be approximately two-thirds the length of the x axis. The grid marks (dashes) on the axes denote the units of measurement. If changes on the axes are disproportionate, the differences will be distorted. Thus, the curve or slant of the line must accurately depict the data. Notice the double slash on the axes in Figure 13.1. This indicates that the origin of the coordinates is not zero.

Bar Graphs. Bar graphs are easy to read and construct (see Figure 13.2). Solid vertical or horizontal bars present one kind of data. There are also subdivided bar graphs (each bar shows two or more kinds of data); multiple bar graphs (whole bars represent different variables in one data set); and sliding bar graphs (bars are split by a vertical line that serves as the reference for each bar).

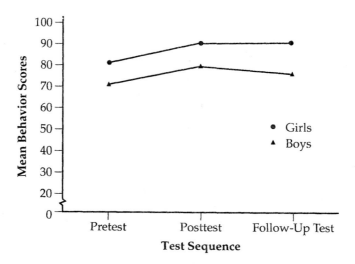

FIGURE 13.1 Example of Line Graph

Circle Graphs. Circle or pie graphs show percentages and proportions (see Figure 13.3). A general rule to follow, for clarity, is to depict only five or fewer items. The segments should be ordered from large to small, with the largest segment beginning at the 12:00 position and moving clockwise to the smallest. The differences in segments should be highlighted from light to dark, with the smallest portion being the darkest. Using different patterns of lines and dots shows the shaded patterns.

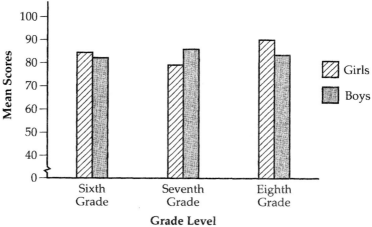

FIGURE 13.2 Example of Bar Graph

Time Alloted for Health Science Classes
Newbury High School, 1978–1987

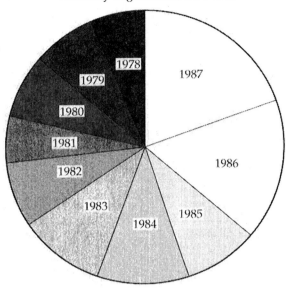

FIGURE 13.3   Example of Circle Graph

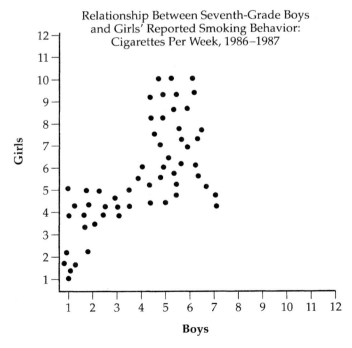

Relationship Between Seventh-Grade Boys
and Girls' Reported Smoking Behavior:
Cigarettes Per Week, 1986–1987

FIGURE 13.4   Example of Scatter Graph

Scatter Graphs. Scatter graphs consist of single dots that are plotted as on a line graph, but the dots are not joined together (see Figure 13.4). The dots represent where the variables intersect, and a cluster of dots along a diagonal indicates a correlation.

Charts. Charts can describe relationships between group segments in the sequence of operations in a process. These are usually depicted by boxes that are connected by lines. Examples include charts of organizations (see Figure 13.5), flow charts that show a step-by-step process, and schematics that show components in a system (e.g., a television circuit board).

Drawings. Drawings are usually prepared by a professional artist because they are difficult to accomplish. The drawing should be as simple as possible so that the author's idea can be easily conveyed. A drawing enables the author to augment the

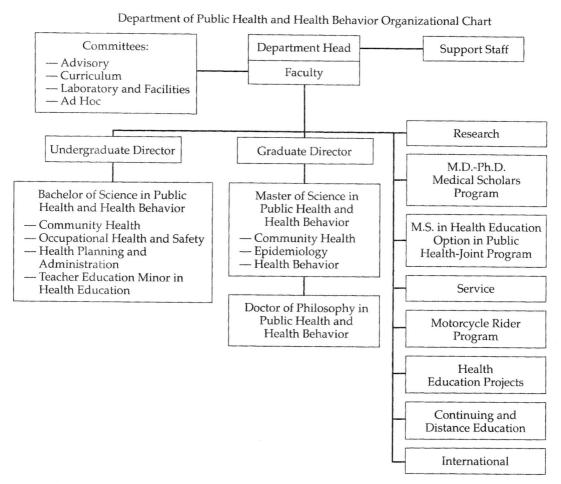

FIGURE 13.5 Example of Organizational Chart

manuscript by providing ideas and images from different viewpoints: two-dimensional and side views.

Photographs.   Professional photography is important when photographs are used in a manuscript. They can provide focus and interest points and add something of value to the words in a manuscript. Inform the photographer that there should be a strong contrast between the subject and the background. The use of black-and-white film is mandatory because color prints are difficult to reproduce accurately. When photographing people, attempt to get a signed consent form from those people. When using a photograph from another source (book, journal, or other), obtain the original picture (because photographs of photographs do not reproduce adequately). You must also obtain written permission to reprint from the copyright holder and must acknowledge the holder in the figure caption (APA, 1994).

Citing of Figures

When using a figure, it should be placed as close as possible to the first reference made to it in the manuscript. The figures should be consecutively numbered with arabic numerals in the order as they are mentioned (e.g., *Figure 1, Figure 2, Figure 3*). They can be linked to a chapter number, if appropriate. The number should be written lightly in pencil on the back of the figure, near to the edge. In addition, note the top (top) of the figure and write the figure's title (again, lightly). In the manuscript refer to figures by numbers; for example:

> Figure 1 shows . . .
> The data are related (see Figure 1)

Avoid writing "see the figure above or below" on a specific page. This is because the placement of figures cannot be determined until the manuscript is typeset. The printer should be apprised of the approximate placement of the figure by a break in the text and a note:

Insert Figure 1 about here

The same procedure is used for noting the placement of tables.

Captions and Legends

The *caption* is the explanation of the figure and is placed below it. The caption describes the contents of the figure in a sentence or a phrase.

Example of Figure Caption

Figure 1. Time and set point between attitude and behavior surveys.

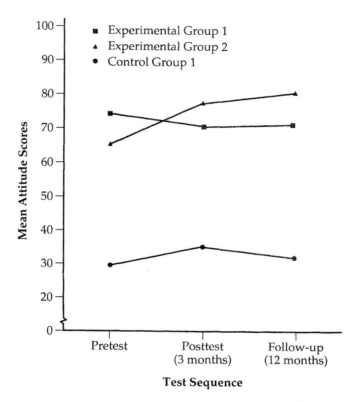

FIGURE 13.6 Mean Attitude Scores of Eighth-Grade Students Over 12 Months

Information that is needed to clarify the limits of measurement should be placed in the caption in parentheses after the caption. It is important that all terminology used in the text and the figures agree.

The *legend* is a key to the symbols in the figure. There are some standard legend symbols: ■, ●, and ▲. Figure 13.6 is an example of a figure with a legend. The legend is put into the figure and should have the same kind and size of lettering that is utilized in the figure.

All figure captions should be typed (double-spaced) on a separate page. The notation *Figure Captions* should appear in the top center of the page, and each caption should be flush to the left margin. Underline *Figure* as well as the number, a period, and the text of the caption. Capitalize only the first word and proper names. Double-space if there is more than one line, for example: *Figure 1. The relationship of skills and attitudes to health science knowledge.*

Instructions for Preparing Figures

The following list provides some general instructions for preparing figures for manuscripts, reports, term papers, theses, dissertations, and so on:

1. Place each figure on a separate page measuring $8\frac{1}{2} \times 11"$. Sometimes you will have to use larger paper. In these cases, check with your local format procedures.
2. Check to make sure that the figure is necessary.
3. Do not type letters; employ a professional or use a lettering stencil.
4. Minimize the number of lines and check to see if the data are plotted properly.
5. Make sure all words are correctly spelled.
6. Check the legend to ensure that it is clear.
7. Use arabic numerals, and be sure that all figures are mentioned in the text.
8. In pencil, lightly write *TOP* on the back of each figure.
9. Identify all figures by lightly writing on the back of each in pencil.
10. Receive written permissions for all figures for which they are necessary and include them in the package.
11. Write all figure captions on a separate page.

Graphics and the Computer

Computers have given researchers distinct advantages: speed and accuracy. Computer programs allow us to use word processors to prepare reports, theses, and dissertations. We can also use the computer to help prepare figures and tables. This section will give a brief overview of computer graphics. We recommend that you consult computer experts on your campus and microcomputer software programs for a specific review of graphics for your own computer.

The Impact of Computer Graphics

Pictures, charts, and graphs have always added to the written word by enhancing or explaining sometimes complex thoughts and ideas. With the advent of computer graphics, we have more efficient ways of producing these enhancements. When preparing a manuscript, thesis, or dissertation, a computer graphics program becomes indispensable.

Applications of Computer Graphics

Many fields such as engineering, business, art, education, chemical and biological sciences, and medicine utilize computer graphics. Engineers use the computer to provide graphics in five areas: design, analysis, drawing, manufacturing/construction/processing, and quality control. Chemical scientists who study the structure of chemical substances use X rays to determine the location of atoms in molecular structures. Using computer graphics allows chemical scientists to complete more complicated structure determinations and provides a faster way to determine the structures (Demel & Miller, 1994).

In the business world, computer graphics have enabled companies to send reports to management that aid in making decisions concerning selling, buying, or expansion. Graphics can be presented in color or black and white and integrated with the text, which saves time when producing a report. Computers have also provided businesses with *modeling,* which is a type of program that simulates the action of the marketplace.

In the field of art, computer graphics are utilized for illustration, for the creation of images and repetitive patterns, for animation, and for dynamic displays. When the many and repetitive drawings animators have to make to merely change the movement of a leg are considered, the computer certainly has offered an opportunity for the artist to be more efficient and productive in his or her work.

Education has benefited from computer graphics in that the learner can interact with the computer, and dynamic motion enables complicated concepts to be more easily presented. Objects appear more realistic and three-dimensional, which enhances the learning of students. New graphics systems can provide pictures of real objects for the user to point to or select. These are called *icons;* for example, a picture of a trash can to indicate the action of throwing something away. The icon allows the user to think in real terms about the electronic information and its actions.

Computer graphics have played a very important role in making medical diagnoses and in planning and performing surgery. Surgeons use graphics to guide instruments to remove or repair tissues and organs. Diagnostics has played a large role in creating magnetic resonance imaging (MRI), where three-dimensional representations of body organs can be manipulated to reveal details about an organ's condition. Another computer graphics application, known as optical biopsy, shows three-dimensional plots of data obtained by illuminating living tissue with laser light (Foley, Van Dam, Feuer, Hughes, & Phillips, 1994).

The benefits of computer graphics are wide and varied. They enhance productivity, allow for greater creativity, and speed up the process. While some graphics programs may still be expensive, their use is becoming commonplace, and many are relatively inexpensive.

Computers Using Graphics

Several types of computers have the capacity for using graphics. These include mainframes, minicomputers, and microcomputers. *Mainframe* computers are large and can accommodate several users at once. These types of computers are usually found in large universities, financial institutions, large companies, hospitals, and other multiuser places of employment. The *minicomputer* is smaller than a mainframe and usually slower. It is lower-priced, simpler to operate, and can be assembled in different ways for various applications. These attributes enabled the minicomputer to lead the way in computer graphics. *Microcomputers* are even smaller and lower-priced than the minicomputer. The microcomputer has been a big boon for computer graphics because many software programs are available for these computers. Both IBM-compatible and Macintosh computers have excellent software for computer graphics.

Case Discussion

Caleb, in working through his project, would need to consider the objective(s) of his study, the nature of his data and findings, and his audience (for the report or presentation), and then select the best mode of presentation. If he has access to a computer with a statistics and graphics package, he should be able to generate several different types of tables, graphs, and charts. However, he must be careful not to "overkill" his presentation; instead, he must keep it simple and to the point.

Summary

This chapter gave an overview of how to present tables and figures in a term paper, research report, thesis, or dissertation. Each student should check with his or her college's or university's required format before embarking upon writing. The use of a guide makes writing and working with tables and figures much easier.

Tables are usually representative of quantitative material. However, words may be used in a table to present qualitative comparisons or descriptive information. When deciding to utilize a table, make sure that the table enhances the manuscript and gives the reader a clearer understanding and comprehension of the numbers mentioned in the manuscript. A good table *supplements* the text and must be mentioned or referred to in the body of the paper.

There are several types of tables that you may need to use in a paper: single variable, percentage, contingency (bivariable), and multivariable. Regardless of the type, the format is the same for any kind of table. Formatting is dependent upon the particular style you or your institution adheres to and should be carefully followed. Several guidelines in constructing a table were mentioned.

Figures are more difficult to construct because they require professional lettering and spacing. Figures include charts, graphs, drawings, maps, and photographs. A cautionary note: Make sure that the figure is necessary and that it augments the text. When submitting figures along with a manuscript, include a separate page listing the figures because this ensures correct captions. Each figure should be titled in light pencil on its reverse, along with a notation as to which end is the top. Legends denote the symbols used in the figure. Symbols are used to differentiate between groups, sexes, and so on. It is important that these symbols remain consistent within and between the figures in the manuscript. The final part of Chapter 13 dealt with computer graphics. There have been many applications for graphics, especially in the fields of engineering, chemical sciences, arts, education, and business. Computer graphics are available for a large variety of computers: mainframes, minicomputers, and microcomputers. Graphics enhance the text, allow for faster productivity, and can include a variety of interactive activities.

Suggested Activities

1. Prepare the following types of tables, using data from any journal article: single variable, percentage, contingency, and multivariable.

2. Using a different article than the one you used in Activity 1, prepare a figure to illustrate an apparent trend.

3. Use the computer graphics program on your PC to prepare one table and one graph.

4. Search the Web for the CDC home page and find two topics that interest you. Utilize the appropriate website and find one table for each topic. Attempt to interpret each table, and critique (both positively and negatively) the tables. How would you improve upon the presentation of the material?

5. Determine how a chart differs from a table or graph. Use the Web to find a chart and then rework it into a table or graph. Explain how the content of the material might change once you have accomplished this activity.

References

American Psychological Association. (1994). *Publication manual of the American Psychological Association* (4th ed.). Washington, D.C.

Demel, J., & Miller, M. (1994). *Introduction to computer graphics* (3d ed.). Belmont, CA: Wadsworth.

Foley, J., Van Dam, A., Feuer, S., Hughes, J., & Phillips, R. (1994). *Introduction to computer graphics*. New York: Addison-Wesley.

Mullins, C. (1983). *A guide to writing and publishing in the social and behavioral sciences* (2d ed.). New York: Wiley.

Slade, C., Campbell, W., & Ballou, S. (2000). *Form and style* (2d ed.). Geneva, IL: Houghton Mifflin.

Chapter *14*

Writing a
Research Report

The preceding chapters have dealt with the many aspects of conducting research. Once the research study is complete, the project needs to be communicated to other interested professionals. The communication may take the form of a term paper, research report, manuscript for a journal article, master's thesis, or doctoral dissertation. This chapter will provide some guidelines to help you prepare the research report. Keep in mind, however, that style manuals, university and college requirements, and each journal require different types of written preparation. Make sure to check the format that is required *before* you embark upon the writing of your study.

The Report as a Communication Document

Health science is exactly that: a science you have learned through many years of schooling. A good health scientist begins with a theory, devises hypotheses based on that theory, designs and carries out an investigation to test the stated hypotheses, and analyzes the collected data to ascertain if these hypotheses can be accepted (or rejected). The last step, which can be the most exciting, is to communicate this process to other health scientists and interested people. The study has been well planned and thought out, and carried through as expected. Usually, several obstacles have been faced and successfully dealt with. These obstacles and other problems undoubtedly alter the search process, therefore causing unexpected results. This is the exciting part! If the research project had progressed as smoothly as planned, the report could have been written before the study was conducted. When you begin to think about writing the research report, you should probably start by thinking about the data you have collected and what these results actually mean. This process leads to finding unexpected results, which may lead to new, exciting, and extremely relevant information for the field of health science. Some researchers are reluctant to report negative results or results that do not support their theories. All good research should be communicated; we have a responsibility to our colleagues to inform, reaffirm, and present new findings related to human health behavior. It is this communication that encourages others to conduct investigations that will help the growth of the health sciences.

The research report is generally divided into the following sections:

1. *Introduction:* An explanation of the problem and why it is important.
2. *Review of the literature:* A review of relevant studies focusing on the theory and its importance and implication for the study.
3. *Methodology:* A description of the procedures, subjects, and instruments employed in the study.
4. *Presentation and analysis of the data:* A discussion of the method used to analyze the data, a presentation of the findings, and a discussion of what the findings mean.
5. *Conclusions and summary:* Conclusions and a brief summary close the report.
6. *References:* All cited sources are included here.
7. *Appendix:* If appropriate, this section may include instruments, letters of commitment, etc.

We cannot emphasize one point too strongly: Remember, all journals have their own format, as do several style manuals used by different colleges and universities. The following material will enable you to write the research report, regardless of the format, because the information can always be rearranged to suit a particular format.

Preliminaries

We have outlined the many parts to the research report. However, certain *preliminary* pages might be necessary for a manuscript, journal article, thesis, or dissertation.

Title Page

The first page of the report is called the title page. The page usually includes the title of the paper, author, relationship of the report to either a course or degree requirement, name of the institution to which the report is submitted, and date of submission. The title of the report should be brief but specific in terms of describing the project. For example, if you were to conduct an experiment to compare the behavioral changes of diabetes patients who completed a new patient education course as compared to the behavioral changes of a matched group who were exposed to the regular patient education instruction, a good title might be: "A Comparison of Experimental and Regular Diabetes Patient Education Instruction on the Behavioral

A COMPARISON OF EXPERIMENTAL

AND

REGULAR DIABETES PATIENT EDUCATION

INSTRUCTION ON THE

BEHAVIORAL CHANGES OF

DIABETES PATIENTS

by

SUSAN JONES

A Term Paper Submitted in Partial Fulfillment

of the Requirements in

CHLTH 440: Health Behavior:

Theoretical Perspectives

University of Illinois

March 6, 2001

FIGURE 14.1 Title Page

Changes of Diabetes Patients." A second choice—"Behavioral Changes of Diabetes Patients"—is too short and does not really describe the experiment.

The title should be typed in capital letters, single-spaced, and centered. If there is more than one line in the title, it is divided so that each successive line is shorter, forming an inverse pyramid. Figure 14.1 is an example of a title page.

Copyright

Most doctoral dissertations have a copyright. Theses and other reports may also be copyrighted, if you wish. To initiate this, the author must obtain a copyright authorization form (usually available from university or college business offices), complete it, pay the fee, and include a copyright notice at the front of the dissertation or report. The notice appears, centered on a single page, as follows:

© Copyright by
(author's name)
(date)

If the author has received a great deal of assistance from a person or persons, an acknowledgment page is included at the beginning of the thesis or dissertation. This page should be kept simple and to the point. Usually, the student's committee members and family members are mentioned. In addition, it is considered correct to give mention to the participants and other site personnel. If you are preparing a report or journal article, and there are groups or individuals who should be acknowledged, you can do so by providing a note to be placed on the first page (at the bottom) of the manuscript. The guidelines for acknowledgments here are slightly different from those used for theses or dissertations. The author would not acknowledge committee or family members but might mention those who have helped in the data collection process or those who have reviewed the manuscript previous to its being submitted for publication.

Table of Contents

The table of contents provides an outline of the contents of the paper. The major headings and subheadings are included along with the page number of each. Figure 14.2 shows a table of contents for a research report. The table of contents for theses and dissertations will vary according to the style utilized by individual institutions.

List of Tables and Figures

When writing a report you may utilize figures and or tables to supplement the manuscript. If you do, a separate list for each (tables and figures) should be included after the table of contents. The exact table titles and numbers used in the report are presented along with the pages on which they are located.

Abstract

The abstract is a brief summary of the problems, methods, results, and conclusions of the study, which gives a short rendition of the manuscript. This enables the reader to determine if it is necessary to continue reading the remainder of the report or article. Abstracts for theses and dissertations are usually presented after the table of contents. They are paginated in lower-case roman numerals, as are all preliminary materials mentioned in this section. An example of an abstract is shown in Figure 14.3.

Text or Main Body of the Report

The main portion of the report consists of an introduction, review of the literature, methodology, presentation and analysis of the data, and conclusions and summary. Each of these sections serves as a communication of the study.

TABLE OF CONTENTS

FIGURE 14.2 Table of Contents

Introduction

The introduction serves to state the problem and coordinate that problem to the literature that has been published. It also enables the writer to make the argument for the study. Hypotheses or research questions are formed from reviewing the relevant literature. Delimitations, definition of terms, and assumptions are also part of the introduction. Finally, the importance of the research is described.

THE RELATIONSHIP BETWEEN SELF-EFFICACY THEORY AND
EXERCISE COMPLIANCE IN A CARDIAC POPULATION

Patricia Marie Vidmar, Ph.D.
Department of Health and Safety Studies
University of Illinois at Urbana-Champaign, 1991
L. Rubinson, Advisor

This investigation utilized a cross-sectional study design in order to examine the relationship between self-efficacy theory and exercise compliance in a cardiac population. The study sample was comprised of 20 females and 118 males who had completed a Phase II cardiac rehabilitation program. Of the sample, 43 were enrolled in a Phase III program, while 77 reportedly were exercising on their own, at the time of data collection. Only 18 of the respondents reportedly did not exercise at all.

Exercise compliance/behavior was assessed according to guidelines developed by the American College of Sports Medicine (1986). Frequency, intensity, and duration of exercise were assessed and then combined to produce the dependent variable (exercise behavior). Two measures were utilized to assess self-efficacy: the aggregation of six self-efficacy activity scales (total self-efficacy) and the aggregation of 16 perceived barriers to exercise (exercise barriers efficacy measure).

Based on ACSM (1986) guidelines, exercise compliance for this particular population was similar to that delineated in previous studies (44%) (Barnard, Guzy, Rosenberg, & O'Brien, 1983; Bengtsson, 1983; Oldridge & Jones, 1983). A positive correlation was observed between the exercise behavior measure and the exercise barriers efficacy measure ($r = .6727$, $p < .001$). The exercise barriers efficacy measure was found to be the most significant predictor of exercise behavior ($R^2 = .270$, $p < .001$), although total self-efficacy was also found to be a significant predictor of exercise behavior ($R^2 = .180$, $p < .005$).

Since exercise barriers efficacy was found to be the most predictive of exercise behavior, it was suggested that preceived barriers be assessed of all graduates of the formal program (Phase II) and periodically of those enrolled in Phase III. Once these barriers have been identified, the sources of self-efficacy can be employed in an effort to alter and/or negate the barrier(s). Methodologies for implementing the sources of self-efficacy were offered. Future research is recommended which would assess compliance with other long-term treatment regimens (dietary changes, smoking cessation, and stress management) and their relationships with self-efficacy following completion of a Phase II program.

FIGURE 14.3 Abstract

Statement of the Problem

The problem statement occurs within the first or second paragraph, setting up a rationale for the ensuing background literature. The writer should be sure that the problem is clearly and concisely stated, so that readers who may not be informed about the problem get a true conceptual notion about the problem. When stating the problem, the author should cite those sources that have direct bearing on it and follow up with an in-depth review of the literature in a later section. This part of the introduction should begin with broad statements that become more specific until the study is introduced by means of stating the hypotheses or research questions.

Hypotheses or Research Questions

The next step in writing the research report is to formulate and state the hypothesis or research questions. Dependent upon the particular format you are required to use, the review of literature can precede the hypotheses, or serve as a rationale and hence be stated after the review of literature. In any case, the hypotheses should be reasonable and simply stated, consistent with known facts or theories, be able to be tested, and express the relationship between two variables.

There are some studies that do not lend themselves to formulation of research hypotheses. These are generally investigations that do not have experimental and control groups but are considered experimental anyway.

Example of Research Questions

These research questions were taken from a study in which self-efficacy was used as a predictor of attrition for clients in a treatment program for poly-drug abuse:

1. Will self-efficacy scores allow prediction of likelihood of attrition for subjects of low socioeconomic status who enter an intensive program for poly-drug abuse treatment?
2. Will self-efficacy scores allow prediction of the likelihood of attrition for client subgroups of different ethnic background and gender?
3. Will subjects who complete the program successfully show significantly different self-efficacy profiles from those who drop out? (Steinhoff-Thornton, 1994, p. 8)

Limitations

Studies are usually conducted within certain boundaries, and the results cannot be extrapolated to other populations. These are the limitations. For example, in a study entitled "Contraceptive Self-Efficacy in Adolescents: A Comparative Study of Male and Female Contraceptive Behavior," the authors stated:

> This study focused on older adolescents. More specifically, the sample was drawn from college student volunteers. As such, results of this research cannot be generalized to the entire adolescent population. Furthermore, past research on college students' sexual behavior has shown that college students tend to have more liberal attitudes, and tend to be more permissive than others in their age group. (Rubinson & Van den Bossche, 1997, p. 32)

Definition of Terms

Some terms used in the literature and in studies may be ambiguous and thus cause confusion for the reader. To be sure that the reader does not misinterpret any terms, the writer devises a definition wherein the term provides a frame of reference for the reader. In addition, the variables that are being studied should be defined in operational terms. The following definition of terms was taken from a study that examined areas of vulnerability for runaways utilizing self-efficacy theory:

> **Runaway.** A child or youth, ages 10 to 17, by self-report, who left home without parental permission.
> **Throwaway.** A child or youth, ages 10 to 17, by self-report, who has left home against his or her wishes after being told to leave by parents or parental figures. (Kaliski et al., 1990, p. 10)

Assumptions

There are some facts concerning the study that are established, but the writer cannot prove these facts. In a study entitled *The Health Belief Model and Contraceptive Behavior Among College Females*, the following were listed as assumptions:

1. The design of the instrument would yield responses that were valid and reliable.
2. That self-report, as in the case of a self-administered questionnaire, is an accurate measure of actual behavior.
3. That individuals are able to project themselves into hypothetical situations and accurately assess their probable feelings and actions. ((Robertson, 1983, p. 30)

Significance of the Problem

The major purpose of conducting any study is to provide knowledge and insight into a particular theory or provide relevance for practitioners. In this section, the writer presents the possible implications of what the results of the study will mean to the specific area under investigation. A discussion of how these results will be useful in solving problems and answering questions in the general field is also included (Ary, Jacobs, & Razevieh, 1996). The significance of the problem should additionally include the applications of the results of the study to health science practitioners, if applicable. That is, if the findings of the investigation will benefit those in the field, then this should be stated. The problem's significance convinces the reader that the experiment is worthy and should be carried out by the investigator.

Review of the Literature

The literature review was discussed in detail in Chapter 3. Here we will explain, briefly, the importance of the review of literature, a suggested process for carrying out the task, and a summary of this particular section.

The review of the literature is intended to give the reader an understanding of *why* you have chosen to conduct your study. The relevant information is put together to give purpose to a question that is important, or that you may believe to be important. The writer uses mainly primary sources to support the previously stated hypotheses or research questions. The general themes to concentrate on in the writing of the review include: What previous theories are relevant to your problem? What is your knowledge about those previous works?

The process of conducting the search can at first look unwieldy and forbidding, especially if you have chosen a problem on which there has been much previous research. A good starting point, as was described in Chapter 2, is to conduct the search using note cards, prepare an outline of the major topics you have reviewed, and then provide order to those topics. You may have as many as 20 cards per topic, and this is where the *writing* of the review of literature becomes difficult. Too often, writers abstract each source (article, book, and so on) and just write it down, paragraph after paragraph. This is *not* a good way to write the review: it is boring and provides no insight from the writer. Some studies that are considered the classics pertaining to your topic should be described in detail. Other projects should be mentioned and grouped together to provide a coherent, well-integrated review. There are ways to handle this in your paper. You might write, "Findings of the above studies have been largely supported by a number of other studies that have employed similar approaches" (Gall, Gall, & Borg, 1999). Then you can reference those other studies. Or you might write, "There are several other studies that support this notion" (name, 1996; name, 1997; name, 2001).

As the literature review takes shape (i.e., when the topics are well researched and referenced properly), you need to develop for the reader a sense of integration and insight into the knowledge that you have amassed. This is difficult because you must be thoroughly familiar with and have a complete understanding of the relevant literature. Interpretation of the findings of all of these studies becomes the most important part of the literature review.

The summary of the literature review should include a brief discussion of the findings and their implications for the study being proposed by the writer. These implications should indicate those areas of agreement and disagreement relevant to the problem, as well as any gaps in the existing literature.

Methodology

The methodology section includes a plan of how the study will be conducted so that the hypotheses or research questions can be ascertained. We have discussed in previous chapters the many research designs that are available for almost any type of study. The writer would choose one that best suits the hypotheses or research questions. The methodology section also includes a description of the subjects, the exact procedures utilized to collect the data, and an explanation of the instruments employed in the conduct of the study.

Subjects

The methodology usually begins with a description of the sample used in the study. Detailed description is necessary so that the reader can determine if the research sample is representative and can be generalized to other, similar populations. If the reader knows this then he or she may be able to apply the results to another study, or even replicate the study. Information such as sex, age, educational level, social economic status, place of residence (urban, rural), and the like are important and should be included. In addition, a discussion of how the subjects were selected should be integrated into this section. Here, the population from which the sample was drawn should be described and methods of selection mentioned, such as randomization or matching. These methods must be very carefully detailed and include the criteria, the number of lost cases, and the effect these lost cases might have on the study. The following is an example of the subjects' section from a master's thesis:

> The population defined for the purpose of this study included 412 cases from school unit superintendents and principals of middle, junior high school, and senior high school attendance centers in the state of Illinois in 1975. Only 412 questionnaires were used from the original 871 cases collected by the Illinois Office of Education because the information on some of the questionnaires could not be accurately interpreted. (Tunyavanich, 1975, p. 21)

Procedures

In the procedures section of the paper, a detailed description of the procedures is written. A synopsis of the subjects, the setting, and the variables studied begins the section. One way to organize this part is to present the procedures in chronological order. You might begin by describing the research design with enough detail so that a replication of the work could be attempted. Next, the writer gives a review of how the data were collected, again describing in detail any events that were unusual or that affected the study. A discussion of any steps taken to control or even to reduce errors (e.g., administering measures to all groups at the same time) should be delineated for the reader (Gall, Gall, & Borg, 1999). This is necessary so that the reader will be able to reconstruct the study and perhaps avoid pitfalls that you encountered. All is done in the name of progress! If the procedures were complicated and had many variables, groups, and data collection methodologies, you can end this section with a one-paragraph summary, as the following example demonstrates:

Procedure

> The instructor of each section of the sex education and family life course administered the questionnaire on the first day of class to the students. The course was held on weekday evenings in the meeting rooms of university housing. The instructors were asked to have the students complete the questionnaire at the very beginning of the first class, prior to any instruction or introduction of materials for the course. Instructors were also asked to follow a guideline given to them when administering the questionnaire. Participation in completing the questionnaire was voluntary and anonymous. Students were asked to place the questionnaire, whether completed or not, in an envelope located in the center of the room. The last student was requested to seal the

envelope. The sealed envelope was then returned to the mailbox of the investigator. (Harmata, 1980, p. 56) (See Appendix B [of thesis].)

Instruments

In a research project, independent variables are manipulated and then studied for their relationship with the dependent variables. In order to accomplish this task, instruments or measures are used to assess achievement, behavior change, attitude, or some other construct. In this section of the report, a detailed description of instruments used to collect the data is given. If the instruments are standardized tests, then the description should be brief and include a description of the scores, a review of reliability and validity measures, a mention of each variable that was measured by the scores, and a statement of the relationship of the measure to the hypotheses or research questions (Gall, Gall, & Borg, 1999).

Instruments can also be new or adapted from other standardized measures. If this is the case with your study, then the instrumentation section of the paper must be more detailed. Here the first construction phase must be explained. Types of items used are shown as examples; reliability and validity scores that have been obtained in pilot testing are revealed; and an explanation of the way the measure was constructed is offered. Finally, you should include, by example, the way in which the measure was scored. Usually, a copy of the instrument along with a key or instructions for scoring are included in the appendix of the paper or report.

Presentation and Analysis of Results

The presentation and analysis of the results of a study may be written together or separately. This depends upon format style and the type of paper, report, or thesis. In articles, again dependent upon the journal's format, the results and analysis (sometimes called discussion) sections are combined. In longer, more complicated studies, the results may be separated from the analysis, although the integration of the two is necessary throughout either section.

Introduction. At the beginning of the results and analysis section, the writer should present evidence that the study procedures actually tested the stated hypotheses or research questions. If, for example, you sent out a survey and obtained a low response rate, this may have influenced the results of the study. This fact must be mentioned in the results and analysis section. Also, if you had experimental and control groups, you should be sure to indicate their homogeneity. If the groups did differ, then explain the procedures you took to deal with these differences. The next paragraph or so should explain the method of data analysis (the coding procedures, how the raw scores were converted, combining responses, patterns of response, and so on). Included here should also be a discussion of the statistical analyses used. If you used ordinary or often-used methods, then the description should be brief, as in the case of analysis of variance. However, if you used more complicated and unusual analyses, then you need to fully explain the analyses and give a rationale for their use. (This is accomplished by citing a source for the reader.)

At the end of this introduction section, it is recommended that you tell the reader how the results and analysis will be presented. One good method of organizing this section is to use the hypothesis or research questions as organizers. Each hypothesis is restated, one at a time, and the results and subsequent analysis regarding that hypothesis are discussed. This is an easy method to use, but certainly not the only one. You should discuss this matter with an advisor or someone who has had experience in writing reports or theses; their insights will prove helpful to you.

Presenting the Findings. When presenting the findings, you must be careful not to present so many numbers and tables that your results section is ignored. One method is to state the basic finding (related to a hypothesis or research questions) first, and then work to the more specific findings. The result should be communicated with words first, then with numbers and statistics. It is also a good idea to provide brief summaries throughout the section because this maintains coherence and clarity for the reader.

Presenting the Analysis (or Discussion). This section on presenting the analysis has three main components: interpretation of the findings, implications of those findings, and application of the findings to practice. If this section is centered around the hypotheses or research questions and is combined with the results section, you do not have to restate the questions or hypotheses. You can begin by accepting or rejecting the hypothesis or giving the answers to the research questions. Here the writer should make some inferences from the findings and interpret the results in relationship to the theory and other research. This section is where the writer compares his or her results to other studies and states the possible flaws in the research. Reasonable explanations are expected; keep them brief and sensible. If, on the other hand, you might have developed a new theory, or link to a new or even old theory, you should explain that phenomenon as well. Again, even if this discussion is the most exciting event in your life, keep it brief and to the point.

The second part of this section deals with the implications that the results may have for the general field encompassed within your study. For example, you may have found that self-efficacy was a major predictor of smoking behavior among adolescents, but what are the implications for the health science field? Is self-efficacy, as a part of social learning theory, a good mechanism for determining program interventions in antismoking campaigns? These implications should suggest additions to theories and further research that may follow from the present study.

The final section of presenting the analysis should attempt to illustrate how these findings can be used by the practitioners in the field. Will these results provide a new administrative style, teaching method, or community organizer?

Conclusions and Summary

The last section of the paper or the final chapter of a thesis or dissertation is probably the one most often read. It provides a brief review of the investigation and clearly discusses the conclusions reached by the investigator. Many journals no longer require a summary because the material is covered in the abstract. Nonetheless, research papers, reports, theses, and dissertations still require, for the most part, final conclusions and a summary.

Conclusions. In the conclusions, the investigator should indicate whether the findings support or do not support the hypotheses or what the findings mean in relationship to the research questions. The conclusions are actually the major *inferences* of the study based on the results of the experiment. For example, in one of our case studies, Jayne found that the new health science curriculum, "No Smoke" produced more changes in students' behavior regarding smoking than the old health science curriculum, "Smoking's Bad." This is an observed result based upon measurement scores and observations of students. Jayne could then conclude by inference that the "No Smoke" curriculum is more effective in changing smoking behavior than the "Smoking's Bad" curriculum. This section may also include recommendations for further research and a discussion of new research questions that may have arisen.

Summary. The summary is usually the last section of the report and should briefly restate the problem, describe the procedures, and discuss the principal findings. The writer must be sure not to add anything new here because it is an account of what has already been written in the report.

References

All material that was cited in your report or article must appear in the reference list. The list begins with the word *References* centered at the top of the page. The works are arranged alphabetically by author's last name. The style manual that your institution has selected will provide exact details as to how to prepare the reference list. In this textbook, we have used the American Psychological Association's style manual, but there are others you can utilize, including the following:

Slade, C. (2000). *Form and style* (11th ed.). Boston: Houghton Mifflin.
The Chicago manual of style. (1993). 14th rev. ed. Chicago: University of Chicago Press.

Appendixes

The appendixes include materials that were not appropriate to be included in the body of the paper, but will be useful to the reader. These materials usually include copies of instruments, keys to those instruments, raw data scores, instructions to subjects, letters of support, and long tables or printouts of secondary data analyses.

The appendix is usually noted by having a piece of paper precede it with the word *APPENDIX*, capitalized and centered. The first page of the first appendix is titled *Appendix A,* centered at the top, and is numbered consecutively from the last pages of the manuscript. Each subsequent piece of material constitutes an appendix and is designated by *B, C, D,* and so on. Make sure to check your specific style requirements, because they may differ from our instructions.

Writing Style

The report, article, thesis, or dissertation need not be pedantic and dull, as so many have been. You should keep your writing to a minimum; it should be clear, concise, simple, and coherent. The main points to strive for when writing are clarity and accuracy (Judd, Smith, & Kidder, 1991). Anything you add to enhance the text, such as humor, is acceptable if it is done in a professional manner. Many new writers want to make their reports flowery, including similes and alliterations. This type of writing style should be avoided in the writing of scientific papers.

Voice and Tense

Because scientific writing is supposed to be objective, writers have traditionally used the impersonal form of expression. For example, they say "the investigator observed" in place of "I observed." The good news is that many journals and style manuals for thesis and dissertations have relaxed this rule to enable the writer to have a more personal style. For example, writers may say "I instructed the data collectors" instead of "The data collectors were instructed." Though personal pronouns are now acceptable, do not overuse them in your report. The term *we* should be used if "we" really collaborated on the study. You may also use *we* occasionally when referring to yourself and the reader, as in "We can see from Table 16. . . ."

The experiment must have been completed if you are now writing the report. Therefore, utilize the past tense throughout the paper. Be especially careful in the review of literature section, where there is a tendency to write "Smith notes" instead of "Smith noted." The studies have been completed, therefore they should be reported in the past tense (Slade, 2000). There are occasions within the report where you can use the present tense, such as "Table 16 shows the relationship." In addition, when discussing the implications of your study you might write, "The data from the present investigation suggest."

Nonsexist Terminology

We are supposed to be an enlightened society and free from stereotypes. To reinforce this idea, writers are not to use sexist language, because it might convey attitudes and sex roles that perpetuate stereotypes. Therefore, in 1977 the American Psychological Association published guidelines for nonsexist journal writing. The manual does provide ways to use alternatives, such as the following:

> *Improper:* The health scientist is the best judge of his attitude toward smoking.
>
> *Proper:* Health scientists are the best judges of their attitudes toward smoking.

In this example the use of the plural was used as an alternative to sexist language. At times, you might have to refer to an individual; this may be accomplished by using "he or she" or "him or her," if it is not done too often.

When describing your subjects, however, you must report numbers of males and females. This is done by using either male or female pronouns. Attempt to find sex-neutral terms—*flight attendant* rather than *stewardess, parenting* rather than *mothering,* and so on—to describe persons in your study. In addition, we should all attempt to avoid sex-role stereotyping when using examples (Judd, Smith, & Kidder, 1991). Not all physicians are male, nor all dental hygienists female.

Rewriting the Report

When you first begin writing research reports, it will seem an arduous and impossible task. But, as with anything else, the harder one tackles the problem, the less insurmountable that task becomes. This is very true with writing. As you write, you will find it helpful to have peers or faculty members review the drafts. Usually their comments will prove to be helpful, and you will learn something about the necessity for rewriting the original draft. Most if not nearly all writers never submit a first draft but rewrite various portions of a manuscript several times. This may seem tiresome, and it is, but it does produce good results.

The first draft is often written as quickly as possible, so that time and energy are saved for subsequent rewrites. You may realize after reviewing the draft (using the input of others as well) that the report needs more literature review or data analysis to support your arguments. Again, this is a difficult process. You may have to almost begin again, but you will be much more satisfied with the results of your extraordinary efforts.

Summary

The research report, term paper, journal article, thesis, or dissertation is really a method of communication. As a health scientist, you have the obligation to report the results of your investigation in a clear and concise manner. To accomplish this we have suggested that you first check with your local authority as to the type of style or manual that you should utilize. The second step in preparing a manuscript for a journal article is to research that journal's specific style requirements.

A research report consists of several parts: introduction, review of the literature, methodology, presentation and analysis of the data, and summary and conclusions.

Each section has several subheadings, which require attention to detail, clear and concise writing, and logical interpretations of the results of your study.

The writing style you grow into and eventually adopt will depend upon what you read and how often you read the literature, journal articles, theses, and dissertations. The style should be free of clichés, personal or sarcastic remarks, asides, and sexist language. Having others review your work before submitting it will be extremely helpful to you in preparing the manuscript. The finished product, with your name affixed to it, is well worth all the effort!

Suggested Activities

1. Determine the style manual your college or university requires you to utilize.

2. Prepare a detailed outline of a research report you are going to submit this semester.

3. Differentiate between hypotheses and research questions. Give examples of each.

4. Utilizing any Web-based library access program, identify five style sources that you would incorporate into writing a research report. Explain how you would use these materials.

5. Access a thesis or dissertation via your computer, and critique the style that the writer utilized. How could you improve upon the report?

References

Ary, D., Jacobs, L., & Razevieh, A. (1996). *Introduction to research.* New York: Harcourt.

Gall, J., Gall, M., & Borg, W. (1999). *Applying educational research* (4th ed.). New York: Longman.

Harmata, J. (1980). Differentiation between actual and preceived sexual behavior among college students. Unpublished master's thesis, University of Illinois.

Judd, C., Smith, E., & Kidder, L. (1991). *Research methods in social relations.* New York: Holt, Rinehart, and Winston.

Kaliski, E., Rubinson, L., Lawrance, L., & Levy, S. (1990). AIDS, runaway behavior and self-efficacy. *Journal of Family and Community Health, 13*(1), 65–72.

Robertson, N. (1983). The health belief model and contraceptive behavior among college females. Unpublished master's thesis, University of Illinois.

Rubinson, L., & Van den Bossche, F. (1997). Contraceptive self-efficacy in adolescents: A comparative study of male and female contraceptive behaviors. *Journal of Sex Education and Therapy, 22*(2), 23–29.

Slade, C. (2000). *Form and style* (11th ed.). Boston: Houghton Mifflin.

Steinhoff-Thornton, R. (1994). Self-efficacy as a predictor of attrition for African American and white client populations in treatment for polydrug abuse. Unpublished doctoral dissertation, University of Illinois.

Tunyanavich, N. (1975). The status of health instruction in Illinois public schools. Unpublished master's thesis, University of Illinois.

Common Statistical Procedures

The procedures are listed alphabetically.

Procedure	Common Usage
Analysis of covariance (ANCOVA)	Describes the relationship (difference) between a continous dependent variable and one or more nominal independent variables (like ANOVA), but also controls for the effect of one or more continuous independent variables.
Analysis of variance (ANOVA)	Used to analyze the means among a number of groups. It is a generalization of the *t*-test and is used for two or more groups. Generally, the dependent variable is interval level and continuous, and the independent variable(s) are nominal. Assumes homogeneity within group variation and normal distribution. When groups can be classified in a 2×2 contingency table and the response under study is a continuous normal distribution, a two-way analysis of variance is used.
Bartlett's test	This test is for homogeneity of variance over k groups. The F-test is for two groups, whereas this test is for more than two. Useful in deciding whether to use ANOVA.
Chi-square test	Compares the frequency count of what is theoretically expected versus what is actually observed. This test can be used to determine (1) an association between two variables, (2) homogeneity of subgroups, (3) significant difference between proportions, and (4) how well observed data fit a specific model. Yates correction factor can be used when cell numbers are ≤ 5. Nonparametric test.

Continued

Procedure	Common Usage
F-test	Used to test for the equality of two variances. If they are not significantly different, the general rule of thumb is to use a two-sample *t*-test with equal variances. If the difference is significant, use a two-sample *t*-test with unequal variances.
Factor analysis	Used to arrive at one or more composite variables (i.e., factors) from other reduced variables. All variables are classically continuous, but in practice almost all types have been used.
Fisher's exact test	Used for a two-sample problem with binominal distribution and independent samples; all values are expected to be ≤ 5. Nonparametric test.
Friedman's ANOVA	Used to determine if a significant difference exists among more than two dependent groups. Nonparametric test.
Kappa statistic	For use with categorical variables to measure reproducibility. An example would be to check the reproducibility of a categorical variable in two surveys. The Kappa statistic quantifies the association.
Kruskal-Wallis test	Used to compare the means among more than two samples, when either the data are ordinal or the distribution is not normal. This is a nonparametric alternative to the one-way ANOVA. When there are only two groups, it is equivalent to the Mann-Whitney *U*-test.
Linear structural relation analysis (LISREL)	Most often used to test causal relationship, similar to path analysis, but can be used as an approach to factor analysis. This analysis is generally better than path analysis because it does not have to meet so many assumptions.
Mann-Whitney *U*-test	This is the ordinal equivalent of the *t*-test (difference between means) and is generally equal to or greater in power than the *t*-test. This test is equivalent to the Wilcoxon rank-sum test since the same *p*-value is obtained by applying either test.
Mantel-Haenszel test	In epidemiology, used to assess the association between a dichotomous disease and a dichotomous exposure when confounding is present. Used for estimating the common odds ratio for stratified data.
McNemar's test	Used for a two-sample problem wherein the distribution is binominal and the samples are related. In short, this is a two-sample test for binominal proportions for matched-pair data. Nonparametric test.
Multiple logistic regression (logit analysis)	Used to analyze relationships between multiple independent variables and a dependent variable that is nominal (i.e., categorical). The independent variables are classically continuous, but in practice a mixture of variables has been used. Logistic regression can be used to generate odds ratios.
Multiple regression	Examines the strength, direction, and extent of a relationship between a continuous dependent variable and several independent variables. The latter are usually, but not always, continuous. This is an extension of simple linear regression.

Procedure	Common Usage
Multivariate analysis of variance (MANOVA)	Used to test for prespecified relationships between multiple independent variables and two or more dependent variables. Dependent variables should be at the interval level; interactions are permitted. Tests of significance for MANOVA are usually Wilk's lambda, Roy's greatest root criterion, or Pillai-Bartlett V-tests.
Newman-Keuls multiple comparison	Used to determine which of k means in a one-way ANOVA are significantly different. Newman-Keuls is preferred when pairs of means are contrasted. Multiple comparison procedures may be better than t-tests if there are many groups and not all comparisons between groups have been well thought out in advance.
Path analysis	Regression-based method applied to a specific model based on theory and prior knowledge. For example, it can be used to test relationships based on the Health Belief Model.
Pearson correlation	This correlation is used to show the relationship between two variables (X and Y) that have an underlying normal distribution.
Scheffé's multiple comparison	Used instead of Newman-Keuls for multiple comparisons in a one-way ANOVA when linear contrasts are more complex than simple contrasts of pairs of means. As with Newman-Keuls, this test helps protect from declaring too many significant differences. This method is preferred for multiple comparisons from a one-way ANOVA when linear contrasts are compared (rather than means).
Simple linear regression	Looks at the linear relationship between two variables and is used to predict the dependent variable (Y) from the independent variable (X).
Spearman rank correlation	This is a correlation coefficient based on ranks. It shows the association between two variables (X and Y), which are not normally distributed.
t-test	With one sample it can be used to test the sample mean against some specified value. With two samples, the t-test can be used to compare means. The samples can be independent or paired; if used for the latter, it is sometimes called a dependent t-test. The formula will vary with the nature of the test. Normal distributions are assumed. The test can be one-tailed or two-tailed. Parametric test.
Wilcoxon matched-pairs test	The most common nonparametric test for the two-sampled repeated measures design. Assumes an ordinal dependent variable, ordinal, continuous distribution, and random sampling. This test is sometimes called the Wilcoxon signed-rank test.
Wilcoxon rank-sum test	Used with two independent samples and is based on ranks. Similar to a t-test, except no assumptions as to normal distribution or equal variances are necessary. This test is equivalent to the Mann-Whitney U-test.
Wilcoxon signed-rank test for ordinal data	Used with two dependent samples, using differences between the individual pairs of observations. Similar to a paired t-test except for nonparametric data.

The following references were used for this table and provide further explanations.

Cleary, P. D., & Angel. R. (1984). The analysis of relationships involving dichotomous dependent variables. *Journal of Health and Social Behavior, 25,* 334–348.

Cooley, W. W., & Lohnes, P. R. (1971). *Multivariate data analysis.* New York: Wiley.

Hayduk, L. A. (1987). *Structural equation modeling with LISREL: Essentials and advances.* Baltimore: Johns Hopkins University Press.

Kleinbaum, D. G., Kupper, L. L., & Muller, K. E. (1988). *Applied regression analysis and other multivariate methods* (2d ed.). Boston: PWS-Kent.

Kuzma, J. (1984). *Basic statistics for the health sciences.* Palo Alto, CA: Mayfield.

Morrison, D. F. (1976). *Multivariate statistical methods* (2d ed.). New York: McGraw-Hill.

Rosner, B. (1990). *Fundamentals of biostatistics* (3d ed.). Boston: PWS-Kent.

Appendix *B*

World Wide Web Research

The World Wide Web (www) offers innumerable sites for research activity. Some government sites provide basic health information about disease and wellness, while others offer databases that can be used in research efforts. There are statistical sites that can analyze your data and assist in determining sample size for your study. More recently, sites have been added that address evidenced-based health care for use by researchers, educators, and policymakers. From a recreational standpoint, some sites provide humor made especially for researchers. Of course there are many more sites than those listed below, and you are encouraged to use your browser to seek other sites. If you find an interesting link in any of the sites in this appendix, you are encouraged to follow it.

Statistical Sites

Title	Address
The World Wide Web Virtual Library: Biostatistics—Focuses on statistical support for medicine, environmental science, public health, and related fields.	http://www.biostat.washington.edu/Xvlib/
York University in Toronto—Provides great resources links to consulting services.	http://www.math.yorku.ca/
Fed Stats—The gateway to statistics from over 100 U.S. federal agencies.	http://www.fedstats.gov/

Continued

Statistical Sites (cont.)

Title	Address
SAS Institute Main Entry Point—Offers information on the newer wireless techniques.	http://www.sas.com/
SPSS Entry Point	http://www.spss.com/
S-Plus for Exploratory Data Analysis	http://www.splus.mathsoft.com/
Mathematica—Provides statistical packages for students and teachers, with special editions for elementary and secondary school teachers.	http://www.wri.com/
Minitab Statistical Packages	http://www.minitab.com/
Power Calculator—A UCLA site that provides assistance with sample size and more.	http://ebook.stat.ucla.edu/textbook/calculators/powercalc/
Two-Sample Test Calculator—When you input two sets of numbers, it gives a one-sided or two-sided t-test for paired or independent samples. It can either look up the p value for t, or compute the p value using the randomization distribution.	http://ebook.stat.ucla.edu/textbook/calculators/twosamp/
Sample Size—Computes sample size needed for a given confidence and a given maximum allowable deviation; currently used for means, proportions, and totals.	http://ebook.stat.ucla.edu/textbook/calculators/sampsize.phtml
K–12 Statistics—Provides projects and problems to teach statistical concepts.	http://www.mste.uiuc.edu/stat/
Electronic Statistics—The Electronic Textbook— Begins with an overview of the relevant elementary concepts and progresses to a more in-depth exploration of specific areas of statistics (ANCOVA/MANCOVA, discriminant analysis, nonparametric statistics, distribution fitting, factor analysis, multidimensional scaling, reliability/item analysis, cluster analysis, log-linear analysis, nonlinear estimation, canonical analysis, survival analysis, time series analysis, structural equation modeling, etc.) Provides a glossary of statistical terms and a list of references for further study.	http://www/statsoft.com/textbook/stathome.html
Statistical Humor	http://baserv.uci.hun.nl/~johnh/useful/stathum.html
Statistician Jokes	http://info.business.utah.edu/~bebrblf/statjoke.html

Evidence-Based Health Care Sites

Title	Address
Center for Evidence-Based Medicine—National Health Service in Great Britain—Has links to several sites and a PowerPoint presentation about EBM.	http://cebm.jr2.ox.ac.uk/
Pediatric and Related Resources for Practicing Evidence-Based Medicine—Lists excellent readings for all aspects of EBM; offers links to databases and searches.	http://pedsccm.wustl.edu/EBJ/EB_Resources.html
National Institute of Child Health and Development Cochrane Collection on Neonatal Health	http://www/nichd.nih.gov/cochraneneonatal/
PERRY—Provides youth and adolescent information on the six risk behaviors outlined by CDC.	Go to the CDC website. No listing at the time of publication.
Database of Abstracts of Reviews of Effectiveness (DARE)—Contains systematic reviews; one of the databases of the Cochrane Library.	http://nhscrd.york.ac.uk/darehp.htm
Natioal Guideline Clearinghouse™ (NGC)—A public resource for evidence-based clinical practice guidelines.	http://www.guideline.gov/index.asp
The Cochrane Collaboration—Provides systematic reviews.	http://hiru.mcmaster.ca/cochrane/cochrane/cc-broch.htm
The Evidence-based Medicine Resource Center—New York Academy of Medicine and American College of Physicians in New York.	http://www.ebmny.org/thecentr2.html
Netting the Evidence—Offers EBM practice on the Internet; provides excellent resources and links.	http://www.shef.ac.uk/~scharr/ir/netting/
Trawling the Net—Lists and describes free-access databases for EBM.	http://www.shef.ac.uk/~scharr/ir/trawling.html
The Health Information Research Unit (HIRU) at McMaster University—Conducts research in health information science.	http://hiru.mcmaster.ca
Center for Evidence-Based Child Health—Offers short courses, resources, and networking.	http://www.ich.bpmf.ac.uk/ebm/framcent.htm
Pediatric Evidence-Based Medicine—Offers critically appraised topics (CATs).	http://depts.washington.edu/pedebm/

Continued

Evidence-Based Health Care Sites (cont.)

Title	Address
Centres for Health Evidence-Canada—Focuses on presenting and disseminating health knowledge in ways that facilitate its optimum use.	http://www.cche.net/
Centre for Evidence-based Mental Health	http://www.psychiatry.ox.ac.uk/cebmh/index.html
Herbal Medicine—Provides hyperlinked access to the scientific data underlying the use of herbs for health. It is somewhat of an evidence-based information resource.	http://www.herbmed.org

Government Sites

Title	Address
CDC—Adolescent and School Health Division—Offers YRBSS data and much more.	http://www.cdc.gov/nccdphp/dash/
Centers for Disease Control—Offers a variety of information for research; check the data and statistics section for scientific, surveillance, laboratory, and health statistics.	http://www.cdc.gov/
National Center for Health Statistics—Offers data on surveys and collection systems (NHIS, NHANES, NIS, NSFG, NHCS, SLAITS, trend data, state data).	http://www.cdc.gov/nchswww/
Statistical Export and Tabulation System—Provides tools to handle large data sets on your PC; check the NCHS for available data sets as well as other CDC sites.	http://www.cdc.gov/nchs/sets.htm
NCHS Data Warehouse—Provides both tabulated and microdata at national and state levels.	http://www.cdc.gov/nchs/datawh.htm
CDC National Prevention and Information Network—Provides data on HIV, AIDS, and TB.	http://www.cdcnpin.org/
searchgov.com.—Provides links to executive, independent, and state and local agencies.	http://www.searchgov.com/
U.S. Department of Education—Prescribes funding opportunities and provides and other educational information.	http://www.ed.gov/

Government Sites (cont.)

Title	Address
healthfinder.gov.—Serves as a gateway to selected information from libraries and databases to listservs and self-help groups.	http://www.healthfinder.gov/moretools/
National Cancer Institute	http://www.nci.nih.gov/
Department of Health and Human Services—Offers grant information.	http://www.os.dhhs.gov/ http://www.os.dhhs.gov/agencies/grants.html
Office of Population Affairs—Provides information on adolescents, parenting, and sexuality.	http://www.hhs.gov/progorg/opa/index.html
DHHS Grants Net—Offers an electronic road map to grants.	http://www.hhs.gov/grantsnet/
National Institutes of Health—Leads to information about NIH grant and fellowship programs as well as research contracts.	http://grants.nih.gov/grants/index.cfm
Substance Abuse & Mental Health Services Administration—Provides grant information.	http://www.samhsa.gov/
Agency for Healthcare Research and Quality—Provides information on funding, research findings, and fact sheets.	http://www.ahrq.gov/fund/grantix/htm

Name Index

Abdelnoor, M., 234
Aday, L. A., 102, 103, 153, 155, 158
Ahren, A., 236
Anderson, R. M., 130
Anderson, S., 212, 215, 219
Angel, R., 240
Angstrom, T., 236
Annemans, L., 131
Ary, D., 3, 4, 238, 283, 318

Bailey, K. D., 15, 68, 115, 179
Baker, E., 212, 213, 214
Ball, S., 212, 215, 219
Balou, S., 290, 291
Baranowski, T., 196
Barribal, K. L., 108
Beauchamp, T. C., 61
Becker, H., 184
Becker, M., 5
Beecher, H. K., 57, 69
Bennett, J., 40
Berg, B. L., 110, 111, 171, 172
Bergman, F., 236
Best, J., 6, 11
Bettcher, D. W., 131
Bickman, L., 169, 170
Biklin, S., 163, 165, 168, 182, 184, 185, 188, 189
Bilodeau, B. A., 124
Binet, A., 201
Bloom, B., 201
Bogdan, R., 163, 165, 168, 182, 184, 185, 187, 188, 189
Bogdewic, S., 177
Bohneneblust, S., 273
Boniface, R., 272
Borenstein, M., 152

Borg, W., 173, 279, 280, 282, 319, 320, 321
Box, G., 94
Bracht, G., 85, 86
Brandt, A., 54
Brewer, M., 195
Britan, G., 225
Brogan, D., 232
Buchler, J., 2
Burns, N., 110

Campbell, D., 82, 84, 85, 91, 92, 94, 200
Campbell, W., 290, 291
Capron, A., 60
Chave, E., 122, 123
Chelimsky, E., 196
Childress, J. F., 61
Chok, B., 232
Christiansen, C. L., 232
Clark, H., 86
Clark, N., 196
Clark, T., 54
Cleary, P. D., 240
Clegg, D., 128
Clinton, W. J., 55
Cohen, J., 151, 152
Cohen, L., 2
Conant, J., 3
Conklin, K. A., 111
Cook, D. J., 41, 42, 43, 46
Cook, R. J., 46
Cook, S., 107, 108
Cook, T., 94, 200
Cooper, R., 221, 222, 223
Copernicus, 8
Cristol. D. S., 108

Cummings, S. S., 130
Cutter, G., 196

Dalkey, N., 131
Daly, J., 287
Daniels, D. S., 232
Davison, B. J., 124
Degner, L. F., 124
Demel, J., 306
Denzin, N., 174
Deutsch, M., 107, 108
Dillner, J., 236
Dolan, M. S., 42
Donald, A., 40

Ebbutt, D., 130
Eisner, E., 207, 208
Eleazer, K., 40

Fan, X., 115
Farewell, V. T., 240
Ferguson, L., 124
Feuer, S., 307
Fleiss, J. L., 245, 247
Fletcher, R. H., 232
Foley, J., 307
Forthofer, W., 153
Fowler, F.J., 111
Freeman, H. E., 195, 203
Frey, J. H., 113
Fromer, M. J., 56
Furlong, D. K., 112

Gall, J., 173, 319, 320, 321
Gall, M., 173, 279, 280, 282, 319, 320, 321
Gallagher, P. M., 111
Garcia, R., 130

337

Subject Index

Abstracting and indexing services, 35–37
Accreditation model, 209–210
Actuarial estimates, 240
AIDS education case study, 271, 287
Analysis of covariance (ANCOVA), 79, 239, 282, 327
Analysis of variance (ANOVA), 278–279, 294, 327, 328
Analysis of variance, Friedman two-way, 264, 328
ANCOVA (analysis of covariance), 79, 239, 282, 327
Anecdotal records, 170
Anonymity, 65, 111, 128. *See also* Privacy rights
ANOVA (analysis of variance), 278–279, 294, 327, 328
API (aptitude-treatment interaction) research, 86
Applied research, 6
Area sampling, 145–146
Assumptions in problem statements, 20
Attitude scale construction, 120–122. *See also* Scaling
Attrition, 84
Audiotapes/audiotaping, 65–66, 173, 183

Bartlett's test, 327
Basic research, 5–6
Behavioral objectives model, 201–202
Bias
  attrition and, 84
  confounding, 236
  contamination, 84–85

as error type, 235–236
goal-free evaluation and, 206–207
information, 236
interviewer, 116
in mail surveys, 108
selection, 84, 236
in statistical records, 186
in study design, 41–42
value-free research and, 16
Bibliography index, 34
Blood pressure case study, 139, 141, 158–159
Body language, 167, 172
Branching questions, 119
Budget considerations. *See* Costs

CAPI (computer-assisted personal interviewing), 112
Cardiac rehabilitation case study, 195, 225
Case-control investigations in epidemiology, 230–232, 233–234, 245–247, 250
Case study
  in evaluation research, 221
  model, 208–209
  one-shot design, 88
Case study examples
  AIDS education, 271, 287
  blood pressure, 139, 141, 158–159
  cardiac rehabilitation, 195, 225
  cervical cancer, 229, 249–250
  cervical dysplasia, 53–54, 73–74
  health science curriculum, 77, 96
  immunization education, 139–140, 141, 158–159
  outreach education, 101, 132–133
  research course, 289, 308

suicide, 229, 249
teen pregnancy, 253, 269
wellness center, 163, 191
CATI (computer-assisted telephone interviewing), 111–112
Causation establishment in epidemiology, 235
Cause and effect, 219, 263
Central tendency measures, 256–258
Cervical cancer case study, 229, 249–250
Charts in presentations, 303
Children, as research subjects, 57–60, 62, 72
Chi-square test, 280, 327
CI (confidence interval), 247–249, 271–272
CIPP model, 204
Cluster sampling, 145–146
Cochrane Library, 47
Coding in data analysis, 187–188
Coefficient of variation (CV), 261–262
Cohort studies in epidemiology, 230–233, 243–245, 250
Combined form questionnaire, 117
Committee on research participation (CRP), 72. *See also* Institutional Review Board role
Computer assistance
  computer-assisted personal interviewing (CAPI), 112
  computer-assisted telephone interviewing (CATI), 111–112
  computerized self-administered questionnaire (CSAQ), 112
  in literature searches, 37–40
  in statistical analysis, 281–282